Drug Problems

Cross-Cultural Policy and Program Development

Edited by
Richard Isralowitz, Mohammed Afifi, and Richard Rawson

Auburn House
Westport, Connecticut • London

Library of Congress Cataloging-in-Publication Data

Drug problems: cross-cultural policy and program development /
edited by Richard Isralowitz, Mohammed Afifi, and Richard Rawson.
p. cm.
A collection of 19 scholarly contributions, the majority dealing with Israel and Palestine.
Includes bibliographical references and index.
ISBN 0–86569–299–8 (alk. paper)
1. Drug abuse—Middle East—Cross-cultural studies. 2. Drug abuse—Middle East—Prevention—Cross-cultural studies. 3. Drug abuse—Treatment—Middle East—Cross-cultural studies. 4. Drug abuse—Government policy—Middle East—Cross-cultural studies. 5. Middle East—Social conditions. I. Isralowitz, Richard. II. Afifi, Mohammed. III. Rawson, Richard A.

HV5840.M628 D78 2002
362.29′18′0956—dc21 2001046352

British Library Cataloguing in Publication Data is available.

Library of Congress Catalog Card Number: 2001046352
ISBN: 0–86569–299–8

First published in 2002

Auburn House, 88 Post Road West, Westport, CT 06881
An imprint of Greenwood Publishing Group, Inc.
www.greenwood.com

Printed in the United States of America

The paper used in this book complies with the
Permanent Paper Standard issued by the National
Information Standards Organization (Z39.48–1984).

10 9 8 7 6 5 4 3 2 1

Contents

Foreword

Patrick F. Bogan

Drug abuse is a problem that ignores language, boundaries, political strife, social class, and economic status. The United States is a nation with immense criminal justice resources, public health expertise, and scientific knowledge; however, it is one of the major consumer nations of illicit drugs. Few in the United States are satisfied with the current state of affairs in the never-ending "war on drugs." Whether one talks about the crack cocaine problem in America's cities, the escalating problem of high-grade heroin in east coast urban centers, the methamphetamine epidemic in western and midwestern rural areas and suburban communities, or the explosion of ecstasy (methylenedioxymethamphetamine [MDMA]) and "club drugs" among teens and young adults, no one is claiming victory in America's drug war.

In many other countries with far fewer resources and wealth, drug use, abuse, and addiction destroy lives, ruin families, and erode basic institutions. Illicit drug use is not solely a problem of the rich, nor of the poor. It can destroy the life of a wealthy Beverly Hills movie star as readily as it can degrade and debase the poorest and most under-privileged person in any third world nation. It can devastate the inner core of major U.S. cities as readily as it can destabilize the governments of developing democracies. No vaccine has been developed to inoculate any social class or society from the impact of illicit drug abuse.

At present, one of the best weapons against the problem of illicit drug use is accurate information. It is folly for societies to create high-tech interdiction efforts, prevention programs, and treatment systems without knowing the nature of the problem. As with any public health and criminal justice problem, before a meaningful societal response can be developed, one must first know the specific nature of the problem, which segments of the population and number of people affected, and which agencies can help provide information about the people being impacted. Only by first gaining insight into these issues can a society mount a rational, effective response to the problem of illicit drug use.

The Middle East is a region associated with some of the world's most splendid achievements and some of the world's most challenging problems. The establishment of Israel in 1948 is viewed by some as a considerable accomplishment; for others it is viewed as a source of injustice. There are many issues that divide the citizens of Israel and their Palestinian neighbors. Land, water, religion, culture, justice, identity, economics, and history are all topics that come to mind when discussions of the Israeli-Palestinian conflict occur. It is easy to forget that in the midst of these global, centuries-old issues, there are millions of people who spend their lives struggling with the same day-to-day problems that face citizens of other less newsworthy parts of the world.

It is highly unlikely that drug use, abuse, and addiction would be listed among the "top ten" concerns if world leaders were asked about the most important issues in the Middle East. It would probably surprise many people to know that in this "center stage" of world politics, the problem of drug abuse is as real a concern to mothers, fathers, and other family members as it is in the rest of the world. Criminal justice and public health agencies across the region strive to create communities where drug use and the consequences of drug use are reduced to the lowest possible levels. However, as in the United States, it would be difficult in this part of the Middle East to find many people who are satisfied that illicit drug use has been eradicated.

In the mid-1990s, a group of Israeli and Palestinian public health and criminal justice leaders began to discuss their mutual concerns about the problem of drug use in Israeli and Palestinian communities. There were few, if any, channels of communication between the two groups that could be used to support this effort. There was no established model for how these joint concerns could be addressed. And there were many questions about whether it was even a good idea for the two groups to discuss such a controversial and politically charged issue as illegal drug use. The only good reason for the two groups to discuss this topic was that both groups believed that it was important to know the extent of the drug problem they faced and what kinds of activities could best reduce the existing problems.

Support for this effort has come from numerous agencies and individuals. Israeli and Palestinian nongovernment organizations and the U.S. Department of State have helped bring people together and support this process. Grants from the Dutch and Israeli governments, the cooperation of the World Health Organization, as well as support from private foundations and individuals have helped the process move forward. However, the most important contributions have been made by the Palestinian and Israeli participants who have attended meetings, collected data, written articles, and stayed with the effort through periods of peace and periods of conflict in the region. Their commitment to the health and well-being of their communities has been the glue that has held the initiative together.

Friends Research Institute, Inc., and Matrix Institute on Addictions, including their respective boards of directors, are proud to have provided support to the efforts that brought Israeli, Palestinian, and U.S. drug abuse experts together to plan a course of action to address the drug problem in the region. These institutes are proud to have been involved with the development of the work described in this book.

We hope that this book will promote communication, cooperation, and coordination among those involved regarding the problem of drug use, and we plan to continue our support and involvement with this important endeavor.

Introduction

*Richard Isralowitz, Mohammed Afifi,
and Richard Rawson*

Illicit substance use and its consequences, including crime and violence, government action in the form of military and police intervention, lost work, family destruction, property confiscation, and massive allocations of funding resources for treatment and health maintenance, constitute a major public concern. Substance use is a deeply embedded characteristic of society. This is true for well-established, modern Western democracies as well as developing nations and regions throughout the world, such as the Middle East.

In spite of the attention that the drug issue generates, there is a limited history of policy addressing the production and use of illegal substances from an international perspective. For example, the United Nations (U.N.) General Assembly has held only one special session devoted to this issue since its beginning in 1946. That special session was held in 1990 to address the drug control issue. Eight years later, its current secretary general, Kofi Annan, stated that "the sad reality . . . is that the problem of illicit drugs remains with us, and the trends are not slowing. Drug trafficking has become a multi-billion dollar industry, a clandestine, criminal, cartel-driven enterprise, leaving no country unscathed. Addiction is similarly indiscriminate, crossing lines of class, gender, religion and ethnicity" (Annan, 1998).

In U.N.-sponsored meetings held in Vienna and New York (1998), representatives from 130 governments agreed to a political declaration calling for a drastic reduction of both the illicit supply and demand for drugs by the year 2008. Additionally, the main themes for the members' discussion and consideration included: precursor chemicals used to manufacture illicit drugs; the manufacture, trafficking, and abuse of amphetamine-type stimulants, which are the most abused synthetic drugs manufactured clandestinely; judicial cooperation, such as strengthening the legal framework to improve application of drug control laws regarding extradition and illicit traffic by sea; the laundering of money derived from illicit drug trafficking and other serious crimes; and the elimination of illicit crops and the promotion of alternative crop development (Annan, 1998).

Within the Middle East, the focus of this book, Jewish and Arab people have been in a declared or de facto state of war since before the establishment of Israel in 1948. In this region, neither the U.N., the European Union, nor any other organizing body has had much clout in building a broad-based infrastructure able to address common drug-related concerns and problems or organizational needs, including drug control through law enforcement information sharing, research, and the training of personnel.

DRUGS IN THE MIDDLE EAST: STATUS IN THE 1950s

The history of addressing illicit drug use in the Middle East reveals one noteworthy initiative during the last 50 years or so. After World War II, the U.N. Commission on Narcotic Drugs was established. Following the inception of the commission, sources continually reported that opium was coming out of the Middle East through the Mediterranean and going to other parts of the world, especially North America. Specifically, in 1951, there were reports that the manufacture of opium into crude morphine and diacetylmorphine (heroin) was increasing within the Middle East. There was also considerable evidence of heavy traffic in cannabis (hashish) directed to a large and growing market within the Middle East itself. During the thirteenth session of the commission in 1958, several delegations believed conditions in the Middle East warranted an exploratory mission to the region. One year later, the Middle East Narcotics Survey Mission was in place to familiarize itself with the situation, make suggestions on the ways in which technical assistance might be utilized to curb the traffic of illicit drugs, and guide the commission on the best ways in which the difficulties of governments facing a drug problem could be met. The mission was informed of the illicit drug traffic in the region by reports of governments, recommendations and resolutions of the U.N. and the International Criminal Police Organisation (Interpol), and reports of the Permanent Anti-Narcotics Bureau of the League of Arab States. In the countries it visited, including Israel, Jordan, Lebanon, and Egypt, the mission consulted with numerous officials and examined the issues of drug control, including the modus operandi of smugglers and traffickers (Bulletin on Narcotics, 1960).

The mission approached illicit drug traffic in the Middle East as a serious regional problem. It found substantial cannabis (hashish) production and consumption; that there was substantial opium production and growing levels of consumption; and that opium derivatives, particularly crude morphine, traveled from the Middle East to other parts of the world, particularly Europe and North America. The mission found no evidence of significant importation of illicit drugs into the Middle East. The regional traffic followed all routes, by land, sea, and air. An important land route for the hashish traffic passed through the Syrian province of the United Arab Republic, Jordan, and Israel, and into Egypt. The opium traffic to Egypt also followed this land route to a significant extent. Opium was converted to crude morphine to facilitate its transport via Syria, Lebanon, or Turkey into European countries such as France and Italy for refining; from there it was transported to North America. The mission noted that along the main routes and in the border areas, cultural and legal features worked to the smuggler's advantage. At that time there were tribes, some of them nomadic, that spanned frontiers and whose members had loyalty to the tribe rather than to any particular country. Regulations in some border areas permitted residents to move freely within a specified distance on either side of the frontier. There were families and groups that had engaged in smuggling for generations and looked upon it as a way of life rather than a criminal undertaking. Some of these groups did not hesitate to resist by armed force if threatened with apprehension (Bulletin on Narcotics, 1960).

Several suggestions for improving the situation were proposed to the mission or originated within the mission itself. For example, a number of countries advocated greater cooperation at the working level, especially along frontiers. The mission noted that to improve cooperation at the working level, broad and comprehensive agreements between neighboring countries were essential. The mission emphasized the necessity for a strong national policy and machinery to control illicit trafficking: "Generally speaking, it seems beyond dispute that a fundamental requirement for good enforcement in any area is determination of national governments to eradicate the illicit narcotics traffic fully within their borders. Where such a determination exists and is coupled with a readiness to cooperate fully and whole-heartedly with neighboring states, the narcotic problem will be kept under control. There must be strong, honest, and well-directed administrative and enforcement machinery in each country to apply the legislation and carry out the policy of the government. Where such machinery is found, not only is the standard of national enforcement high, but international agreements may be applied fully and effectively" (Bulletin on Narcotics, 1960).

The mission proposed other recommendations to help governments in the region and the Narcotics Commission address drug use problems. These included measures related to laws and regulation, administrative provisions, national policy, international obligations, and cooperation with existing agencies (e.g., Interpol). Also, the mission urged that the great value of bilateral agreements between governments be recognized and that on the basis of these agreements every possible action be taken to encourage and improve direct liaison between enforcement agencies and others working on the problem.

THE PRESENT: WHAT DO THE MIDDLE EAST COUNTRIES SAY TODAY?

The Bureau for International Narcotics and Law Enforcement Affairs of the U.S. Department of State annually publishes an *International Narcotics Control Strategy*

Report (U.S. Department of State, 1999). Each country involved in the report prepares a description of drug-related issues, conditions, and problems. The following excerpts provide an overview of the drug situation in a formidable portion of the region: Israel, Jordan, Lebanon, and Egypt (selected on the basis of shared borders and their relation to Palestinians). (Editors' Note: Because questions may exist regarding the veracity of the information provided by the countries to the U.S. Department of State for its report, each country's situation and regional status regarding the drug problem should be interpreted cautiously.)

Israel

Demand for drugs is growing in Israel, use is becoming more accepted, and users begin drug use at increasingly younger ages. Drug prices have remained stable or decreased, suggesting significant supplies of illicit drugs are available to users. Drug users generally fall into one of two groups: one where use of amphetamines dominates, and the second where use of cannabis dominates. . . . It seems that heroin is a secondary drug of abuse. Israel is neither a major [shipping] point nor a major producer of drugs or precursor chemicals. . . . Indeed, drug cultivation in Israel doesn't even meet [the country's] own illicit demand.

Cooperative efforts with Egypt, Jordan, and the Palestinians remain important for the interdiction of some drugs coming to Israel . . . [and] cordial relations exist between [the] counterparts; however, there is little to no operational assistance. . . . Israel . . . offers little assistance to any of them [and there] is no benefit yet from the improving relationships for [better] narcotics interdiction. . . . Israeli authorities believe the majority of cannabis and heroin consumed in Israel originates in Turkey, Egypt, and elsewhere and enters Israel across borders with Lebanon, Jordan, and Egypt . . . and [through] the growing use of express mail to move amphetamines, LSD, and other drugs, . . . [which] often originate from Europe. . . . Other drugs come to Israel from the United States and South America.

Most law enforcement officials believe that a significant amount of money is laundered through Israel because money laundering is not a crime [in this country]. Money laundering legislation is pending in the Knesset [the Israeli parliament]. Should it become law, Israel hopes to become a party to the 1988 U.N. Drug Convention.

Among recent immigrants, Russian and Ethiopian youths have significantly higher drug use rates [and there are government-supported studies that report that] drug use in the Israeli-Arab community is three times that of the rest of the county. Age of first use among youth is dropping to 12–14, and the percentage of Israelis who find recreational drug use culturally acceptable [has risen] from 10 percent to 20–25 percent in the last 4 years. . . . Use of ecstasy has increased more than tenfold over the past 3 years.

Jordan

The country's domestic drug abuse problem is small largely due to law enforcement and the cultural and religious norms which help limit use of illegal drugs. . . . The Ministry of Moslem Affairs and Holy Places manages a program of religious speeches, lessons, and lectures on awareness of drugs and their effects.

Jordan has been in the past, and remains today, a transit country [not a narcotics-producing one] for illicit drugs . . . due to its pivotal location between drug producing countries to the north, and drug consuming countries to the south and west. [There is] law enforcement [cooperation] with Syria and Lebanon, and cooperation with Israel has intensified with movement in the Middle East peace process. [Nevertheless], Jordan's most challenging burden to eliminate trafficking remains the long, open and often desolate borders with neighboring countries to the north; the vast array of nomadic tribes associated with trafficking often elude even the most sophisticated efforts of interdiction. . . . [Also], according to enforcement officials, [there are incidents when] family members from Jordan [attempt] to smuggle heroin through Jordan and over the western border to family members in the West Bank.

Jordan still remains a country without a money laundering law. Law enforcement sources fear the lack of such a law will ultimately open the borders to more aggressive trafficking with potential for money laundering.

Seizure statistics for 1999 suggest a reduction of the amount of hashish that transits Jordan; heroin seizures indicate no significant increase, but opium seizures have increased . . . due to an increase of drugs from Turkey, making their way to and through Jordan.

Egypt

Egypt is not a significant producer or consumer of narcotics or precursor chemicals, though opium and cannabis are grown in parts of the country. . . . Opium poppy is grown in the southern Sinai part of the year, and cannabis is grown year round in the northern and southern Sinai and in parts of upper Egypt. . . . A program of crop substitution in the Sinai has been largely unsuccessful. . . . Cannabis and stimulants are the most commonly abused drugs in Egypt. . . . According to the United Nations International Drug Control Programme (UNDCP), opium production in Egypt is declining while cannabis production is increasing. . . . No heroin processing labs have been discovered in Egypt in the last 10 years. . . . Some methamphetamine has been reported in Egypt, and a handful of labs are thought to be operating clandestinely.

The country is a transit point for heroin and cannabis. The flow of drugs through Egypt has decreased recently . . . [perhaps] due to increased border surveillance and interdiction activity as well as the opening of alternative smuggling routes from South Asia through countries of the former Soviet Union. Nonetheless, the lead agency for fighting narcotics trafficking in Egypt (Anti-Narcotics General Administration—ANGA) continues to intercept shipments of hashish and heroin heading to Western Europe and North America from such producers as Lebanon, Pakistan, and Afghanistan.

Egypt does not have a serious problem with money laundering; [nevertheless], a bill specifically criminalizing money laundering is under discussion in [the country's parliament].

Lebanon

Lebanon is not a major illicit drug producing [country]. Three types of drugs are available in Lebanon: hashish, heroin, and cocaine. Hashish and heroin are no longer available in large quantities; sales of user quantities continue at the local level. The Government of Lebanon (GOL) forcefully [combats] illegal crop cultivation. . . . In cooperation with Syrian authorities, [the GOL] continues to suppress the illicit cultivation of opium and cannabis in the Biqa' Valley. . . . GOL authorities maintain that as a result of destruction of hashish and poppy plantations, the production of hashish and heroin [has been nearly] eliminated, although small quantities of morphine and heroin are smuggled overland from Turkey for local use. Local cannabis production is insignificant and there is practically no lab processing. South American cocaine is smuggled into Lebanon primarily via air and sea route connections with Europe, Jordan, and Syria. Lebanese nationals living in South America in concert with resident Lebanese traffickers often finance these operations.

Drug trafficking across the Lebanese-Syrian border has been substantially diminished as a result of Lebanese and Syrian efforts to deter illicit cultivation and smuggling activity. Lebanon is no longer a major transit country; any transit is done by amateurs outside the major drug trafficking networks. Established smuggling routes have been substantially weakened. The transport of hashish across the Syrian-Lebanese border was drastically reduced in quality and value in 1999. This is attributable to the general attitude of both the Lebanese and the Syrian governments toward fighting drug trafficking.

There is no significant money laundering and banks comply with self-regulatory . . . guidelines. Lebanon is a party to the 1988 U.N. Drug Convention.

ABOUT THIS BOOK

Presenting the drug problem by means of an edited book, regardless of its focus, may be likened to craftsmanship. The task of collecting and organizing information from government and nongovernmental authorities, policymakers, researchers, educators, and others who have knowledge of drug issues or who have developed ways to address drug abuse is no simple feat. To generate a final product that provides a coherent body of usable knowledge requires skill—it is a time-consuming process that involves communication, cooperation, and coordination among contributors and others involved in preparing the book.

This book, *Drug Problems: Cross-Cultural Policy and Program Development,* began in 1997 with promoting human relations among Israeli and Palestinian people as well as organizing regional and international experts on the drug problem and its amelioration. In many respects, this book is a valuable source of practical knowledge for policy development and drug prevention and treatment strategies in the Middle East and elsewhere.

The co-editors made no effort to impose comparative perspectives upon contributors. Rather, we, the co-editors, propose that the juxtaposition of Israeli, Palestinian, and international contributors generates a broad knowledge base for multiple applications. The chapters in this book are grouped under four themes: The Social Context of Reality: Perspectives of Drug Use and Abuse among Palestinian and Israeli People; People in Transition; Toward an Understanding of Drug Prevalence Estimation and Evaluation for Palestinian and Israeli Populations; and Perspectives of Drug Services: Needs and Intervention Strategies.

The first section of the book, The Social Context of Reality: Perspectives of Drug Use and Abuse among Palestinian and Israeli People, begins by defining culture and how it shapes the meaning of and responses to substances such as marijuana and heroin over time and across locations. This chapter is followed by a contribution that examines a unique effort that has brought Palestinians and Israelis together by addressing the common problem of substance use. Through this effort, mutual respect and understanding among Palestinians and Israelis were generated, contributing to the promotion of peace in the region.

The Middle East is in constant transition. In this context, five chapters have been prepared for the second section, People in Transition, that examine: the drug situation in Palestine, covering Gaza, the West Bank, and the Arab-populated section of Jerusalem; substance use among Jews and Arabs in Israel; alcohol use among Arabs in the region; Russian immigrant heroin addicts; and patterns and problems of substance use among Bedouins.

The third section of the book, Toward an Understanding of Drug Prevalence Estimation and Evaluation for Palestinian and Israeli Populations, presents perspectives by international experts who consult with the U.S. National Institute on Drug Abuse and the World Health Organization based in Geneva, Switzerland. Specifically, their works address issues related to the development of drug prevalence data collection instruments, rapid assessment of substance use and abuse problems, and the development of data collection from a drug abuse early warning network. These chapters are particularly valuable to countries that are at initial and developmental stages of drug services organization and service provision.

Finally, under the heading of Perspectives of Drug Services: Needs and Intervention Strategies, five chapters are devoted to issues of: drug treatment in Israel (Note: An appendix profiling services that have evolved in Israel for the treatment of drug addiction is provided to complement this chapter); the development of a manualized treatment protocol among Palestinian and Israeli service providers; alcohol and drug use from an Islamic perspective; drug addicts anonymous self-help group treatment; and evaluation of drug treatment.

ACKNOWLEDGMENTS

This effort has been supported with a grant provided by the United States Agency for International Development (USAID) Regional Professional Technical Assistance Program. We are grateful for the support and cooperation provided by USAID personnel responsible for Israeli and Palestinian activities, William Crane and Boaz Ayalon.

The editors of this book express appreciation to our editors, Kris Langabeer and Maggi Davidson, and gratitude to our colleagues for their contributions to this unique collection of information about the problem of substance use. Also, we acknowledge the expertise and cooperation demonstrated by our publisher and its employees specifically our acquisitions editor, Jane Garry, of Greenwood Publishing Group, as well as Terri Jennings, production editor.

We dedicate this effort to our children in the hope of peace and an environment free of harmful, addictive substances.

REFERENCES

Annan, K. (1998). Perils without passports. *United Nations Chronicle, 35*(2), 1–2.

Bulletin on Narcotics (1960). The Middle East narcotics survey mission (September–October, 1959) of the United Nations. *Bulletin on Narcotics, 4*, 1–9.

U.S. Department of State. (1999). *International narcotics control strategy report.* Washington, DC: Bureau for International Narcotics and Law Enforcement Affairs.

Part I

The Social Context of Reality: Perspectives of Drug Use and Abuse among Palestinian and Israeli People

1

The Social Context of Reality: Substance Use in the Middle East

Richard Isralowitz

INTRODUCTION

The use of licit and illicit addictive substances is not a new phenomenon. Throughout history, the meaning of substance use has been grounded in social context, which includes the customs, beliefs, values, knowledge, and skills of a people—attributes that tend to vary over time and geographic location (Berne, 1964; Linton, 1947; Orlandi, 1995). The type of drug used and its use, the social strata of society that use it, the kinds of situations in which it is used, and the publicity and public opinion regarding its use are included in the social context of drug use. As Goode (1989) states, "How a drug is regarded—by the public, the law, its users, and even the medical profession—depends as much on irrational cultural factors as on its objective properties."

According to the Center for Substance Abuse Prevention (CSAP) of the U.S. Substance Abuse and Mental Health Services Administration, "[c]ulture provides people with a design for living and for interpreting their environment. . . . [It] has been defined as 'the shared values, traditions, norms, customs, arts, history, folklore, and institutions of a group of people.' Culture shapes how people see the world and structure their community and family life. A person's cultural affiliation often determines the person's values and attitudes about health issues, responses to messages, and even the use of alcohol, tobacco and other drugs. . . . A cultural group consciously or unconsciously shares identifiable values, norms, symbols, and ways of living that are repeated and transmitted from one generation to another. . . . Race and ethnicity are often thought to be dominant elements of culture. But the definition of culture is actually broader than this. People often belong to one or more subgroups that affect the way they think and how they behave. Factors such as geographic location, lifestyle, and age are also important in shaping what people value and hold dear" (Wright, 1994).

The relation between culture and substance use for ethnic and racial communities is relatively well documented in Western countries, as evidenced by publications of CSAP and professional research journals. In the Middle East, documentation of such relationships is less developed. There is a growing body of knowledge from the Middle East, however, that contributes to a cross-cultural understanding of the patterns and problems of substance use in terms of particular groups as well as in an international comparative context. For example, it has been found that the loss of cultural identity plays an important role in the substance use and drug-dealing behavior of youth and young adults. Transitions in living environments (e.g., pastoral to urban) have been linked to patterns of substance use (Abu Saad, 2002). Also, cultural influences have been linked to attitudes and behavior regarding the type of substances used and the pattern of use among different groups, including the association between opiate use and ethnicity (e.g., heroin use among Russian-speaking immigrants from the former Soviet Union and Israeli-born citizens with a Sephardic heritage from countries such as Morocco and Tunisia); gender among high school youth; religious and secular adults; and university students (Isralowitz, Abu Saad, & Telias, 1996; Isralowitz & Peleg, 1996; Isralowitz, Telias, & Abu Saad, 1994; Isralowitz, Telias, & Zighelbaum, 1992; Isralowitz & Troestler, 1996). In their examination of substance use studies among Arabs in Israel, Jordan, and Palestine, Weiss and colleagues conclude that secularization and the exposure to the alcohol and drug consumption patterns of Israel and of Western culture in general (through television, tourists, etc.) resulted in unexpectedly high levels of alcohol and other drug consumption patterns among these traditional, predominantly Moslem populations (Weiss, Sawa, Abdeen, & Yanai, 1999).

Culture is a powerful factor influencing attitudes and behavior related to substance use. Culture, however, is not a factor that evolves in a vacuum. Culture is shaped over time and is influenced by social, political, and economic forces, the same forces that are used to formulate policy, determine funding for projects, and enforce regulations. Brief histories of marijuana and heroin, the two most commonly used illegal substances in the Middle East, are presented as examples of how historical context and other factors interact to form the social context of substance use.

MARIJUANA

Historical Perspective

No substance in the world has generated more controversy and, perhaps, investigation in terms of impact on individual behavior and society than marijuana. As Grinspoon and Bakalar state in their 1993 book, *Marijuana: The Forbidden Medicine*:

The marijuana, cannabis, or hemp plant is one of the oldest psychoactive plants known to humanity. It is botanically classified as a member of the family *Cannabaceae* and the genus *Cannabis* . . . [and] grows as [a] weed and cultivated plant all over the world in a variety of climates and soils. The fiber has been used for cloth and paper for centuries and was the most important source of rope until the development of synthetic fibers. The seeds (or, strictly speaking, akenes—small hard fruits) have been used as bird feed and sometimes as human food. The oil contained in the seeds was once used for lighting and soap and is sometimes employed in the manufacture of varnish, linoleum, and artists' paints. . . . The chemical compounds responsible for the intoxicating and medicinal effects are found mainly in a sticky golden resin excluded from the flowers on the female plants. . . . The plants highest in resin . . . grow in hot regions like Mexico, the Middle East, and India. . . . The three varieties are known as bhang, ganja, and charas. The least potent and cheapest preparation, bhang, is produced from the dried and crushed leaves, seeds, and stems. Ganja, prepared from the flowering tops of cultivated female plants, is two or three times as strong as bhang; the difference is somewhat akin to the difference between beer and fine scotch. Charas is the pure resin, also known as hashish in the Middle East. Any of these preparations can be smoked, eaten or mixed in drinks. (Grinspoon & Bakalar, 1993)

"Cannabis may have been cultivated as long as ten thousand years ago. It was grown in China by 4000 B.C. and in Turkestan by 3000 B.C.; also, it has long been used as a medicine in India, China, the Middle East, Southeast Asia, South Africa and South America" (Grinspoon & Bakalar, 1993). The earliest reference to cannabis is in a pharmacy book written in 2737 B.C. by the Chinese emperor Shen Nung. Referring to the euphoriant effects of the substance, he called it the "liberator of Sin." The plant was used medicinally to treat "female weakness, gout, rheumatism, malaria, beriberi, constipation and absent mindedness" (Ray & Ksir, 1990; Snyder, 1970). By 1000 A.D., the social use of the plant spread to the Moslem world and North Africa. In the Middle East its use was associated with a religious cult that committed murder for political reasons. The cult was called Hashishiyya, from which the word "assassin" developed. Stories related to the substance involving intrigue, sex, and murder spread throughout Europe for centuries. French soldiers with Napoleon's campaign in Egypt used hashish, as did many other Frenchmen who worked for the government or traveled in the Near East during the nineteenth century.

A considerable amount of medical attention was given to cannabis from 1840 to 1900, during which time it was recommended for a variety of illnesses and discomforts. Among its recommended uses were as an analgesic (in the form of tincture of hemp—a solution of cannabis in alcohol taken orally); as a topical anesthetic for the mouth and tongue; and for problems and discomfort related to tetanus, neuralgia, dysmenorrhea (painful menstruation), convulsions, rheumatic and childbirth pain, asthma, postpartum psychosis, gonorrhea, chronic bronchitis, migraine attacks, certain kinds of epilepsy, depression, asthma, rheumatism, gastric ulcer, and drug addiction, particularly to morphine and other opiate substances (Makuriya, 1973). By 1890, the medical use of cannabis declined because, among other reasons, the potency of the preparations was too variable and the invention of the hypodermic syringe in the 1850s made opiates the more effective pain reliever because hemp products are insoluble in water and cannot be easily administered by injection. Also, synthetic drugs such as aspirin, chloral hydrate, and barbiturates, which are chemically more stable, became attractive for medicinal purposes in spite of their disadvantages.

In the 1930s, marijuana received considerable negative attention in the United States. For example, it was said that the substance "would cause users to go crazy and become violent; men would rape and kill under the influence, and women would become promiscuous." Publications from the period had titles such as "Marijuana—Sex-Crazy Drug Menace," "Marijuana—The Weed of Madness," and "Marijuana: Assassin of Youth." Today these supposed effects receive no attention even in the most vigorous anti-marijuana polemics (Mann, 1985; Nahas, 1975). "Almost no observer argues that, in a single episode of use, marijuana generates psychosis, violence, or sexual 'excess' in the typical user. These issues are simply no longer the focus of controversy. . . . While the acute effects were emphasized in the 1930s, it is the chronic effects that have become the center of attention today" (Goode, 1989).

Considerable information regarding the politics of marijuana in the United States has been detailed (Gray, 1998; Isralowitz & Telias, 1998). Despite the ongoing polemics regarding this substance, the health facts have tended to remain the same for decades (Ray & Ksir, 1990). In a detailed analysis of the negative consequences of marijuana, Sussman and colleagues report that "the most well-confirmed danger from marijuana use is lung damage (and probably lung cancer). . . . A second potential negative consequence is that marijuana use appears to reduce the effectiveness of the immune system, although it may be a temporary reduction and may or may not be a medical concern among regular users. . . . Third, it apparently impairs biosynthesis of nucleic acids and proteins which may disrupt selective attention and long-term memory encoding if used over several years. . . . A fourth potential consequence includes pregnancy-related effects such as low birth weight and prematurity, although the data are equivocal. . . . Fifth, very high doses produce a toxic delirium, (especially if eaten), the symptoms of which include confusion, agitation, disorientation, loss of coordination, and hallucinations. [However,] there have not been any reports of deaths from overdoses. . . . A sixth potential, but unconfirmed, consequence of chronic marijuana use is that it reduces one's motivation to accomplish goals. . . . [Seventh, marijuana] has been found to be associated with a lower sperm count; however, this association may be temporary. . . . An eighth consequence is that adult users report subjective difficulties. These difficulties, which may or may not have empirically observable behavioral or functional correlates, include impairment of memory, concentration, motivation, self-esteem, interpersonal relationships, health, employment and finances, safety, and pregnancy. . . . Ninth, marijuana use also has been investigated as a stepping stone drug. A number of studies indicate that marijuana users are at relatively high risk for use of hard drugs and their related negative consequences. . . . A tenth potential consequence is that marijuana may be addictive. Psychological dependence (e.g., conditioning effects) appears to be more important than physical dependence regarding withdrawal of use. . . . Finally, [the substance] affects coordination, [which] may place users at risk for accidents. THC [trans-delta-tetrahydrocannabinol, which is the primary psychoactive agent in marijuana] is found in the blood of more than 30 percent of fatally injured drivers, and more than 50 percent of persons stopped for reckless driving show detectable levels of marijuana, or marijuana and another drug, [in their] urine" (Sussman, Stacy, Dent, Simon, & Johnson, 1996).

A substantial amount of evidence has accumulated about the relatively benign consequences of marijuana use. Additionally, the significant benefits of marijuana use in the treatment of cancer, AIDS, and other serious illnesses are widely acknowledged. In spite of the body of knowledge available about marijuana and the few instances of legislation allowing the use of marijuana for medical purposes, many governments, including Israel and Palestine, continue to oppose decriminalization of marijuana use.

Social, Political, and Economic Factors: Thoughts for Regional Policy Development

The social, political, and economic factors associated with marijuana, over time and across nations, raise a number of interesting and somewhat puzzling concerns. Among them is the attitude of narcotic and government officials that marijuana use should remain punishable by law. Seemingly, such policies toward marijuana use have not been based on well-documented and researched information; instead, there are a number of possible reasons why policies for outlawing any kind of marijuana use have prevailed for many years. Among the possible reasons are: (a) to control labor conditions, including the spread of migrant workers, the marijuana "problem" is pinned on minority groups, as evidenced in the 1930s after the Great Depression in the United States; (b) the substance poses a threat to the alcohol industry, the profits for which go into government coffers; (c) marijuana is a cheap analgesic that could pose a threat to pharmaceutical companies engaged in the manufacture of new medicinal products for profit; (d) drug dealers themselves may consider the legalization of marijuana as a threat to their profits and livelihood; and (e) perhaps law enforcement and government bodies, in their steadfast stance against legislation or even decriminalization of the substance, want to maintain their legitimization to manage and control resources (funds), status, and power.

In spite of this situation and the fact that prospects for reevaluation and reform look dim (Bertram & Sharpe, 1996), history shows that the legal and moral status of psychoactive drugs constantly changes. "During the seventeenth century the sale and use of tobacco were punished by death in much of Europe, Russia, China, and Japan. For centuries many of the same Muslim domains that forbade the sale and consumption of alcohol, at the same time, tolerated and even regulated the sale of opium and cannabis" (Nadelmann, 1993).

In the Middle East, especially in Israel, the benefits of marijuana are being discussed. Such discussions, however, tend to reach no conclusions since there is no broad-based coalition of respectable special interest groups and community-based organizations to move drug policy and practices to a more rational and pragmatic level. Certainly, if such an organization does not develop, there is always the issue of economic realities and constraints—neither Israelis nor Palestinians are keen on using limited government resources or paying more taxes to enforce laws against a relatively benign substance whose use could be addressed through controlled regulation. The door is open for change by both nations in terms of how the problem of marijuana use is to be addressed; the only questions are when and how that change will occur. Getting there will not be easy, and the effort should be taken incrementally. Such gradualism would allow for a necessary shift in values so that more socially and economically pragmatic policies can be formulated and enacted (Shopping for a Drugs Policy, 1997). For some, such legislation may be a leap in the dark. Indeed, there will be unpredictable consequences as well as predictable ones. But that does not argue for taking no action, or for tough talk that is empty in terms of action and outcomes.

HEROIN: THE "KING" OF ILLEGAL DRUGS

Historical Perspective

If one substance were to be labeled the "king" of illegal drugs, most people would say it is heroin. Since the late nineteenth century, when it was created, heroin has virtually defined the drug problem (Kaplan, 1983).

> Disapproval of any level of use is higher for heroin than it is for any other drug; opposition to legalization is higher for heroin than it is for any other drug; and heroin addicts are the most stigmatized of all drug users. Heroin is the epitome of the illicit street drug. Its association in the public mind with street crime, in spite of strong competition from crack, is stronger than for any other drug. The stereotype of the "junkie" is that [of a] dweller in the underworld, an unsavory, untrustworthy character to be avoided at almost any cost. (Goode, 1989)

Heroin is chemically derived from morphine, which comes from the opium poppy grown primarily in the Golden Crescent, an area of Afghanistan, Pakistan, and Iran; the Golden Triangle, located in parts of Thailand, Laos, and Burma (now Myanmar), the Middle East, most notably, Lebanon; and Latin American countries, including Colombia and Mexico. Opium is the product of the poppy plant, *Papaver somniferum,* a rather undistinguished annual plant with a long-stemmed flower that is usually either purple or white but sometimes scarlet depending on the species. The plant grows in mountainous areas, although not at very high altitudes. Once the flower opens, the bulb is slashed or punctured with a three-pronged knife and the flowing juice, once dried by the wind, is collected. This dried substance is then boiled until it becomes a mass of raw opium called "black." Black is then refined to a morphine base, which is later transformed into heroin. Each successive step requires more sophisticated laboratory techniques, although the first steps can be accomplished directly in the fields, where a good part of the opium is often eaten by natives.

The word "opium" is derived from the Greek word for juice, and literary critics have suggested that the sailors who accompanied Ulysses in the *Odyssey*, whom Homer described in the ninth century B.C. as eating lotus, were actually consuming opium; the Country of the Lotophagi would, according to this version, be located in the Far East: "The first historical reference to opium is on a wall plaque from 2000 B.C. found in Kurgia, Turkey. The four edges of the plaque are decorated with opium poppy pods. The first written description of the use of opium is on a papyrus called the *ibis papyrus*, dated between 1550 and 1600 B.C. The papyrus points out some of the salient therapeutic uses of opium, even in those days, for pain and for constipation" (Harris, 1993). Opium and the opium poppy had been known to the Chinese well before the year 1000 A.D., when it was primarily used by a select, elite group. Over the years, the Chinese developed the habit of smoking tobacco and eating opium. Eventually, these two pleasures became one (that is, in the form of smoking) and opium became the substance of choice (Ray & Ksir, 1990). Arab merchants trading in the Silk Route knew it as "amdak," and they introduced it to the West as a medicinal plant in the seventh and eighth centuries A.D. The Chinese name for the substance was "chandu," or "yen" (this is the origin of the English word "yearn"), and it became "akbari" when introduced to India. Opium preparations were part of the armamentarium of every self-respecting Arab doctor in a period when Arab medicine was probably the best in the world. Opium over time has been used against malaria, colitis, and pain (Telias, 1991).

By 1729, the use of opium in China was so prevalent that a law was introduced mandating that opium shop owners were to be strangled. Once opium for nonmedical purposes was outlawed, it was necessary for the drug to be smuggled in from India, where poppy plantations were abundant (Scott, 1969). The economic stakes were high for those involved; smugglers included British adventurers and members of the East India Company. It has been noted that "the British had very little success with introducing alcohol either in India or the Far East. A certain percentage of the Asian population have enzyme systems that cause them to have severe side effects from the ingestion of alcohol. Thus, until recently, alcohol was not popular in [that region of the world]. The British decided to go into the opium business, and they were joined by all the other Western powers. They grew opium in India and exported it to China" (Harris, 1993). When an effort was made in 1839 to suppress the smuggling of opium into China, relations among nations and peoples became strained, resulting in the Opium War of 1839, which lasted about two years. "As victors, the British were given the island of Hong Kong, broad trading rights, and $6 million to reimburse the merchants whose opium had been destroyed" (Ray & Ksir, 1990).

Not until 1906, through the British parliament, was legislative action taken to stem the opium trade, but by that time, problem behavior related to opium addiction was no secret, especially among those who were provided the substance. "There were at the end of the Second World War, hundreds of thousands of opiate dependent individuals in the People's Republic of China. These by and large disappeared from view, at least until very recently, when there has been a resurgence in opiate use" (Harris, 1993).

In 1806, a young German scientist by the name of Frederich Sertürner published a report on his isolation of the primary active ingredient in opium—an ingredient 10 times more potent than opium itself. Sertürner named it "morphium" after Morpheus, the god of dreams. Two major developments during the nineteenth century promoted the widespread use of morphine. First, in 1853 the hypodermic syringe was perfected by Dr. Alexander Wood, making it possible to introduce morphine directly into the bloodstream or body tissue rather than the slower process of eating opium or morphine and waiting for it to be absorbed through the gastrointestinal tract. The second factor was the use of morphine as a pain relief agent for casualties of the American Civil War (1861–1865), the Prussian-Austrian War (1866), and the Franco-Prussian War (1870). The percentage of returning veterans from those wars addicted to morphine was high enough that the illness was later called "soldier's disease," or the "army disease" (Lindesmith, 1965; Weisberger, 1993).

In 1874, a chemical bonding process for morphine was discovered that produced heroin—a substance about three times as potent as morphine. Initially marketed by Bayer Laboratories of Germany in 1898 as a nonaddictive substitute for codeine derived from opium, it took nearly a decade of research to find that heroin was the most addictive of the opiates, able to affect brain functioning faster than anything yet known.

Despite the growing problem of opiate dependence arising from unrestrained distribution of opium derivatives within the medical system in the United States, it was the street use of the opiates and cocaine that generated public and professional interest in their habit-forming properties. After the U.S. Civil War, a host of conditions arose that led to various city, state, and federal attempts to legislatively control the spread of drug use. Among these factors were: increased Chinese immigration on the West Coast, which was linked to opium smoking, the possession of opium pipes, and the maintenance of opium dens; the addicted Civil War soldiers; and the widespread use of patent medicines for the relief of aches, pains, and anxiety that contained alcohol and/or opiates such as opium or morphine, and which could be legally purchased at a store or through mail order firms like Sears, Roebuck and Company (Musto, 1973).

Although estimates varied, it was generally believed that the total number of addicts never exceeded a quarter of a million, divided evenly between medical and street dependence. Increased awareness, brought about by crusades waged among law enforcement officials against the street use of opiates and cocaine, aroused public anxiety about a narcotics problem of major proportions. The movement for national alcohol prohibition further sensitized the public to a need for national drug prohibitions. The culmination was the passage of the Harrison Narcotics Act of 1914 in the United States (Ray & Ksir, 1990). "This act outlawed non-medical use of opiates, and Supreme Court decisions during the next seven years further narrowed even the medical uses of opium products. With the Harrison Act, people who had become dependent on opiates had to seek alternative sources for drugs containing opiates. This elimination of the medical supply of opiates and the criminalization of opiate use shifted narcotic addiction from the medical arena to the legal arena. At the same time, this law precipitated the need for treatments to assist those who were addicted to opiates but could no longer obtain them from their physicians" (McCann, Rawson, Obert, & Hasson, 1994). Following World War II, "the enactment of anti-opium laws in many parts of Asia in which opium use was traditional—India, Hong Kong, Thailand, Laos, Iran—effectively suppressed the availability of opium at the cost of stimulating the creation of domestic heroin industries and substantial increases in heroin use. The same tradition had occurred in the United States following Congress's ban on opium imports in 1909" (Nadelmann, 1993). It has been noted that at the turn of the century

> despite the virtual absence of any controls on availability, the proportion of Americans addicted to opiates was only two to three times greater than today. . . . The typical addict was not a young black ghetto resident but a middle-class white Southern woman or a West Coast Chinese immigrant. The violence, death, disease, and crime that we today associate with drug use barely existed, and many medical authorities regarded opiate addiction as far less destructive than alcoholism (some doctors even prescribed the former as treatment for the latter). Many opiate addicts, perhaps most, managed to lead relatively normal lives and kept their addictions secret even from close friends and relatives. That they were able to do so was largely a function of the legal status of their drug use. (Nadelmann, 1993)

With a ban on opiates, new forces entered the market, namely, the illegal organizations interested in making a quick profit. Those organizations succeeded in popularizing the opiates in the United States and Europe much faster than the British had succeeded in China. Until the mid-1960s, laboratory facilities that could transform morphine base into heroin were available only in Europe and the United States. This meant that most of the product had to be transported to be refined, and the refining process put a great deal of money into Western hands. In the mid-1960s two apparently unrelated episodes changed the situation. On one hand, under American pressure, the Turkish government agreed to close most of the illegal fields in that country, reserving a small portion of the product for legal medicinal purposes. On the other hand, Hong Kong–based drug entrepreneurs succeeded in establishing a series of laboratories along the Mekong River and refined the product locally.

> [It is rumored that] those organizations foresaw the massive American intervention in the Vietnam War and readied themselves to profit from the American soldiers coming to the area. Others claim that the Vietcong foresaw American intervention and assisted the Chinese

in establishing the laboratories, so that heroin could be easily available in order to support the war effort. . . . Also, it is claimed that the political changes undergone by Vietnam at the time were related, at least partially, to the war for the domination of the heroin market. (Telias, 1991)

In the United States, evidence tends to show no significant rise in opiate and heroin addiction, despite the general impression to the contrary (Johnston, O'Malley, & Bachman, 1987; Martz, 1990). For example, about 1 percent of all Americans have tried heroin at least once in their lives, but among those who have used any illegal drug, fewer than 3 percent have tried or used heroin (National Institute on Drug Abuse, 1986; SAMHSA, 2000: 61). Among all episodes of illegal drug use only 1 percent involve heroin (Goode, 1989). Based on a nationally representative probability sample of hospitals located throughout the United States, the 1997 Drug Abuse Warning Network (DAWN) survey shows that 1.3 percent of males compared with 0.6 percent of females ever used heroin, and 0.4 percent of males compared with 0.2 percent females used heroin during the year prior to the survey. DAWN data for 1998 show that women account for 20 percent of all heroin/morphine mentions and about 26 percent of drug abuse deaths.

From the European perspective, surveys reveal that illegal drug use is on the rise, especially among young people. According to the European Monitoring Center on Drugs and Drug Addiction, the most alarming trend is in heroin use. "It has long been the biggest source of Europe's drug-related crime and medical problems, including AIDS and hepatitis from shared needles. Now its availability and popularity are growing" (Dickey & Underhill, 1996). In the early 1990s the European addict population, estimated at between 500,000 and a million, seemed to stabilize. Now, in most places, heroin has become cheaper, purer, and easier to purchase. For example, the price of heroin has dropped to a level that has made it cheap enough to smoke or snort instead of inject, making it attractive to those who want to experiment. One reason for this is geopolitics. Drug profits have been financing some of the religious and ethnic conflicts that have arisen since the end of the Cold War. According to the International Criminal Police Organization (Interpol), "the warlords have become the drug lords. . . . [T]he collapse of the Soviet Empire opened up new supply routes and spawned smuggling rings from Burma to Estonia. The opening of borders in the European Union afforded unprecedented access to a vast untapped market. Aggressive criminal gangs in Africa and South America have been quick to seize the initiative, too. Capitalizing on skills in dealing marijuana or cocaine, they have expanded their product lines to include heroin . . . with a significant amount being South America heroin which was virtually unknown five years ago. In 1994 it accounted for 32 percent of the heroin seized in America; last year (1995) it was up to a staggering 62 percent" (Dickey & Underhill, 1996).[1]

CROSS-CULTURAL PERSPECTIVE OF HEROIN ADDICTS

The use of illegal substances such as heroin may be the result of a number of factors including those of a personal, social, or cultural nature. From a cross-cultural perspective, one question that arises is to what extent addicts from different countries have common attitudes toward the use and abuse of heroin. To assess such a question, an adequate selection of countries must be made, and relevant factors, including economic, political, cultural, need to be considered. While drug use has seldom been systematically studied in a cross-national or cross-cultural manner, considerable exploratory work is necessary, and there can be no guarantee that the most rigorous research will provide definitive results.

Exploratory research has been conducted on Russian-speaking addicts in Israel (see Chapter 6 in this book). Comparative research has been conducted on heroin addicts from Singapore and Israel to test whether culture is related to their attitudes, norms, and behavior (Ong, 1989; Ong & Isralowitz, 1996). Results regarding the psychological characteristics of the heroin addicts revealed that those from Singapore, compared with their Israeli counterparts, have a more positive profile in terms of interpersonal relations, self-concept, personal values, and motivation. The Singapore heroin addicts also tended to be more pleasure seeking, risk taking, and inclined to continue using illegal drugs. The only characteristic shared among the addicts from both countries was rebelliousness. While the findings of this study are exploratory, which limits their generalizability, a number of interesting response patterns emerged, relating to culture and the social context of substance use that are worthy of further investigation. First, Singapore is a small but dynamic society dominated by a rather homogeneous Chinese culture and heritage that strongly endorses positive personal and familial values (Ong & Isralowitz, 1996). It is not surprising, therefore, that the study participants from that island nation, regardless of their drug use status, report more positive attitudes than those from Israel, which is much more culturally diverse. How these results would compare with those of a different socioeconomic group such as Israelis who have a Northern and Eastern European background or Palestinians from the West Bank and Gaza is open to further query. The results of this exploratory binational comparison show that heroin addicts from different cultures tend to have few psychological characteristics in common, and the differences tend to be influenced by the prevailing social and cultural norms of the society in which they reside (Ong & Isralowitz, 1996). Such findings have implications for the nature of future treatment programs.

CONCLUSION

Much of what has been presented here, while culturally and geographically specific to the United States, has considerable relevance to Israelis and Palestinians for a number of reasons. First, the United States is a major exporter of its culture through the mass media and other means, which tends to shape the attitudes and behavior of young people exposed to it. Second, the United States, through grants and other forms of assistance, has a major influence on other nations, such as those in the Middle East, in terms of policy and program decision making regarding substance use. Both factors tend to be reflected by Israeli and Palestinian governments and nongovernmental agencies addressing the drug problem through control over production and distribution and primary prevention and treatment intervention.

Many of the attitudes and behavior patterns that prevailed regarding the spread of marijuana and opiate use in the United States, in terms of racial and ethnic finger pointing, tend to exist also in the Middle East. In a series of recent conferences sponsored by Israeli and Palestinian nongovernmental agencies, substance abuse experts from each side accused the other of creating and spreading the problem. The one factor that representatives from both sides readily agreed to is that those involved with promoting the distribution, sale, and use of illicit substances in the region have better methods of communication, cooperation, and coordination than those responsible for combating the problem.

NOTE

1. Consumption of illicit drugs in Latin America does not approach the levels in the United States, which are by far the largest in the world. The percentage of drug users in Latin America, however, is growing fast. While the following information may not be specific to heroin use, it does reflect the present nature of the problem. One report from Brazil estimates that the cost of medical care for drug addiction soared to $2.9 billion in 1997 from $902 million in 1993. In Buenos Aires, Mexico City, Peru (mainly Lima), and Colombia, rates of illicit drug use are on the rise and the cost of illicit substances has gone down since the 1980s (Faiola, 1999).

REFERENCES

Abu Saad, I. (2002). Social change and substance use among the Bedouin Arabs in southern Israel. In R. Isralowitz, M. Afifi, & R. Rawson (Eds.), *Drug problems: Cross-Cultural Policy and Program Development*. Westport, CT: Praeger.

Berne, E. (1964). *Games people play*. New York: Mentor Books.

Bertram, E., & Sharpe, K. (1996). The unwinnable drug war: What Clausewitz would tell us. *World Policy Journal, 13*(4), 41.

Dickey, C., & Underhill, W. (1996, October 14). The drug threat. *Newsweek, 128*, 41–47.

Faiola, A. (1999, September 16). For Latin America, a boomerang effect on illegal drugs. *International Herald Tribune*, p. 2.

Goode, E. (1989). *Drugs in American society* (3rd ed.). New York: Knopf.

Gray, M. (1998). *Drug crazy.* New York: Random House.

Grinspoon, L., & Bakalar, J. (1993). *Marijuana: The forbidden medicine.* New Haven, CT: Yale University Press (and the Lindesmith Center).

Harris, L. (1993). Opiates: A history of opiates and their use in treatment. In C. Hartel (Ed.), *Biomedical approaches in illicit drug demand reduction* (p. 85). Rockville, MD: National Institute on Drug Abuse.

Isralowitz, R., Abu Saad, I., & Telias, D. (1996). Work values among heroin addicts: A status model perspective. *Journal of Offender Rehabilitation, 24*(1/2), 141–154.

Isralowitz, R., & Peleg, A. (1996). Israeli college student alcohol use: The association of background characteristics and regular drinking patterns. *Drug and Alcohol Dependence, 42*, 147–153.

Isralowitz, R., & Telias, D. (1998). *Drug use, policy and management* (pp. 95–109). Westport, CT: Praeger.

Isralowitz, R., Telias, D., & Abu Saad, I. (1994). Psychological characteristics of heroin addicts and non-drug users in Israel: A status model comparison. *Journal of Social Psychology, 134*(3), 399–401.

Isralowitz, R., Telias, D., & Zighelbaum, Y. (1992). Heroin addiction in Israel: A comparison of addicts in prison, community-based facilities, and non-drug users based on selected psychological factors. *International Journal of Offender Therapy and Comparative Criminology, 36*(1), 62–72.

Isralowitz, R., & Troestler, N. (1996). Substance use: Toward an understanding of its relation to nutrition-related attitudes and behavior among Israeli high school youth. *Journal of Adolescent Health, 19*(3), 184–189.

Johnston L., O'Malley, P., & Bachman, J. (1987). *National trends in drug use and related factors among American high school students and young adults 1975–1986.* Rockville, MD: National Institute on Drug Abuse.

Kaplan, J. (1983). *The hardest drug: Heroin and public policy.* Chicago: University of Chicago Press.

Lindesmith, A. (1965). *The addict and the law.* Bloomington: Indiana University Press.

Linton, R. (1947). *The study of man.* New York: Appleton.

Makuriya, T. (Ed.). (1973). *Marijuana: Medical papers, 1839–1972.* Oakland, CA: Medi-Comp.

Mann, P. (1985). *Marijuana alert.* New York: McGraw-Hill.

Martz, L. (1990, February 19). A dirty drug secret: Hyping instant addiction doesn't help. *Newsweek, 115*(8), 74.

McCann, M., Rawson, R., Obert, J., & Hasson, A. (1994). *Treatment of opiate addiction with methadone* (p. 2). Rockville, MD: U.S. Department of Health and Human Services.

Musto, D. (1973). *The American disease: Origins of narcotic control.* New Haven, CT: Yale University Press.

Nadelmann, E. (1993). Should we legalize drugs? History answers. *American Heritage, 44*(1), 41–48.

Nahas, G. (1975). *Marijuana—Deceptive weed.* New York: Raven Press.

National Institute on Drug Abuse. (1986). *Highlights of the 1985 National Household Survey on Drug Abuse.* Rockville, MD: National Institute on Drug Abuse.

Ong, T. (1989). *Drug abuse in Singapore: A psychological perspective.* Singapore: Hillview.

Ong, T. H., & Isralowitz, R. (1996). *Substance use in Singapore: Illegal drugs, inhalants and alcohol* (pp. 135–144). Singapore: Toppan.

Orlandi, M. (1995). The challenge of evaluating community-based prevention programs: A cross-cultural perspective. In M. Orlandi (Ed.), *Cultural Competence for Evaluators.*

(U.S. Department of Health and Human Services Pub. No. SMA 95-3066). Rockville, MD: U.S. Government Printing Office.

Ray, O., & Ksir, C. (1990). *Drugs, society and human behavior.* St. Louis, MO: Times Mirror/Mosby.

SAMHSA (Substance Abuse and Mental Health Services Administration). (2000). *National Household Survey on Drug Abuse Main Findings 1998.* (U.S. Department of Health and Human Services Pub. No. SMA 00-3381). Rockville, MD: U.S. Government Printing Office.

Scott, J. (1969). *The white poppy: A history of opium.* New York: Funk and Wagnalls.

Shopping for a Drugs Policy. (1997, August 16). *The Economist, 344*(8030), 43–44.

Snyder, S. (1970, December 13). What have we forgotten about pot? *New York Times Magazine*, pp. 27, 121, 124, 130.

Sussman, S., Stacy, A., Dent, C., Simon, T., & Johnson, C. (1996). Marijuana use: Current issues and new research directions. *Journal of Drug Issues, 26*(4), 700–702.

Telias, D. (1991). *The world of 'H'*. Tel Aviv: Freund Publishing House.

Weisberger, B. (1993, February–March). The Chinese must go. *American Heritage*, *44*(1), 24–25.

Weiss, S., Sawa, G. H., Abdeen, Z., & Yanai, J. (1999). Substance abuse studies and prevention efforts among Arabs in the 1990s in Israel, Jordan and the Palestinian Authority—A literature review. *Addiction, 94*(2), 177–198.

Wright, P. (1994). Following specific guidelines will help you assess cultural competence in program design, application and management. *Prevention works: Technical assistance bulletin*. Rockville, MD: National Clearinghouse for Alcohol and Drug Information.

2

Drugs and Peace: New Meanings, Old Metaphors–The Palestinian-Israeli People against Substance Abuse (PIPASA) Experience

Gary Sussman

INTRODUCTION

The predominant metaphor that springs to mind when we speak of drugs is that of war—both cause destruction and claim victims, though on different scales. A former soldier, retired General Barry R. McCaffrey,[1] and the U.S. administration waged a war in the 1990s of unprecedented dimensions against drugs, particularly in terms of supply. The drug trade is also a central aspect of civil wars, funding and fueling ethnic and political conflicts in Asia, Africa, and Latin America. Colombia is a stark example of a country severely affected by a civil war funded by drugs (McDonald, 1997).[2] Since 1987, about 35,000 civilians have been killed or "disappeared" in this civil war. In 1999, 1,000 combat-related killings were recorded and some 300,000 people were displaced as a result of the conflict (Salinas, 2000). Critics of the U.S. government's "war on drugs" suggest that the effort to reduce the supply of drugs—and not the demand for drugs—exacerbate this civil war.[3] In history, the drug-related conflicts we are perhaps most familiar with are the Opium Wars (1839–1843, 1856–1860) between China and Britain.[4]

This chapter examines the conflict in the Middle East, where a unique effort among Israelis and Palestinians has been undertaken to link the war on drugs with the struggle for peace. This was done by building bridges between substance abuse professionals and academicians from the two societies. This experience, led by peace organizations and professional agencies, with important input from international substance abuse experts, created an anti-drug/pro-peace initiative known as the "Palestinian and Israeli People against Substance Abuse" (PIPASA). Recounted here from the perspective of one of the implementers, the experience of the development of PIPASA is assessed in the context of conflict resolution[5] and with the tragic events beginning in the last part of the year 2000 in mind.[6]

CONFLICT RESOLUTION: A THEORETICAL OVERVIEW

Scholars of conflict resolution distinguish between the concepts of *peace making* and *peace building*. Peace making is associated with efforts of diplomats and others, including non-political actors, to bring about a cessation of hostilities by ensuring cease-fires and clinching peace agreements. Peace building represents long-term efforts designed to transform the nature of relations between conflicting parties. In so doing, these efforts are designed to prevent conflict from erupting again (Ryan, 1995).[7] Peace making and peace building represent, therefore, different aspects and phases of conflict resolution and require different strategies. If these two components of the peace process are compared to drug treatment, we can liken peace making to a curative process, whereas peace building is similar to a long-term preventive and treatment approach. The emphasis in peace building is on transforming the nature of relations between ethnic groups or ideological and political movements embroiled in a conflict. To achieve this transformation, John Lederach suggests creating a comprehensive framework that "legitimates and integrates multiple levels of the population affected, in terms of both input in the peace process and its implementation" (Lederach, 1995). Lederach's comprehensive framework for ensuring "conflict transformation" incorporates three main components. The first component is the adoption of an integrated perspective that combines both short- and long-term transformations. The former refers to efforts aimed at initiating the peace process and peace making. This requires taking care of immediate issues such as cease-fires, amnesty, and mutual recognition. Addressing the so-called long-term transformation involves providing a framework to address the long-term agenda. The long-term process includes the second and third components, establishing an infrastructure for peace and building a peace constituency.[8]

The participants in the PIPASA experience were not politicians. They were professionals and academics, and as such they were not in a position to contribute to efforts that could provide a short- or long-term political framework for solving the Palestinian-Israeli conflict. Such a framework was provided by the Oslo peace process and put into practice through its Interim Agreements. Nevertheless, the work that was conducted in the framework of this project contributed in a modest way to creating an infrastructure for peace and building a peace constituency. By an *infrastructure for peace*, Lederach refers to the creation of personal and institutional relationships—bridges—that contribute to new and positive relations between two peoples embroiled in a protracted conflict. Indeed, assessed in the context of the "macro situation," namely, the scant progress in the implementation of the interim peace agreements and in the negotiations regarding a permanent status accord, the PIPASA experience, along with the multitude of people-to-people activities that were undertaken during this period, provided a safety net for Palestinian-Israeli relations. Also, by catalyzing and facilitating contacts through "building bridges," the PIPASA process contributed to the gradual expansion of the peace-building constituency. The project attempted, moreover, to provide evidence that cooperation and coexistence are possible. In sum, this effort to address substance abuse was essentially a "bottom-up" peace-building effort, similar to other initiatives taking place in the Palestinian-Israeli context.

The role of international nongovernmental organizations (NGOs), such as the International Red Cross and Médecins Sans Frontières (MSF), in delivering humanitarian assistance in conflict settings has been documented. Insufficient attention has been paid, however, to the role of health care workers in promoting peace in general and within the Palestinian-Israeli context in particular (Barnea, Ziaad, et al., 2000).[9] One important effort to introduce a typology of Health-Peace Initiatives (HPIs) was presented by MacQueen, McCutcheon, and Santa Barbara (1997).[10] They identify a typology of nine categories of HPIs, according to their mode of operation.

The first of these nine categories encompasses the role of health care workers in communicating knowledge or "truth telling" about the consequences of conflict. In this regard, the authors cite the role of the Nobel Prize–winning organization, the International Physicians for the Prevention of Nuclear War (IPPNW). IPPNW was instrumental in presenting the harrowing consequences of nuclear war in health terms and contributing to a change in public opinion regarding nuclear weapons.[11] The second mode of operation is the role of health care workers in the "evocation and broadening of altruism." Here the authors refer to activities that are designed to counter the depersonalization, and at times demonization, of the enemy. The third mode of operation by which HPIs contribute to peace initiatives is via the "construction of superordinate goals," in which HPIs create joint projects that unite adversaries in the pursuit of a common goal. The authors provide several examples of such projects in Latin America, including the 1985–1992 UNICEF-sponsored "Days of Peace" cease-fires in El Salvador. These cease-fires not only allowed for the vaccination of children[12] but also provided a confidence-building mechanism between the two adversaries. The fourth contribution of HPIs is the "extension of solidarity." Here the authors refer to the role of health workers in working and identifying with victims of war, such as displaced persons or the maimed. Such solidarity activities are instrumental in drawing attention to the plight of victims of conflict through the health workers' domestic and international contacts. The fifth category of HPIs are those activities that facilitate the strengthening of communities. In this regard, the authors argue that attempting to maintain a health system during armed conflict and rebuilding it afterward help to give people a sense of security and normality. Essentially, creating a functioning health service infrastructure is instrumental in encouraging refugees to return to their former homes. "To the extent that it is equally accessable to all, health care will lessen feelings of persecution and denial of needs, and will reduce competition for resources." In this regard, the role of the health worker is therefore to create a tangible "peace dividend" and reassure both protagonists and victims that the peace process is working. The sixth contribution of the HPI is that of social and individual healing. This involves initiatives that bring together physically and emotionally disabled combatants from both sides of the conflict in an effort to integrate them. The seventh form of an HPI that MacQueen, McCutcheon, and Santa Barbara identify is noncooperation and dissent by health care workers in a conflict setting. The eighth type of HPI is the involvement of health professionals in diplomacy as track two diplomats and intermediaries. The last of the nine HPIs is the role of health care professionals in redefining a conflict situation. In this regard, health care workers and other professionals can reframe the parameters of debate over a particular conflict. By portraying nonpolitical dimensions of the conflict, health professionals can open valuable space for an informed public debate on the conflict. Again the authors highlight the role of the IPPNW in reframing the public debate, and as a result, the public's perception of nuclear war. The authors emphasize that the effectiveness of HPIs and health workers is accounted for by the fact that "physicians have a high degree of social legitimacy and tend to be trusted (probably more than politicians) by the public." This particular assumption motivated the Israeli-based Economic Cooperation Foundation (ECF) and the Palestine Council of Health (PCH) to pursue cooperation among health care professionals (MacQueen et al., 1997).[13] It is also worth mentioning that Dr. Hikmat Ajjuri of the PCH, who was involved in the PIPASA process, is an active member of the IPPNW.

In this chapter, the PIPASA experience is examined in terms of Lederach's principles of building a peace constituency and infrastructure. Specifically, this chapter will show the extent to which this experience conformed to the categories of the various HPIs noted above and provided an "Anti-Drugs/Pro-Peace Initiative."

PROJECT BACKGROUND AND HISTORY

This project was initiated through the ECF and the PCH, which work in coalition in the region. On the Israeli side, professional substance abuse leadership was provided by the Regional Alcohol and Drug Abuse Resources (RADAR) Center of Ben-Gurion University, which operates through the Department of Social Work. The key Palestinian substance abuse professionals were affiliated with the Child and Family Consultation Center (CFCC) and the Gaza-based Child Health and Community Research Association (CHCR).

The history of the ECF and PCH cooperation has been well documented in their comprehensive annual reports and, as such, will not be recounted here.[14] Briefly, though, the essence of this partnership has been to create and facilitate opportunities for health professionals to meet and interact. This has involved facilitating study visits to Palestinian and Israeli institutions, and arranging workshops and assisting with the promotion and implementation of joint projects that have emerged from these interactions. This process has not been a simple one, and Palestinian and Israeli organizations that engage in these activities confront many practical obstacles.[15] Beyond the everyday obstacles, the broader peace process greatly influences the dialogue process. In the absence of tangible progress and Israeli settlement expansion, many Palestinian participants view such activities as legitimating the status quo and being insufficiently political. Moreover, as recently witnessed, the tragic violence that has been part and parcel of the process at times leads participants to question the validity of the process.

Based on their success in the area of health, the two organizations made a strategic decision in mid-1997 to broaden this cooperation to include providers of social services. This decision, coupled with an ever-widening network of contacts with Palestinian and Israeli NGOs and the diplomatic community, led to a referral that resulted from a unique proposal made to the ECF and PCH. Dan Sreebny, a Tel Aviv–based American diplomat, contacted the ECF inquiring if the organization could assist a Ben-Gurion University faculty member to identify a Palestinian partner for joint research and program development on substance abuse. Thus, the ECF and the PCH, having made a strategic decision to address broader social welfare issues, were linked to someone able to translate this decision into concrete action, Professor Richard Isralowitz.

The obvious synergy and potential for a Palestinian-Israeli dialogue was apparent from the first meeting held with Professor Isralowitz in the PCH's East Jerusalem office. Following several brainstorming sessions, it was decided that the ECF and PCH, together with the Ben-Gurion University-RADAR Center, CFCC, and CHCR—incorporated by the PCH—would stage a first workshop on substance abuse. As Palestinian agencies, public and nongovernmental, are unable to effectively operate in both the West Bank and Gaza because of Israeli-imposed travel restrictions, it was decided to engage NGOs that worked in the Gaza Strip and the West Bank. The CFCC is based in Bethlehem and CHCR in Gaza City.

The objective of this workshop was to simply facilitate a meeting of professionals concerned with the issue from both societies and gauge the potential for cooperation. It was agreed that the workshop would be held in Beer Sheva and that it was desirable to invite an international expert from the United States. Dr. Richard Rawson, director of the Matrix Institute on Addictions in Los Angeles and associate director of the University of California, Los Angeles, Drug Abuse Research Center (now the UCLA Integrated Substance Abuse Programs), was chosen.[16]

The agenda of Dr. Rawson's visit was widened to include a series of lectures in Gaza and the West Bank for Palestinian professionals, prior to the joint workshop in Beer Sheva. One of the main reasons for this expanded agenda was to ensure that his trip did not depend solely on the joint workshop, which was in danger of being postponed because Israeli border crossings with Gaza and the West Bank had been closed. When Dr. Rawson successfully completed the trips to the West Bank and Gaza, efforts were focused on the first joint two-day workshop, entitled "Palestinian and Israeli People Against Substance Abuse: A Cooperative Effort to Address the Problem through Communication, Cooperation and Coordination." As was common during that time period, travel permits for Palestinians to enter into Israel were a problem for the workshop that was to be held November 4 and 5, 1997. Only two-thirds of the Gaza workshop participants were granted permits. On the West

Bank, two of the key participants were refused entry permits, which prompted the frustrated 18-person West Bank delegation to threaten to boycott the event. Eventually, at the end of a long day of persistent negotiation by the ECF management and staff with the Israeli security establishment, permits were secured for all the West Bank participants. The permits, however, did not include sleepover permission for all, and as a result, the West Bankers arrived on the second day of the workshop.

Despite the workshop getting off to a difficult start as a result of the permit problems, the second day produced a stimulating debate. The participants soon realized that the area of substance abuse encompassed numerous facets and offered diverse opportunities for dialogue and cooperation. Moreover, it became evident that the drug issue was a source of major tension and mistrust. One of the issues repeatedly raised at the workshop was the Palestinian claim that Israel was deliberately encouraging the flow of drugs to Palestinian areas. The perceived Israeli objective of encouraging the flow of drugs into Palestinian areas was to undermine the moral and social fabric of Palestinian society. This perception was influenced by two factors. The first was the perceived collaboration between the Israeli General Security Service and some Palestinian criminals, often drug dealers and prostitutes.[17] A second factor contributing to this perception was that drug dealers holding Israeli identification cards who were arrested for selling drugs in Palestinian areas were seen back on the streets not long after being transferred to the Israeli authorities. However, it emerged that the Israeli authorities often had no choice but to release these people because the authorities lacked the evidence for conviction.[18] The workshop provided a valuable framework to address these perceptions. Improved cooperation in addressing drug use and the supply of drugs was therefore recognized by the participants as a priority. Indeed, participants noted the ease with which Israeli and Palestinian criminals cooperated to spread drugs (Isralowitz, 1998a). The participants also stressed the importance of joint research, including an assessment of Palestinian needs in drug abuse education and training among those treating substance abusers. It is worth noting that Dr. Rawson played a central role in this workshop and its discussions by providing a neutral third-party perspective, particularly at junctures when sensitive issues seemed to shift the focus of the workshop to a series of mutual recriminations. The role of a third party in such a dialogue cannot be sufficiently underscored, especially when there is an element of mistrust and when each party has its own perspective. A stenographer recorded these and other workshop proceedings, which were edited by Professor Isralowitz and prepared for publication in booklet form by the ECF and the PCH.

The initial Israeli-Palestinian substance abuse workshop fulfilled several important functions. First, the workshop opened channels of communication, which were essential in establishing cooperation and coordination. Specifically, the Beer Sheva workshop provided an opportunity for participants to establish personal and professional contacts on matters involving substance abuse policy development, treatment, education, and research. Also, the workshop served to generate a few concrete ways of promoting further cooperation; as such, the event served to ensured that the process and cooperation were demand driven. This was crucial because such dialogues may evolve into exercises where one side imposes their will and agenda on the other side. From these discussions, several superordinate tasks were identified as well, including the need for human resource development, research programs, information dissemination, resource centers, and training workshops. Finally, the forum provided an opportunity to dispel a number of misperceptions about the drug problem and reinforce the mutual nature of the problem. In sum, the first workshop made significant progress in humanizing the "other side" and challenging prejudices. To use an old cliche, the participants recognized that drugs know no boundaries.

Building on the first workshop, a second effort focused on community-based initiatives. With cooperation from the U.S. Information Agency, James Copple of the National Crime Prevention Council in the United States was invited to attend the workshop. The workshop, entitled "Prevention and Beyond: A Workshop on Community Based Initiatives," was held in Bethlehem.[19] The workshop was logistically much easier to organize because permits for participants from the West Bank were not required. Over 60 persons attended. A variety of new NGO representatives and representatives of various government ministries attended from both the Israeli and Palestinian sides, expanding the network of contacts. The participation of the government representatives was particularly significant at the time, considering that government-to-government contacts had tapered off because of the impasse in the peace process. In addition to the professional interactions, the evening saw the Israelis, who slept over in Bethlehem, visiting local coffee shops with the Palestinian participants.[20] Again, as in the first workshop, Palestinians expressed the belief that Israel was "flooding" Palestinian streets with drugs. For the police force of Bethlehem, the sight of recently arrested Israeli drug peddlers on their streets was a source of anger and frustration (Isralowitz, 1998b).[21] Once more, these matters were discussed and diffused, this time by the numerous police officers attending from both sides. In response to these Palestinian accusations, Dr. Pini Yehezkeli, a senior representative of the Israeli police force, informed Palestinian officers that he, too, faced similar problems in Tel Aviv and other Israeli cities as a result of liberal Israeli arrest laws and procedures (Isralowitz, 1998b). This particular interaction underscored the limits of the formal channels that were in place and the need for a proactive police-to-police dialogue on the drug issue. The Bethlehem workshop, therefore, laid the platform for and legitimized future police-to-police cooperation.

Following the second workshop, Ben-Gurion University secured funding from the Israeli Ministry of Foreign Affair's Center for International Cooperation (MASHAV) for two substance abuse training programs for Palestinian professionals. These programs were organized by Ben-Gurion University in cooperation with its Palestinian partners. Twenty Palestinian professionals participated in the first course (Principles of Prevention and Treatment), which was held in Beer Sheva during the first week of July 1998. The second weeklong course was held in October 1998 and addressed the use of manualized drug treatment protocols. This course was presented by Dr. Richard Rawson and Jeanne Obert of the Matrix Institute and held in conjunction with the Al-Quds (Jerusalem) University. This progress was paralleled by the generation of several research projects, including one from the Palestinian-Netherlands Research Program, supported by the foreign ministries of the Netherlands and Israel, and the establishment of contacts with the World Health Organization (WHO) Substance Abuse Department, based in Geneva, Switzerland.[22] The WHO relationship resulted in a visit by Dr. Maristela Monteiro, who encouraged Palestinian and Israeli researchers to participate in an international WHO research program related to primary prevention of substance abuse. During her visit to the region, Dr. Monteiro joined Dr. Richard Rawson and Jeanne Obert for the third two-day training workshop, entitled "Substance Abuse Disorders: Recent Advances in Treatment," which was held immediately after completion of the Al-Quds University training program. This third workshop was held in Beer Sheva for Israeli and Palestinian participants.

After this blitz of activity, a fourth workshop was to have been held focusing on promoting dialogue among Israeli and Palestinian law enforcement personnel, including judges and police officers, regarding drug problems. This event was, however, postponed on two occasions as the Israeli participants were denied entry into Gaza by the Israeli Defense Force on security grounds. On the occasion of the first attempt, Judge Bernard Leroy, a senior advisor with the United Nations International Drug Control Programme (UNDCP) based in Austria, traveled to the region unaware of the postponement. The core parties, however, did meet with Judge Leroy in Bethlehem and explored ideas for cooperation in this particular area.

Finally, after considerable persistence from the ECF and PCH staff, the fourth workshop, supported by an Israeli foundation, was eventually staged in Ramallah on March 24 and 25, 1999. The activity was attended by officially sanctioned delegations of the Israeli and Palestinian police and legal experts—including the chief prosecutors of the North and South of Israel, representing the Ministry of Justice. Unfortunately, Palestinian judges from Gaza, including supreme court justices, returned home after being delayed at the border. Also attending the workshop were the Deputy Director of the Israeli Anti-Drug Authority and his Palestinian counterpart, which resulted in improved relations between the two anti-drug authorities.

While the previous endeavors created sufficient momentum for a variety of research and development projects, it is clear in retrospect that these efforts were also instrumental in building the confidence and goodwill necessary for this "police-to-police" meeting. The PIPASA framework and process not only legitimized the dialogue but also provided a context for a constructive interaction. To a certain extent, high-ranking Israeli officers were suspicious of an NGO-driven process. These officers felt that the necessary structures for cooperation and coordination were already in place and that there was no need for its personnel to meet with their Palestinian counterparts. However, the frustration voiced at the previous workshops underscored the limitations of these formal channels of cooperation and coordination. It was evident that certain issues were not raised and addressed in these formal channels. Moreover, the reality was that a poor state of relations—characterized by mistrust—prevailed between the Palestinian National Authority (PNA) and the government of Israel, reducing interactions to a bare "reactive" minimum. As a consequence of this political situation, the participation of the Palestinian police was largely facilitated by the involvement of other Palestinian NGOs, who served as both intermediaries and hosts. Again, the Ramallah workshops witnessed a reiteration of the alleged role Israel had in supplying drugs to Palestinians. This time the Israeli Mossad was the focus of accusation (Isralowitz, 1999), resulting in an emotive debate. Tempers flared to such an extent that the Israeli police delegation threatened to leave en masse. Despite these initial heated exchanges, the workshop proved to be a constructive forum for Israeli and Palestinian drug enforcement personnel, including police and legal experts, to discuss common concerns (Isralowitz, 1999).

Among the major problems raised was the inability of the PNA police to freely act in locations referred to as Area B, areas under joint Palestinian and Israeli security forces that require the cooperation of both sides for drug raids. This cumbersome process made the PNA's effort ineffectual and worked to the advantage of the criminals. Moreover, in Area C, which was under full Israeli responsibility, the PNA was unable to act at all. As a result of the lack of effective law enforcement, Areas B and C have been havens for drug smugglers. It was only in the territorially minuscule Area A, which is under full Palestinian control, that the PNA was able to effectively act. It also emerged that in the case of Israelis arrested in PNA-controlled areas, the full seizure of drugs was not always transferred to Israel, making an indictment impossible. Furthermore, it emerged that police officers who were required to give evidence in Israeli courts were often unable to get permits to attend the trials, enabling criminals to avoid conviction.

In April 1999, again with the encouragement of the U.S. Information Agency, Dr. Thomas Babor of the University of Connecticut visited the region to conduct training programs in Gaza and the West Bank. He also led a two-day workshop in Beer Sheva (April 26 and 27, 1999) entitled "Joint Israeli-Palestinian Training on WHO International Substance Abuse Research." Again, the PIPASA partners managed to attract a number of drug treatment center personnel who had not been involved in the process. The challenge of broadening the network and number of participants was a key value shared by all participants. This was the last event organized during the tenure of the author, but this process has been continued in order to maintain relations and allow new contacts.

In addition to the four workshops described above, the PIPASA spawned several programs and initiatives. These included applied social research projects and drug center resource development in Gaza and the West Bank. Moreover, a delegation of Israeli and Palestinian drug personnel attended an international meeting of the National Institute on Drug Abuse's Substance Abuse & Mental Health Administration personnel and RADAR personnel in Irvine, California, on May 3–8, 1999. This latter event was indeed a crowning achievement of the joint effort.

These programs and successful interventions by Ben-Gurion University and ECF to secure funding reflect a small but meaningful way of addressing the asymmetry between the two sides that emerged from 27 years of Israeli military occupation. The ECF and the PCH subsequently focused their energies on the dialogue between the two police forces and, indeed, succeeded to host a regional workshop that included Egyptian and Jordanian representatives. The PIPASA may be considered a model process of addressing peace through substance abuse, but, to the disappointment of this author, efforts to create a joint office or secretariat to manage and coordinate activities were unsuccessful.[23] In retrospect, it was an impossible goal due to the variety of interests, issues, and actors involved that needed to be continuously in a state of balance. Such a structure to promote cross-border cooperation in combating substance abuse does, however, remain an imminently sensible structure to contribute to peace building in a setting for post-permanent-status agreement.

PIPASA IN PERSPECTIVE: CONCLUDING REMARKS

Evaluating projects of this nature is, by definition, difficult, if not impossible. To date no methodological tools to evaluate the success and impact of such projects exist. Evaluating (and sustaining) such activities is even more challenging in light of the recent violence that has affected the region since September 2000. Indeed, the only feasible framework within which to assess the PIPASA initiative is to compare it with other health-peace initiatives and the categories provided by MacQueen and colleagues (1997).

One indicator of success is participation. On average, some 40 professionals, Israeli and Palestinian, met and discussed a matter of mutual professional concern, substance abuse, at four workshops held over a two-year period. In addition, the partners endeavored to ensure maximum participation by inviting new and varied institutions and professionals. As a result, over 100 individuals met and discussed matters of common professional concern with fellow professionals. Academics, social workers, physicians, nurses, psychologists, police officers, lawyers, and other professionals met counterparts from the "other side." This alone ensured that there was a diminishing of the negative stereotyping about the other side. On a basic level, Israelis and Palestinians were in a position to gain firsthand insight into prevailing needs and conditions, both in terms of the particular problem of substance abuse as well as general and personal situations. More Israelis were made aware of their Palestinian counterparts' lack of free movement and resources, as well as the consequences of Israeli occupation in professional and personal terms. The suffering of ordinary Palestinians was brought home to the Israeli participants. Similarly, Palestinian professionals better understood the aspirations and apprehensions of ordinary Israelis. It is also safe to assume that the professionals involved were viewed as credible cue givers by those with whom they worked—fellow professionals and clients. Many participants related their experience to their family and friends. In this sense, the process had a multiplying effect that carried the benefits beyond those who participated.

By "tapping in" to an issue such as substance abuse and by focusing on its professional and academic dimensions, the PIPASA initiative was in a position to appeal to people who were not necessarily "peace camp" constituents in each of the two communities. Indeed, by drawing in representative delegations of the police force, academic departments, treatment centers, and various government ministries, these activities included participants who probably reflected the broader spectrum of public opinion. Indicative of this success is a confession made by a police officer who participated in the Ramallah "Legal and Judicial Aspects" workshop. The officer confided in an ECF staff member that he and his fellow officers never "in their wildest dreams" envisaged themselves participating in an event of this nature. In this respect, the project contributed to broadening the peace constituency by reaching out to new populations. The significance of Israeli professionals, including representatives of the police, courts, education, and other ministries, crossing the "green-line" separating Israel from the West Bank and sleeping over in Ramallah and Bethlehem also cannot be minimized.

Perhaps the greatest achievement of this experience was the successful organization and implementation of cross-cultural workshops in the prevailing Israeli and Palestinian political context. Many of the PIPASA events took place during a prolonged stalemate within the Oslo peace process and in the absence of substantive progress in the implementation of the Interim Accords. Indeed, many Palestinian partners felt uncomfortable engaging in these activities, with many publicly expressing opposition to "normalization." While events of this particular period underscored the dependence of "bottom-up" peace initiatives on the prevailing macro political situation, the PIPASA experience underscored the vital role of NGO frameworks in providing a safety net for promoting and sustaining relations. This was particularly the case for government officials, whose formal contacts were increasingly limited as the hiatus in the formal peace process continued. Perhaps the most illustrative example of this was the dialogue between the police forces. The informal PIPASA setting allowed the police forces to go beyond their formal roles and interactions and become familiar with members of the opposing ranks and their needs. While the Palestinians and Israelis were on a difficult journey from an interim to a permanent status understanding, this particular HPI provided an island of sanity and interaction in the rough political seas. The important role of such activities is not recognized by the MacQueen and colleagues (1997) typology. Indeed, the recent breakdown of formal channels of communication yet again underscores the essential role of informal professional networks and contacts. When this most recent round of tragic violence ends and negotiations are again resumed, these personal and professional contacts will provide an essential foundation for rebuilding relations.

The PIPASA activities provided an important channel for Palestinians to air their perceptions that Israel was encouraging the spread of drugs. Also, they provided Israeli professionals the opportunity to debunk these fears. Such myths and stereotypes complicate and undermine relations. Indeed, the author is of the opinion that the Israeli side was, until these meetings, not fully cognizant of the strength of Palestinian sentiment regarding the alleged Israeli role in the drug trafficking to Palestinians. These meetings have not eradicated this perception, but giant strides were made in raising awareness of its existence and addressing it on certain levels. If anything, that these issues persistently emerged in the informal workshops exposes the limitations of formal channels of communication. In this sense, formal contacts are at best functional, and in a conflict situation politics may indeed precede the professional and personal dimension of intercommunal relations. Many personal and institutional contacts were made possible by this initiative. The contacts and activities reported in this chapter were those conducted by a host of nongovernmental and professional organizations. There is no way of numbering the plethora of other initiatives and contacts that resulted from this process.

The PIPASA experience also underscored the important role of "catalysts." The core PIPASA partners were a well-experienced and highly motivated team, and hence well suited to initiate and support this process. Beyond opening doors and providing opportunities to network with people, the core partners ensured that the initiative was sustained beyond these meetings. Often peace initiatives or HPIs are not sustained. The failure to sustain small opportunities to dialogue may indeed undermine the people's confidence in peace processes, in that failure on the micro level may provide a metaphor for the macro level and the long term. The lesson of PIPASA in particular and the ECF-PCH experience in general is that there is great value in providing specialized and professional structures to support such initiatives.

The PIPASA process allowed for the identification and pursuit of superordinate projects and ensured that the process was based on recognition of the needs of both sides. Perhaps the most salient achievement in this regard was to underscore that substance abuse is a problem that can most effectively be addressed jointly. By training Palestinian professionals and securing resources for a resource center (in Gaza), the process contributed to improving human services and public education programs that address substance abuse issues. The projects that were spawned by the dialogue therefore provided a small dividend in terms of reinforcing cooperation and providing a counterweight to conflict. Indeed, the research projects that emerged from this process are a vital component of a long-term effort to improve services and strengthen communities. The PIPASA experience, therefore, fulfilled three of the modes of operation suggested by MacQueen, McCutcheon, and Santa Barbara (1997), namely: evocation and broadening of altruism, the construction of superordinate goals, and the strengthening of communities. In this particular context, these were perhaps the most important goals.

In terms of the peace-building/peace-making nexus, the most significant contribution of the PIPASA experience was its modest role in providing a "safety net" for Palestinian-Israeli relations at a particularly challenging juncture in the Oslo process. The PIPASA effort, along with the plethora of NGO people-to-people activities, provided an infrastructure for peace that made it easier for Palestinians and Israelis to resume the peace process in mid-1999 relatively near to the status at which it was left off in mid-1996. This said, however, the PIPASA experience and the recent violence underscore the limitations of HPIs and similar "bottom-up" initiatives. These initiatives cannot be a substitute for the formal peace process and real progress in that process. HPIs are only meaningful if progress is made through the formal process. Such initiatives can only contribute to peace building only if there is a real peace process.

Finally, the important role of the international experts in this process needs to be acknowledged. First, the international experts contributed to the professional legitimacy of the process, which was vital in terms of ensuring the involvement of participants from both societies. Second, the international experts were instrumental in focusing the debate and discussion on the issue at hand. Third, the international experts opened up international opportunities and ideas, enabling the two groups to work together in a spirit of cooperation and coordination regarding their mutual interests and concerns about substance abuse. In this latter regard, these experts were instrumental in facilitating the promotion and implementation of superordinate projects. The important role of international experts in supporting HPIs needs to be given greater recognition and consideration.

One last afterthought is to ask aloud whether this experience can be replicated in other settings, particularly where communities are in conflict. Can the problems of drugs, which are often common to divided communities and a source of conflict between them, be used to build bridges? Based on the PIPASA experience, the answer is *yes.* Much, however, depends on the nature and scope of conflict and the formal political process.

NOTES

1. General Barry McCaffrey served as commander of the U.S. Army's Southern Command (Southcom) before being promoted to head of the U.S. Office of National Drug Control Policy.

2. Geraldine McDonald (1997) argues that in the case of Colombia, "political violence between the government and insurgent groups is exacerbated by drugs-related violence, which leads to high levels of domestic violence and so on." Indeed, McDonald views the drug trade as a "barrier to peace-building" as drug money finances paramilitary units, and struggles for trafficking routes raise the stakes in territorial disputes.

3. See, for example, the reports of Human Rights Watch (2001) (http://www.hrw.org/campaigns/colombia/) and the Centre for International Policy (2000) (http://www.icdc.com/~paulwolf/drugwar.htm).

4. The Opium Wars were fought between the British and the Chinese over British merchants' illegal importation of opium into China. The wars resulted in major gains in both trading privileges and territory for the British, including the acquisition of the Chinese territory of Hong Kong.

5. The author previously served as the Israeli project director of a joint Palestinian-Israeli program entitled "Building Bridges through Health." The project is a partnership between the Tel Aviv–based Economic Cooperation Foundation (ECF) and the East Jerusalem–based

Palestine Council of Health (PCH) and was supported by the Swedish International Development Agency. The author would like to acknowledge these two organizations and their senior management and staff. In particular, Dr. Abdel Rahim Abu Saleh, Avivit Ish-Am, Dr. Ron Pundik, and Dr. Hikmat Ajjuri. The author also wishes to thank the representatives of Palestinian and Israeli partner organizations who contributed to this effort, in particular Professor Richard Isralowitz of the Spitzer Department of Social Work at Ben-Gurion University, Dr. Elia Awwad of the Bethlehem-based Child and Family Consultation Center (CFCC), and Dr. Mohammed Afifi of the Gaza-based Child Health and Research Association (CHCR). The author is also grateful to the international experts who made such a significant contribution to the process. Even though the author left the ECF in July 1999, the work is being actively promoted by the ECF and the PCH. This continuity is deeply appreciated.

6. This chapter was first drafted in October 1999, following the election of the "Oslo friendly" Barak government. The events following September 28, 2000, dictate a reassessment of the original article.

7. "Simply put, whereas peace-keeping is about building barriers between groups who want to fight each other, peace-building attempts to build bridges between the parties and allow for positive and creative interaction; and whereas peace-making is concerned with intervention at the elite, decision-making level, peace-building is focused on the social, economic and psychological environments of ordinary people at the grass roots level. As such, peace-building is the conflict resolution strategy most likely to result in conflict transformation" (Ryan, 1995).

8. John Lederach (1995, p. 211) further argues that "an adequate transformative framework must explicitly and intentionally devise mechanisms for integrating and coordinating high-, middle-, and grass roots level strategies, ensuring that they are given space and are legitimized and coordinated. Such an undertaking is directly linked to the idea of building a peace constituency."

9. It is worth noting that recently the Al-Quds University and the Joint Distribution Committee/Brookdale Institute completed comprehensive research on Palestinian-Israeli cooperative health initiatives. See Barnea et al. (2000).

10. More recently MacQueen and Santa Barbara (2000) have streamlined their typology.

11. At the height of the Cold War, a group of Soviet and American doctors founded IPPNW to educate health professionals, political leaders, and the public about the medical consequences of nuclear war. For this effort, which reached millions with the message that nuclear weapons must never be used again, IPPNW received the 1985 Nobel Peace Prize. See http://www.ippnw.org/.

12. The initiative was a joint effort by UNICEF, the Roman Catholic Church, and local organizations. These "days of tranquility" ensured a suspension of hostilities over three-day periods from 1985 until the peace accords were concluded in 1992 to allow for the immunization of children. This period of peace ensured that 300,000 children were annually immunized. See MacQueen and Santa Barbara (2000).

13. The PCH and ECF had, as early as the end of 1996, made a strategic decision to target professionals engaged in providing health services as their focus for people-to-people activities. The reasons for focusing on this target constituency were a mix of practical reasoning (i.e., the PCH was a health organization) and the recognition of the important role that health professionals could play in reshaping Palestinian-Israeli relations. The ECF and PCH found that when people shared a professional language and understanding, dialogue was easier and more effective.

14. For more details on the activities of the "Building Bridges through Health," please contact the ECF and PCH at the following e-mail addresses: ecf@ecf.org.il or pchealth@planet.edu.

15. These include the challenge of arranging travel permits for Palestinian professionals to leave the West Bank and Gaza, to either visit the West Bank or Gaza, and to enter Israel. Often not all applicants are granted permits, and in some situations permits are granted at a relatively late stage of the process and are therefore of no use. Beyond the far-reaching practical implications of this complex procedure on arranging events and the insecurity that it generates, Palestinians view permits and the process of obtaining them as humiliating. The system was introduced by the Israeli government in response to acts of terror, with the express purpose of limiting the entry of Palestinians into Israel. To complicate matters further, Israelis wishing to enter the Gaza Strip are obliged to secure entry permits from the Israeli Defense Force, a process that requires complicated security coordination procedures with the Palestinian security forces. To this we add the enmity and ill-feeling of 30 years of military occupation, land confiscation, and settlement expansion and the historical conflict between two national movements that (with the creation of the State of Israel) led to the exile of what are today millions of Palestinians. Last, but not least, both Palestinians and Israelis have witnessed violent acts of terror against civilians in both societies. The research of Barnea et al. (2000) addresses these and other obstacles.

16. The U.S. Information Agency, in affiliation with the Tel Aviv U.S. Embassy covered his travel expenses. Funding for the workshop was secured from the Charles Bronfman (CRB) Foundation and a German industrialist and philanthropist, Dr. Heinz Horst Deichman.

17. According to Robinson (1997), these "social marginals were given protection by Israel and allowed to practice their trades in exchange for information, and often, cooperation in recruiting fellow Palestinians."

18. According to Article One ("Criminal Jurisdiction") of Annex Four ("Protocol Concerning Legal Matters") of the Interim Agreement, signed on September 28, 1995, Israel has "sole criminal jurisdiction" over offenses committed in Palestinian-controlled territories by Israelis. See the Israeli-Palestinian Interim Agreement on the West Bank and Gaza Strip (1995). (Jerusalem: Ministry of Foreign Affairs) 204.

19. The British embassy's (Tel Aviv) Small Projects Fund supported this second workshop.

20. There is clearly a positive value in Israelis sleeping in a city like Bethlehem and wandering around safely at night. Unfortunately, many Israelis have very negative (personal security) stereotypes of life in Palestinian cities; such visits tend to counter these perceptions and fears.

21. Colonel Mahmoud Al-Zuheiri, who was later to become instrumental in this dialogue, raised these concerns at the Bethlehem workshop.

22. These contacts were facilitated through the good office of Dr. Miriam Hirschfeld, Israel's most senior representative to the WHO and sister of the ECF's Director General, Dr. Yair Hirschfeld.

23. Dr. Yair Hirschfeld (1998) has succinctly promoted the logic and merits of creating such joint structures—referred to as hubs of cooperation—in promoting Palestinian-Israeli cooperation.

REFERENCES

Barnea, T., Ziaad A., et al. (2000). Israeli-Palestinian cooperation in the health field 1994–1998. Jerusalem: JDC-Brookdale Institute, JDC-Israel, AJJDC and Al-Quds University.

Centre for International Policy. (2000). War on drugs and human rights in Colombia. Retrieved May 22, 2001, from the World Wide Web: http://www.icdc.com/~paulwolf/drugwar.htm.

Hirschfeld, Y. (1998). Keeping Oslo alive: Developing a non-governmental peace strategy. In S. Nusseibeh, M. Maoz, & J. Gerster (Eds.), *Is Oslo alive?* Jerusalem: Konrad Adenauer Stiftung, Harry S Truman Institute for the Advancement of Peace, and Palestine Consultancy Group.

Human Rights Watch. (2001). Crisis in Colombia. Retrieved May 22, 2001, from the World Wide Web: http://www.hrw.org/campaigns/colombia/.

Isralowitz, R. (1998a). *Palestinian and Israeli people against substance abuse: A cooperative effort to address the problem through communication, cooperation and coordination: Workshop proceedings*. Beer Sheva, November 4–5, 1997. Tel Aviv and East Jerusalem: Economic Cooperation Foundation and Palestine Council of Health. 5.

———. (1998b). *Palestinian and Israeli people against substance abuse: Prevention and beyond: Workshop proceedings*. Bethlehem, May 25–26, 1998. Tel Aviv and East Jerusalem: Economic Cooperation Foundation and Palestine Council of Health. 15.

———. (1999). *Palestinian and Israeli people against substance abuse: Substance abuse: Legal and judicial aspects: Workshop proceedings*. Ramallah, March 24–25, 1999. Tel Aviv and East Jerusalem: Economic Cooperation Foundation and Palestine Council of Health. 14, 29–35.

Lederach, J. P. (1995). Conflict transformation in protracted internal conflicts: The case for a comprehensive framework. In K. Rupesinghe (Ed.), *Conflict transformation* (p. 207). New York: St. Martin's Press.

MacQueen, G., McCutcheon, R., & Santa Barbara, J. (1997). The use of health initiatives as peace initiatives. *Peace and Change, 22*, 175–197.

MacQueen, G., & Santa Barbara, J. (2000). Conflict and health: Peace building through health initiatives. *British Medical Journal, 321*, 293–296. Retrieved May 22, 2001, from the World Wide Web: http://bmj.com/cgi/content/full/321/7256/293#B20.

McDonald, G. (1997). *Peace building from below: Alternative perspectives on Colombia's peace process*. London: Catholic Institute for International Relations.

Robinson, G. E. (1997). *Building a Palestinian State: The incomplete revolution* (p. 117). Bloomington and Indianapolis: Indiana University Press.

Ryan, S. (1995). Transforming violent inter-communal conflict. In K. Rupesinghe (Ed.), *Conflict transformation* (p. 224). New York: St. Martin's Press.

Salinas, C. (2000). In focus: Colombia in crisis. *Foreign policy in focus. Internet gateway to global affairs*, *5*(5). Retrieved May 22, 2001, from the World Wide Web: http://www.foreignpolicy-infocus.org/briefs/vol5/v5n05col.html.

Part II

People in Transition

3

Drug Abuse: Problems, Policies, and Programs in Palestine

*Mohammed Afifi, Mahmoud Al-Zuheiri, Violet Fasheh, and Salah El-Sousi**

INTRODUCTION

Despite the absence of reliable data, it is clear to those working in the field of substance abuse that the Palestinian people are not immune to the scourge of drug use. In fact, at a time when the Palestinians are engaged in constructing an organizational infrastructure that will support the future State of Palestine, a rapidly growing enterprise in the West Bank and Gaza is the multimillion dollar drug trafficking industry. This phenomenon not only damages individuals and families, but extends its destructive grip to numerous areas of Palestinian community life, thereby threatening the vitality of the emerging new nation.

The problem of Palestinian drug use is viewed as a manifestation, in part, of the difficult living conditions that have prevailed in the region for many years. The following chapter about Gaza, the West Bank, and East Jerusalem indicates that the causes of the Palestinian dilemma are multiple, complex, and interrelated. For much too long the political and economic situation has been characterized by "crisis conditions," universally acknowledged as the ideal breeding ground for the spread of drug abuse. Destabilized by chronic social, economic, and identity crises, Palestinian youth—the very embodiment of hopes and aspirations for the new nation—are especially vulnerable to the highly destructive drug plague.

---

*The Introduction to this chapter was written by Mohammed Afifi and Mahmoud Al-Zuheiri. The section on the West Bank and East Jerusalem was written by Violet Fasheh. And the section on Gaza was written by Mohammed Afifi and Salah El-Sousi.

In response to the problem, the Palestinian Authority has endeavored to provide treatment and rehabilitation facilities for current victims of drug abuse and, in order to get a handle on the future, to do everything in its power to foster a culture of active prevention. During a 1997 conference ("Palestinian and Israeli People against Substance Abuse") that was convened to discuss the drug problem, it was stated that "prevention is the key, the only approach which offers genuine hope of reducing the number of drug addicts in Gaza and the West Bank in the future. The first goal is to create the conditions in society where people will choose not to use illicit drugs. The second is to reduce and eventually eliminate the supply of drugs in Gaza and the West Bank [since] most—if not all—illicit drugs originate from outside the area. [Palestinians] have to establish regional, national, and international cooperation in order to eliminate the supply of and trafficking in illicit drugs. Thirdly, the Palestinian Authority has adopted a program with regard to drug prevention. The program aims to heighten public awareness; to provide support against drug abuse in the home, the community and the workplace; to reduce drug-related crime; and to establish a forensic laboratory for the detection of drug abuse."[1]

Considerable evidence supports the belief that the lower the perceived risk of drug abuse, the more extensive the use of illicit drugs. Advocates of prevention must therefore focus on providing both potential abusers and the community in general with a well-informed understanding of the risks involved. To this end, it is universally agreed that education must play a major role.[2] There is considerable room for improving and expanding existing awareness-raising programs and similar activities in schools and universities as well as in the wider community. Moreover, cooperation and partnership and the exchange of ideas, approaches, and educational materials with other countries and societies are vital.[3] Equally important is a renewed emphasis on training. Wide-ranging, up-to-date programs for educators, health care professionals, and social workers must be made more widely available and promoted within a supportive infrastructure.[4]

In sum, if Palestinians are to achieve tangible success in the struggle against drug abuse, then effective training programs, cooperation and dialogue with other countries, anti-drug activities in educational establishments, dissemination of information via the media, and active community involvement must be generated. Such efforts must be seen as interlocking elements of a preventive strategy for the Palestinian nation.

GAZA, THE WEST BANK, AND EAST JERUSALEM

Background: Land and Demography

Land

Gaza is a narrow area of land bordered on the south by Egypt, west by the Mediterranean Sea, and east and north by Israel. It is 46 kilometers long and 5–12 kilometers wide, with an area of 362 square kilometers. The coast has no natural bays or inlets, the elevation is 0–40 meters above sea level, the climate is subtropical, and the area is very poor in natural resources. Gaza is administratively divided by the Palestinian National Authority into five governorates: North, Gaza, Mid Zone, Khan Younis, and Rafah. It has four towns, fourteen villages, and eight refugee camps.

The West Bank and East Jerusalem are bordered on the north, west, and south by Israel, and on the east by the Jordan River and the Dead Sea, which separates it from the Kingdom of Jordan. The area is 40–65 kilometers long and covers 5,800 square kilometers. It is a hilly region located between the coastal plain in the west and the Jordan Valley in the east, with an average elevation of 800 meters above sea level. The West Bank is divided by the Palestinian Authority into 10 governorates: Jerusalem, Jenin, Tulkarem, Qalqeliah, Nablus, Ramallah, Salfit, Bethlehem, Jerrico, and Hebron. It has 10 towns, 430 villages, and 18 refugee camps.

Demography

The population in Gaza, the West Bank, and East Jerusalem was estimated (mid-year 1998) at 2,897,452, of whom 50.5 percent are males and 49.5 percent females. Of the total, 1,039,580 (36 percent) live in Gaza and 1,857,872 (64 percent) live in the West Bank and East Jerusalem. Nearly half (47 percent) of the total population are under 15 years of age (50.4 percent in Gaza and 45 percent in the West Bank). The population growth was estimated at 4.5 percent in 1994, and gradually dropped to 3.1 percent in 1998, which is extremely high compared to the global growth rate of 1.3 percent, according to United Nations Population Fund statistics. The population in Palestine can be divided into two groups: refugees and original inhabitants. The refugees are those who were outside of the area or departed from their homes when Israel was created in 1948. Most of the refugees are living in camps in both Gaza and the West Bank. The refugees constitute 65.1 percent of the Gaza population and 26.5 percent of the West Bank population. A few thousand Israeli Jewish people live in isolated settlements in Gaza, and an estimated 150,000 Israeli Jewish people live in settlements throughout the West Bank.

The population density in Gaza is very high: 2,871 people per square kilometer, whereas in the West Bank it is 320 people per square kilometer. Because of the large number of young people, 50.3 percent of the Palestinian people have "dependent" status. The birthrate declined from 40.1 per thousand people in 1996 to 34.5 per thousand in 1998. The fertility rate of women, ages 15 to 49, is 5.58, and the average life expectancy was 69.2 years in 1993 and 71.7 years in 1998.

Education

According to a survey conducted in 1996, 10.7 percent of young adults aged 25–34 years had a university degree or more than 16 years of education, 12.5 percent had completed high school with a secondary certificate (12 years of study), 24.3 percent had a preparatory certificate (9 years of study), and 18 percent had an elementary level education (6 years of study). During the period of Israeli occupation and the Intifada, the school drop-out rate was high. After the establishment of the Palestinian Authority and its control over the schools, however, the situation improved considerably. The growing number of school facilities along with improved human resources has had a positive effect on the attitudes of children toward school, as evidenced by better attendance and less problem behavior.

Marriage and Divorce

The median age at first marriage is 18 years for females in Gaza and the West Bank; for males it is 23 years (22 years in Gaza and 24 years in the West Bank). There is a noticeable number of girls who marry at a young age, as young as 15 or 16 years. The prevalence of divorce among Palestinian people is 1.1 percent for females (1 percent in the West Bank and 1.4 percent in Gaza) and 0.3 percent for males in Gaza and the West Bank. The incidence of divorce among newlyweds in Gaza during the first year of marriage is estimated to be 17 percent, involving mostly young women 16 to 19 years old, according to an unpublished study.

Historical Background: A Sociopolitical Framework

The use and abuse of drugs is an age-old phenomenon that has been present in all societies, including Palestinian society in Gaza, the West Bank, and East Jerusalem. In recent years, however, this phenomenon has increased dramatically to alarming proportions, particularly in terms of the so-called "soft drugs" being substituted for more dangerous "hard drugs."[5] Such a substitution, over time, has resulted in an increase in antisocial behavior and the spread of dangerous social diseases that, if allowed to continue, will signal a breakdown of the very foundations of traditional society, which in Palestinian society, means the breakdown of the extended family as its basic unit.

During the last several years, major changes have taken place within the Palestinian community. Those changes have influenced every aspect of Palestinian life and have also created a crisis for Palestinians at the individual and community levels. In addition, the structures of the Palestinian family and other social groups have been affected.[6] Among the reasons for this situation is the intensity of everyday life coupled with the political and economic tensions that confront Palestinians in Gaza, the West Bank, and East Jerusalem. Another reason is the lack of resources, institutions, and specialized services to help individuals deal with the stresses and turmoil that face the Palestinian people, as well as the consequences of such pressures.

Clear manifestations of these crisis conditions are the unhealthy coping mechanisms, reactionary responses, and counterproductive patterns of behavior used by individuals and their families. One example is the rapid spread of alcohol and drug use and abuse among all classes of people in the Palestinian community, but especially among youth. What makes Palestinian youth the most vulnerable group to alcohol and drug use and abuse is the gloomy political and economic situation, which fails to provide them with a stable environment supportive of addressing their identity-seeking and developmental needs in a healthy manner. The availability of alcohol and drugs, in addition to the absence of any local supervision and control over the trafficking and abuse of drugs, reinforces the unhealthy behavior of Palestinian youth.

Four main periods tend to distinguish the significant changes that have taken place regarding Palestinian public awareness and official reaction to the problem of drug addiction. The first period was between 1948 and 1967. During this time, the West Bank and East Jerusalem were under Jordanian rule, and Gaza was under Egyptian Rule. The establishment of Israel in 1948 affected the public and the official approach to the issue of drugs, both within the country as well as beyond its borders. For example, the smuggling of hashish and opium from Jordan to Egypt via Arab Jerusalem and from Lebanon to Egypt via Gaza did not constitute a source of concern for either the Jordanian or Lebanese authorities. On the Israeli side, however, the issue was presented as a worrisome problem. Drug smuggling by Arabs was viewed as a threat to the integrity of Israeli borders and its security. Also, Israelis feared that the drugs would penetrate into the Jewish population, which led to a change in Israeli drug laws in 1952 and an increase of military police activity at the southeastern border of that country (Hasnain, 1993).

The second period was from 1967 to 1982. In 1967, following the Six-Day War, political changes occurred, for example, the application of Israeli rule and law in East Jerusalem. During this period, a public and official perception was created that Arab drug dealers were trying, intentionally, to distribute hashish among Israeli Jewish youth, including high school and university students. At the same time, Palestinians believed that Israeli authorities were trying to distribute drugs among their youth to minimize their participation in the national struggle.

The third time period, associated with the outbreak of the Lebanese War in 1982, was from 1982 to 1987. This period was characterized by changes in the patterns of drug abuse that, in turn, affected the nature of the social reaction to drug use in Israel, the Palestinian territories, and East Jerusalem.

The fourth period was the Intifada, from 1987 to 1993, during which time there was a remarkable decrease in drug use. Such a change resulted in the closure of "drug selling stations" in East Jerusalem and a low point for the illegal drug marketing business. According to police records and unofficial reports, the decrease in Palestinian drug use was due to many factors including: (a) social pressure from political and religious Palestinian leaders; (b) youth abstaining from the drug business and drug use because they became involved with Intifada activities; and (c) the intensified presence of Israeli police, the creation of checkpoints and road blocks, and the personal and property search of Palestinians by Israelis responding in opposition to the Palestinian national struggle against Israeli occupation.

The social problem of escalating drug use cannot easily be ignored in the Israeli-occupied West Bank (now the Palestinian Territories). Records kept by Israeli police (Hasnain, 1993) indicate that there was an increase in the number of convicted drug addicts between 1974 and 1978 and between 1979 and 1983, with arrested drug addicts from East Jerusalem accounting for more than 37 percent of the Israeli and Palestinian Arab arrestees.

Mental health hospital records in Bethlehem and Gaza reveal increased rates of admission for drug addicts during 1991–1992.[7] Approximately 11 percent of all admissions were drug addicts who approached the mental health hospital for residential treatment (Khamis & Habash, 1995). While caution must be exercised in interpreting the available data, it can be said that little has been done to investigate the extent of the drug problem and to follow up on the needs of those needing treatment.

The drug problem among Palestinians in Jerusalem led to unpredicted responses on the part of Palestinian journalists and public figures. From the 1980s on, especially during 1985–1991, local Palestinian journalists began to blame Israeli authorities and the occupation for the increase in drug abuse among Palestinians. Palestinian religious figures began to seek out and mobilize alternatives to police action such as the community control method, especially from the beginning of the Intifada in late 1987. These latter developments were not created in a vacuum but rather in a political framework. This means that politics for both Israelis and Palestinians was a factor in how the drug problem was being addressed.

Prevalence of Substance Use and Abuse

Today, young people throughout the West Bank use mood-altering substances probably more than ever before in Palestinian history. A new culture has developed over the last three decades that endorses recreational use of substances.[8] In the West Bank and East Jerusalem, for example, the majority of drug users come from the Old City of East Jerusalem (i.e., Al-Nassara Street "Christian Quarter" and Al-Waad) and its suburbs (i.e., Al'zarieh "Bethany," Shufat Camp and Al-Ram), and from other cities in the West Bank such as Bethlehem and Ramallah.[9]

Prevalence estimates of drug use and abuse in the Palestinian territories (Gaza, the West Bank, and East Jerusalem) are not reliable or are nonexistent. Figures that do exist tend to rely almost entirely on observation;[10] systematic data collection methods have been nonexistent or extremely limited in terms of the methods used to collect information. Services addressing the needs of drug users lack professional expertise and objective data analysis.

In 1992, the Israel Anti-Drug Authority and the Israel Ministry of Health published statistics indicating that there were 400,000 persons who used substances in that country. Police statistics for 1993 indicated the number of users in Israel to be 250,000. In that same year, the Israeli prime minister, in a speech to the Knesset (parliament), confirmed that number, meaning there was a decline of 37.5 percent from the previous year's statistics. It was also reported that there were 30,000 to 40,000 drug addicts, most of them addicted to heroin. Almost 3,000 to 4,000 of the addicts were Arabs from the Israeli-occupied territories, which accounts for 10 percent of the total number of drug users in the area (i.e., Israel and the occupied territories), or 1.2–1.6 percent of the population were reported to be using drugs but are not necessarily addicted to those substances. A survey carried out by Caritas

Jerusalem on a hundred households in Al-Nassara Street in the Old City of Jerusalem revealed that 20 percent of the study sample had a drug addict in the family (Khamis & Habash, 1995). At a 1999 workshop held at Al-Quds University, Abu Dis Campus, it was reported that there were 2,500 addicts in East Jerusalem, of which 400 lived in the Old City. Those who use marijuana tend to be 9–18 years old, while those who use heroin are older, 18–34 years old. Among Palestinian youth, marijuana is a gateway drug leading to hashish and hallucinogenic drug use. Such substances are seen by youngsters as exciting, and therefore hard to refuse; also, the use of such drugs is seen as a way to escape reality and avoid facing economic, social, political, and personal problems.

While these estimates may provide some information about the Palestinian drug addict population in the Old City of East Jerusalem, it cannot be assumed that similar levels of drug use occur in all subunits of the Israeli-occupied territories, including other cities, villages, and camps. Any reporting methods or statistics of addicts in Gaza, the West Bank, and East Jerusalem are influenced by several factors. First, drug addicts themselves are not likely to disclose their abuse because they fear the social stigma that would result from public declaration. Furthermore, the degree to which different family members are aware of the addiction of their children and its abusive nature is limited. When drug abuse occurs within the Palestinian family, there is usually strong pressure to keep it secret from the outside world. A desire for confidentiality concerning moral issues is felt by Palestinian families and embodied in their codes of behavior, including the need to maintain personal and intergenerational boundaries.

Second, social attitudes and reactions to users of stimulants such as cocaine are sharply different from attitudes and reactions to users of sedatives that have a relaxing effect or induce sleep. Common parlance about the use of socially disapproved or illegal drugs usually conveys the impression that any or all use is abusive and constitutes addiction; conversely, references to socially approved drugs such as tranquilizers usually implies that almost all use, including abuse and addiction, is normal.[11]

Third, the less restrictive environment that resulted from the resignation of Arab police during the Intifada decreased the possibility of drug users and abusers being caught and subsequently convicted. While drug laws in Israel prohibit the import, manufacture, sale, and use of drugs in that country, the interpretation and application of such laws in the Occupied Territories (Gaza, the West Bank, and East Jerusalem) tend to vary, affecting reporting and statistical data-gathering methods.

Finally, the Israeli military occupation increased penalties on Palestinian political activists, not drug users. In the same vein, pharmacists have not been prohibited from selling drugs that endanger the health, safety, and welfare of clients. Any numbers or statistics provided by pharmacists, therefore, are limited.

Factors Affecting the Increase in Drug Use and Abuse among Palestinians

A number of factors (e.g., political, social, cultural, and religious) need to be considered in order to better understand the reasons for the increase of drug use and abuse among Palestinians. They are as follows:

Changes in Values and Family Structure

Palestinian society traditionally has been patriarchal in nature, with extended families catering to the needs and problems of individuals. This pattern has changed drastically over the years, particularly in the cities, where the importance of the extended family has been replaced by an orientation toward a more nuclear family structure. This shift has resulted in the loss of emotional and economic support for many individuals within the family.[12] Many individuals in the larger cities are torn between traditional conservative cultural norms and those of a more liberal, individualistic Western lifestyle as observed in the media and experienced in the daily lives of many, especially those exposed to the modern lifestyle through work and business relations as well as other social and cultural interactions.

Political Factors

Palestinian society has experienced quick and sudden changes due to the wars of 1948, 1967, 1972, and 1982. The consequences of these experiences have resulted in unstable social and cultural attitudes and behavior including feelings of uncertainty, anxiety, and insecurity. Furthermore, the conflicts and crises have resulted in economic deterioration, increased unemployment, poverty, and emigration for Palestinians. A major outcome of these conditions, especially those that resulted from the 1967 Six-Day War, was an environment conducive to the spread of drug use. Easy access of residents of Arab East Jerusalem to Jewish West Jerusalem and their access to Israel proper enhanced the spread of drugs to Palestinians, especially laborers who worked in the Israeli sector. Also, new supply routes opened access to Gaza, through which drugs are smuggled from Egypt, and the country's northern borders, where heavy drugs such as heroin have been smuggled since the 1982 Israeli invasion of Lebanon.

The Intifada uprising, a relatively recent historical event that started in December 1987, had special socioeconomic and political meaning. It created great hopes and expectations that a solution to the Palestinian problem was drawing near. During the Intifada, Palestinians felt that the drug phenomenon threatened the welfare of Palestinian society and the goals that had to be achieved. In certain population centers there were efforts to prevent and combat the problem. In some areas of the Palestinian communities such efforts succeeded. In other areas, however, there was a lack of success, especially where young people came together, such as in prisons, on the streets, at work, and at places of pleasure.

Law and Social Norms

Israeli occupation of Palestinian areas created racial tensions and precipitated policies, regulations, and methods of enforcement that differentiated Palestinian inhabitants living in East Jerusalem, those living in Gaza and the West Bank, and the Palestinian Arabs of 1948 from Israeli Jews. In fact, the most emotionally charged issue of the peace process is the question of whether Jerusalem should be divided into Arab and Israeli sections (the Palestinian position) or remain undivided (the Israeli position) and involves not only political and geographical concerns but considerations related to the world's monotheistic religions of Islam, Judaism, and Christianity. Many of the restrictions imposed on Palestinians made their daily lives difficult and frustrating. Included among the impositions were: closure of all entrances to Jerusalem, separation of East Jerusalem and its inhabitants from the rest of the West Bank, and the Israeli claim of permanent control and sovereignty over all of East Jerusalem, occupied in 1967 (the so-called "unification of Jerusalem"). In addition, residency rights of Palestinians in Jerusalem were challenged through confiscation of their Jerusalem inhabitant identification papers, and other measures were taken to diminish the ability of the city's Palestinian minority to challenge the Israeli claim of sovereignty. Elsewhere on the West Bank and Gaza, tensions and frustration grew among Palestinians as a result of land confiscation by Israelis to build new and extend existing Jewish settlements. This action was taken with little or no regard for Palestinian economic, social, cultural, and legal rights. Also, Palestinians have been forced to live with conditions of high unemployment, labor intensive jobs with salaries lower than those for Israelis doing similar work, closure of commercial markets and export opportunities, and travel restrictions, both within the region and abroad.

During the occupation of the West Bank and Gaza, Israeli authorities followed up on laws to serve their goals of territorial administration. Among them, for example, have been (a) the application of British emergency law used for detention of "troublesome" persons, (b) Jordanian and Egyptian law used for education and cultural purposes, and (c) the Israeli law related to commerce and trade. These difficult social, economic, and political pressures affected the psychosocial well-being of Palestinian people who, because of these laws, lived in a state of ambiguity, controversy, conflict, fear, anxiety, exhaustion, insecurity, and other stressful conditions that promote an environment conducive to drug use.

Finally, the strict laws of enforcement used by the Israeli government to control drug trafficking, use, and abuse among its citizens were not applied in the same manner to Palestinian residents in the occupied territories, including East Jerusalem. This resulted in a spread of drug use, particularly among youth, which diverts them from other causes and purposes including those of a nationalistic nature. During the last two years or so (1998–2000), the Palestinian National Authority has come to address the seriousness of addiction and has made the problem one of its top priorities. Working teams have been formed to define and strengthen law enforcement and control measures as well as pass laws prohibiting the import, manufacture, sale, and use of illegal drugs.[13]

Community

For the most part, the Palestinian community denies the existence of addiction because addiction threatens social norms, values, religious tenets, familial relations, and other guiding principles of acceptable behavior. Drug abuse is a shameful act; it is not acceptable in either the social or religious context. The social stigma of drug addiction frequently results in isolation of the users and abusers as they withdraw from social contacts because of shame and fear of rejection.

In addition to the adverse impact that drugs exert on the psychological and physical functioning of its users are the destructive effects on social relationships in general and marital interactions in particular. Numerous addicts report that their use of drugs is a major cause of marital discord and broken marriages. The quality of relationships within the family is a crucial determinant of any child's future; drug use by a parent or parents can influence their children's use of such substances and their ability to serve as responsible parents.

The increase of drug use and abuse in East Jerusalem and its suburbs, especially those that are heavily populated, has caused a rise in crime as well as antisocial behavior, including prostitution; theft; burglary; a breakdown in social norms, values, and family structure; wife and child abuse; and divorce.[14]

Religion and Spirituality

The value of religion and spirituality in Palestinian culture is an important element that affects drug abuse and its treatment. The treatment process focuses on the physical, mental, psychological, moral, and emotional characteristics of addicts so as to change their attitudes and behavior toward drugs, either at their request or that of a family member or significant other. Religion in the Palestinian culture places moral constraints on the individual, with strong strictures on indulging in drugs in spite of strong motives and pressures to do so. Religion pressures the individual to find ways other than substance use to minimize tensions and frustrations and to resist the temptation to escape reality and responsibilities through substance use.

It is important to address spiritual matters when treating Palestinian drug abusers. Though religion is at the core of Palestinian social norms and is considered a part of daily living, spiritual values emphasize the human aspect of the individual. They help promote and strengthen the internal control of the individual, the weakening of which leads to addiction problems. Some of those who work with Palestinian addicts believe that the discovery of spirituality by the individual can lead to a major character change that is essential to overcoming addiction. Therapists who utilize principles of spirituality in the therapeutic process are probably more effective practitioners.[15]

Organizations and Activities against Substance Abuse

With the establishment of the Palestinian Authority, two main organizations were established, the Palestinian Anti-Narcotics General Administration (PANGA) and the National Committee for Prevention of Crime and Substance Abuse (NCPCS). The main activities of the PANGA are to fight and control the drug dealers (reduction of supply) and carry out the legal and judicial activities against the spread of drugs. The PANGA also participates in awareness activities with other community organizations. On the other hand, the NCPCS is working to coordinate activities, especially the national approach to drug awareness, treatment, and rehabilitation. The NCPCS consists of general directors of relevant government ministries and representatives of nongovernmental organizations. The NCPCS is headed by the minister of social affairs.

Treatment and Rehabilitation

The main facilities to address addiction are governmental psychiatric hospitals, where patients can receive detoxification and chemical treatment. Two hospitals are available, one in the West Bank in Bethlehem, and the other in Gaza. Both hospitals are not specifically prepared to deal with the residential treatment of drug addicts since they care for many other psychiatric conditions. Also, few staff are trained to work with addicts and very little is available for long-term follow up and rehabilitative care of this population.

In the West Bank, there are two other nongovernmental organizations working in the field of treatment and rehabilitation. Bethlehem Drugs Research and Treatment Center specializes in rapid detoxification, which, at a cost of a few thousand dollars, is expensive, and Al Sadeeq Al Tayyeb, which has a residential facility and has adopted the treatment modes of psychotherapy, group therapy, and community-based rehabilitation.

Treatment and rehabilitation in Gaza is a different story; there is not one facility for residential treatment or detoxification. All activities are carried out on an outpatient basis through the psychiatric or the general hospital on an emergency-case basis.

Community-based treatment and rehabilitation (CBTR) is carried out with very limited success by a number of governmental and nongovernmental organizations. The Ministry of Health established a new department called the Department of Community Mental Health, which adopted the policy of CBTR in working with psychiatric cases including substances abusers. There are few trained personnel to carry out these activities and the resources of the department are limited. On the other hand, a number of nongovernmental organizations are working in the field of CBTR treatment and rehabilitation, either as a main activity, as in the case of Al Sadeeq Al Tayyeb in the West Bank, or as a component of a multiservice approach, as carried out by the Community Mental Health Program in Gaza. One recent effort to improve CBTR is the development of the manualized treatment protocol approach to service provision in the Arab language. The method, adopted from the

Matrix Institute for the Treatment of Addictions (USA) technique, is being carried out by Al-Quds University in cooperation with Ben-Gurion University and the Matrix Institute.

Awareness and Information Activities

A limited number of professional personnel are responsible for drug use prevention, and they may be either fully dedicated or only partially engaged in this work. As part of the activities in the schools, the Directorate of Health Promotion and Education in both the Ministry of Health and the Ministry of Education have trained teachers in schools to carry out health and substance abuse education and to facilitate activities of Student Health Groups. A similar activity in United Nations Relief and Works Agency (UNRWA) schools is carried out by specially trained health workers and educators visiting schools. These educators produce and distribute brochures, posters, magazines, and broadcast materials, and stage activities. The Ministry of Education recently started to employ social workers in schools to take care of social and psychiatric activities, including the monitoring and care of drug use.

Additional efforts include the training of doctors, nurses, and health workers in the Ministry of Health, UNRWA, and NGO clinics and community facilities. The media (TV, broadcast, and press) provide intermittent announcements about drug use prevention and "World" days devoted to health issues. A number of community nonprofit organizations are active in drug prevention. In Gaza they include Gaza Community Mental Health Program, Palestinian Anti-Drug Council (Society), Life and Hope Society, Al-Azhar University, the Islamic University, Child Health and Community Research Association, and the Family Planning and Protection Society. In the West Bank they include Al Sadeeq Al Tayyeb, Bethlehem Drugs Research and Treatment Center, Al-Quds University, Bir-Zit University, and Al Najah University. Also, Red Crescent, the Medical Relief Committees, and the Health Work Committees provide drug prevention awareness programs in Gaza and the West Bank.

Research and Information

In the area of information and research, many of the above-mentioned organizations and centers, especially universities, have conducted local studies and research. In regard to drug information resource centers, it is worth mentioning the Child Health and Community Research Center (CHCR) in Gaza and the Regional Alcohol and Drug Abuse Resource (RADAR) Center attached to it. The CHCR has established the only information documentation center in the Gaza for drug and alcohol abuse (RADAR). It is one of the international centers of the U.S. National Clearinghouse for Alcohol and Drug Information (NCADI-USA). The CHCR-RADAR has a working relationship with the Palestinian Anti-Drug Authority, Al-Azhar University (Gaza), Ben-Gurion University (Israel), Matrix Institute (USA), United Nations International Drug Control Programme (UNDCP; Cairo Office), and a number of the local NGOs in the health education and community awareness.

The RADAR Center in Gaza had installed a second station for its documentations in the PADA, and a third one in Al-Azhar University (Gaza). The CHCR-RADAR is working jointly with a number of universities and organizations to develop a practical information system.

CONCLUSION

The causes and consequences of drug use and addiction should be of concern to Palestinians because of the noticeable spread of drug use and its negative effects on the social, political, cultural, and socioeconomic spheres of society. It is essential, therefore, that the problem be perceived, assessed, and responded to in multiple ways that address the needs of the individual, family, and community. Functional policies and programs need to be established that address the needs of Palestinian addicts in the context of prevention, treatment, and rehabilitation. Such programs should focus on demand-reduction techniques and the promotion of positive self-esteem, enabling addicts to address the demands of daily living while resisting peer and social pressures.

While many steps have been and are being taken to address drug addiction, a priority that remains unfulfilled is the need for at least one residential treatment facility in Gaza and another one in the West Bank capable of providing detoxification, residential rehabilitation, and community-based follow-up services. Other important issues that need to be addressed as part of a long-term intervention strategy include the development of (1) human resources through education and training; (2) management leadership skills to promote cooperation and coordination initiatives among service providers; and (3) uniform strategies of psychosocial treatment intervention. From the perspective of research, a need exists for information resource centers where valid and reliable data could be collected and made available to health and social work professionals. In such centers, professionals in the field would be encouraged to assist in generating up-to-date materials for health education. Naturally, to operate most effectively, these centers would have to be equipped with modern information systems. Ongoing financial support for the aforesaid prevention programs and initiatives is essential if the spread of drug abuse is ever to be curtailed.

Future Steps

In order to effectively combat the many problems associated with drug abuse and addiction, a number of further actions are suggested. First, it is necessary to document with reliable data the nature and degree of drug abuse in Gaza, the West Bank, and East Jerusalem, and to identify the most vulnerable age groups. Second, it is vital to establish a treatment and rehabilitation regime whereby detected abusers, instead of being placed in psychiatric hospitals, would be accommodated in special rehabilitation units. In such facilities, they would come under the care of social workers, psychologists, and medical professionals who are specially trained and experienced in the field of drug abuse and addiction. Finally, experience dictates the necessity of developing and providing programs that raise public awareness and promote a cooperative approach to the prevention of drug abuse, drawing on the energies of the total Palestinian community, including volunteers and professionals.

NOTES

Notes are statements made by numerous Palestinian experts at conferences and workshops held from 1997 to 1999. The statements quoted in this chapter as notes were recorded by a professional stenographer and transcribed and published as conference proceedings approved by the conference organizing agencies—the Palestine Council of Health and the Economic Cooperation Foundation (see Isralowitz, 1998a, 1998b, and 1999).

1. Statement attributed to Dr. A. Kharroubi, who is experienced in drug prevention and research.

2. At the 1998 Bethlehem conference (Isralowitz, 1998b), Dr. S. Adwan of Bethlehem University underlined the part played by education. "I think that education has a major role in helping people address the drug problem at both the prevention and cooperation levels. Education is the bottom line in how we internalize reality and how we internalize our problems in daily life through our families, schools, society, universities, etc. . . . We as educators in the Palestinian universities have not been exposed to drug issues as part of our teacher training and that is a challenge we should eventually face. At the same time if we look back to the school textbooks, I have found nothing that mentions awareness of drugs. Now the Ministry of Education is considering appointing school advisers and guidance counselors to address the problem. . . . The role of the school is very important both in formal and informal structures and activities, textbooks and teacher training."

3. For example, at the 1997 Beer Sheva conference (Isralowitz, 1998a), Dr. M. Sansur of Beir-Zeit University emphasized the need "to exchange literature, films, and videotapes. [Among] Arabic-speaking countries, Lebanon is the most advanced in disseminating information on drugs. We could get information in Arabic from Lebanon, which is very advanced in producing anti-drug leaflets, posters, and videotapes." This theme of exchange and cooperation was echoed by Dr. H. Ajjuri, director general of the Palestinian Council of Health, at the 1999 Ramallah Conference (Isralowitz, 1999), "We are two well-educated, healthy societies. We know what we want and how to fight our common enemies. . . . I believe wholeheartedly that we are destined to live with each other under one roof, under two roofs, but as civilized nations . . . we have to exchange views and to learn from each other about how to fight our common enemy [drug abuse]."

4. The concluding recommendations submitted by the delegates to the 1997 Beer Sheva conference (Isralowitz, 1998a) suggested that there should be a focus on preventive education in schools, adolescent services, family problems, health and social services intervention, emergency treatment, secondary and tertiary treatment (including aftercare services for addicts and their families), developing vocational skills, social research development, and voluntary community services such as Narcotics Anonymous. As Dr. Kharroubi (referenced above) indicated, "the training of Palestinians is very important in all areas of drug abuse. Building an infrastructure in the Palestinian community should also be a major goal to start with because we cannot fight or prevent or treat without having the infrastructure."

5. At the introductory session of the 1997 Beer Sheva conference (Isralowitz, 1998a), it was noted that both studies and experience indicate that more deaths, more physical and psychological illnesses, and more disabilities result from drug use than from any other preventable health condition.

6. In the course of his lecture on drug prevention at the 1998 Bethlehem conference (Isralowitz, 1998b), Dr. J. Copple of the U.S. National Crime Prevention Council highlighted the importance of "community cohesion": "On substance abuse prevention we are still trying to figure out what are those . . . things I should do or what are those . . . things in my environment that I can change that will reduce my risk of substance abuse. I have met children who have all the socioeconomic risk factors of substance abuse but never use drugs. I've been to communities and neighborhoods all over the Western Hemisphere, including Colombia and Bolivia, that should be drug-using communities but are not. One wonders, Why? What is different there? There are a number of factors that make the difference and they add up to what is called community cohesion. If the various sectors of the community can create a real cohesiveness, then even in the midst of many negative factors, such as high unemployment and a high incidence of crime, substance abuse may not occur."

7. Until recently many cases of drug abuse were treated under the umbrella of "mental health." Dr. M. Afifi, director of the Child Health and Community Research Center, Gaza, at the 1997 Beer Sheva conference (Isralowitz, 1998a), emphasized that a necessary element of combating the drug problem is to "establish specialized units for dealing with the detected cases. Instead of placing them in psychiatric hospitals we need people to work with them socially, psychologically and medically." In 1999, at the Ramallah conference (Isralowitz, 1999), Colonel Al-Zuheiri indicated: "If an addict needs treatment, we have nothing to offer. We have only private centers. Our detention centers are very poor. When addicts are put here they come out either dead or in a worse situation. . . . We need assistance (to provide) free health centers in which treatment is given, and later rehabilitation, to poor or needy people without cost."

8. Indeed, as noted in the introductory session of the 1998 Bethlehem conference (Isralowitz, 1998b) both Palestinian and Israeli societies now have a significant substance abuse problem. Addicts from each of these communities, particularly youth who could be contributing to the positive development of their respective societies, have instead become a burden to society: they perpetrate criminal acts, sometimes of a violent nature, and frequently demand emergency hospital treatment. Substance abusers are both a drain on the limited resources of society and a menace to the welfare of their fellow citizens.

9. Dr. M. Sansur indicated at the 1998 Bethlehem conference (Isralowitz, 1998b) that "in a pilot study conducted by the Latin Patriarch a few years ago in the Old City (East Jerusalem) it was found that 19 percent of households visited at random had one member either abusing drugs or involved in the pushing or selling of drugs."

10. At the 1997 Beer Sheva conference (Isralowitz, 1998a), Dr. E. Awwad of the Palestinian National Committee for Drug Prevention (director, Child and Family Consultation Center) commented: "In the Palestinian Authority we lack valid statistics on the incidence and prevalence of drug use and abuse. We are starting from below zero." In addition, at the same conference, Dr. M. Afifi noted that "To begin to combat the drug problem we need to identify the actual situation in the community and the affected age group. The only data we have now are from police records and hospitals or other organizations."

11. Dr. S. El-Sousi, professor of pharmacology at Al-Azhar University, at the 1999 Ramallah conference (Isralowitz, 1999) elaborated on the issue of the control of legal drugs. "There are illegal and legal drugs . . . but the legal drugs are more dangerous because they are

permitted and they are imported in organized and legal ways. Trafficking with legal drugs is permitted for the treatment of diseases or for research. . . . [I]f the law is not applied and there is no monitoring and no accountability, and no ways and means of implementing the law, then it will turn into only ink on paper. For example, a merchant comes with all the necessary documentation showing that he brought a certain amount of morphine into the country. Morphine, of course, is a drug used in treatment and is available in all hospitals, and hospitals need it very badly. Therefore, as long as we have official documents, why do we not then follow up to see where these drugs are taken and how they are used?" On the control of pharmacists, Dr. El-Sousi added, "Pharmacies accept legal prescriptions, but sometimes they sell drugs even without prescriptions. Why? Because there is no accountability. The pharmacist should write down all the quantities of morphine used. He should then be given a copy book to fill in. He could have special prescriptions issued by the Ministry of Health and the competent monitoring authorities, and these could be monitored just like a check book."

12. At the 1997 Beer Sheva conference (Isralowitz, 1998a), Dr. M. Sansur of Beir-Zeit University commented as follows: "Unfortunately, we are seeing an increasingly pathological family pattern within our social and family structure and I think that we need to be focusing on [it through rehabilitation programs]."

13. There are two critical areas in which the law fails to effectively address the issue of drugs. First, the varying laws and regulations that apply at present in the Palestinian territories lack the uniformity necessary for universal and effective enforcement of an anti-drug policy. The reasons for this are largely historical. At the 1999 Ramallah conference (Isralowitz, 1999), Professor H. Issa, coordinator, the Palestinian Ministry of Justice, elaborated: "In Tunis on the 21st of April, 1994, President Arafat promulgated a resolution to the effect that in the Palestinian territories the laws which were in effect prior to June 5th, 1967, would remain in force until such time as Palestinian legislation is agreed upon and enacted by the Palestinian Legislative Council. In Gaza there is Egyptian law, in the West Bank Jordanian law. In addition, some Israeli legislation as well as Palestinian legislation in existence since 1936 in one way or another is in force in the Palestinian territories. Although new Palestinian laws are now being adopted and implemented, it is still very difficult as a society to deal not only with the different laws but also with the gaps between these laws."

"Now, following the Oslo Accords, the Ministry of Justice is in the process of drafting new anti-drug legislation for consideration and enactment by the Palestinian Legislative Council. This legislation is long overdue since the current anti-drug laws are obsolete and irrelevant to what is going on today. [The laws] simply were not designed to deal with contemporary drug issues. For example, the Jordanian Law of 1960, the Palestinian Law of 1936, the Revolution [sic] PLO Law of 1979, and Israeli legislation such as Order 858, inter alia, although in force, all fundamentally fail to protect Palestinian society from drug abuse."

Second, to date there has been only limited success in terms of communication and cooperation between the law enforcement agencies in Israel and the Palestinian territories. In the introductory session of the Ramallah conference (Isralowitz, 1999), it was noted that the lack of communication and cooperation between the Palestinian territories and Israel with respect to drug policy as well as legal and judicial matters is "in direct contrast to the cooperative relationships that have developed between the drug traffickers on either side. . . . This very delicate issue lies at the heart of the battle against the use of illegal drugs and their transit across borders: it is only through genuine cooperation that the legal and judicial systems of both societies can be rendered truly effective in this arena."

There is an abundance of distrust and suspicion surrounding Israeli treatment of Palestinian drug traffickers. Indeed the Israeli authorities have been accused by a representative of the Palestinian Police Force's Drug Unit of "deliberately flooding the Palestinian streets with drugs." This accusation was based on a Palestinian police colonel's experience of arresting "Palestinians in possession of Israeli ID cards who were peddling drugs in Ramallah and Bethlehem only to find the same drug traffickers on the street the very next day." The explanation proffered at the Ramallah conference (Isralowitz, 1999) was that when suspects are handed over to the Israeli authorities in accordance with the Interim Agreements, Israeli police officers face the problem of being "unable to hold drug dealers in Israeli prisons due to the relatively liberal arrest and detention laws which exist in Israel."

14. At the Ramallah conference (Isralowitz, 1999), Dr. M. Jaber, president of the Palestinian Committee for Social and Psychological Health, elaborated: "This disease is the most serious social and psychological problem that we face. Therefore, all of us have to be unified to fight against it. We must find ways to reconstruct these families which have been denied their addict fathers and their imprisoned fathers. Israel and the Palestine Authority should not use the term 'criminals' for drug addicts. They are not criminals. They are sick people. The traders, the merchants are criminals. The addicts are really sick people, and the environment, their society, has placed them in such a situation. The main reason really for their addiction is their society. If anyone is to blame it is the government and society. Individuals should not be blamed. They did not know what addiction was, what drugs were. Those children who were separated from their fathers and mothers found people who told them to come and use these drugs and they would experience ecstasy. And this addiction led people to become rapists and to indulge in the world of crime. So now they are considered criminals, but as specialists and doctors we feel that it is a humiliation to describe addicts as criminals."

15. At the 1999 Ramallah conference (Isralowitz, 1999), Dr. M. Jaber stated that "We are in the land . . . of three religions—Islam, Christianity and Judaism. We all have religious people who should play an effective role in reaching the souls of our youngsters. Maybe this would be more effective than the rave culture or the external culture. We live in the Middle East, and I recommend that the police try to secure a prominent role for the religious centers in treating these addicts or criminals."

REFERENCES

Hasnain, S. (1993). *Drugs and politics: A historical analysis of the drug issue in East Jerusalem (1948–1991).* Jerusalem: Institute of Criminology, Hebrew University.

Isralowitz, R. (1998a). *Palestinian and Israeli people against substance abuse: A cooperative effort to address the problem through communication, cooperation and coordination: Workshop proceedings.* Beer Sheva, November 4–5, 1997. Tel Aviv and East Jerusalem: Economic Cooperation Foundation and Palestine Council of Health.

———. (1998b). *Palestinian and Israeli people against substance abuse: Prevention and beyond: Workshop proceedings.* Bethlehem, May 25–26, 1998. Tel Aviv and East Jerusalem: Economic Cooperation Foundation and Palestine Council of Health.

———. (1999). *Palestinian and Israeli people against substance abuse: Substance abuse: Legal and judicial aspects: Workshop proceedings.* Ramallah, March 24–25, 1999. Tel Aviv and East Jerusalem: Economic Cooperation Foundation and Palestine Council of Health.

Khamis, V., & Habash, A. (1995). *Drug addiction among Palestinians in the West Bank: Bethlehem.* Unpublished paper.

4

Psychoactive Substance Use by Jews and Arabs in Israel

Giora Rahav and Meir Teichman

National and ethnic differences and their relation to substance use constitute a major theme for research and discussion. Many attempts to address the problem through controlling production, distribution, and use of harmful substances have stemmed from beliefs, impressions, and anecdotes, as well as local documentation, that are highly susceptible to observational and reporting biases. A common denominator of such reports is that the observer's position within the social systems is bound to affect the observations and the reported behavior.

In Israel, a multiethnic society, the dominant group is Jewish (80 percent of the population) with an Arab minority of slightly less than 20 percent. We designate members of this minority as Arabs rather than Palestinians for two major reasons. First, we wish to avoid terminology that carries, at present, strong political overtones. Second, while we believe that the vast majority of this population sector see themselves as Arabs, it seems unclear to what extent they consider themselves Palestinians. What is unique about the Jewish and Arab populations in Israel is that they differ significantly in terms of their attitudes toward alcohol and other psychoactive substances. Jewish people, for example, tend to project the impression that they have a low level of alcohol consumption. While there are studies that show acculturation tends to affect their drinking patterns (Engs, Hanson, & Isralowitz, 1988), generally it is believed that Jewish people, especially those in the United States, but also those in Canada and Europe, tend to have a lower frequency level of drinking, drink smaller quantities, and suffer less from the adverse consequences of drinking than their non-Jewish counterparts (Bilu & Witztum, 1997; Room, 1968). Numerous explanations and interpretations exist for these patterns (Bales,

1946; Glassner & Berg, 1980; Snyder, 1958) including a recent suggestion that some of the enzymes involved in the processing of alcohol are deficient among Jews as a genetic trait (Neumark, Friedlander, Thomasson, & Ting-Kai, 1998). Nevertheless, culture and its relation to sobriety tend to reflect and support the idea that Jewish people are generally less affected by alcohol than are other ethnic groups. As for the use of illicit drugs, there is no consistent view of Jews as more, or less, prone to using them. It seems reasonable to hypothesize, therefore, that the general attitude of rejection toward intoxication and the traditional emphasis on conscious decision making would be extended to other substances as well. Empirical support for this hypothesis, however, is rather limited.

With respect to the Arab population, alcohol and drug use has been strongly affected by the dominant religion among Arabs, Islam. Islam explicitly prohibits drinking alcohol, a prohibition that is often extended to other intoxicating drugs. While there are several other religious groups among Israeli Arabs (notably Christians and Druze), Islam is a clearly dominant cultural influence. Based on this consideration alone, therefore, we might expect the Arab population to have low rates of alcohol and drug consumption and low or moderate frequency and quantity of consumption among those who do drink or use drugs. Actually, this argument is simplistic. While Islam indeed prohibits alcohol, drinking has been incorporated into Arab life since its early days. Medieval wine songs (like the ones included in the Rubáiyát of Omar Khayyám) have become part and parcel of the classic Arab culture. It is also reasonable to assume that the cultivation of arak as a typical Middle-Eastern drink was not limited to the needs of the non-Moslems. Although we do not purport to summarize Arab attitudes and behavior regarding alcohol and drug use (for a summary see Weiss, Sawa, Abdeen, & Yanai, 1999), it seems that the traditional cultural attitude is one of ambivalence, an attitude that incorporates the dominant ideological demands with "subterranean values" (Matza & Sykes, 1961) influenced by the ongoing contacts with Western culture in general, and Jewish culture in particular. These values are transferred via various interpersonal contacts and the various mass media that reach every home. In certain respects, this is a classic case of culture conflict (Sellin, 1938), a situation known to undermine traditional norms. The Islamic prohibition on intoxicants tends to cover illegal drugs as well. But in that respect, too, religious prohibitions are often ignored. In particular, hashish has been traditionally prevalent in North Africa and the Middle East.

From this brief survey, we can see that Jewish culture encourages limited, moderate drinking, while the traditional Arab approach is either prohibitive or ambivalent. Very little can be deduced from this understanding, however, about the use of other illicit drugs. In this chapter, the substance use patterns of Israeli Jewish and Arab people are examined and discussed.

METHODS

The data used in the present analysis are from two national surveys carried out in 1995 and 1998. Both surveys were conducted by the same investigators using very similar procedures (i.e., sampling procedures, questionnaires, etc.). The sample of Jewish respondents was representative of Jewish communities. In each location, 10 households were approached and one person in the 18-to-40-year age group was selected for an interview (for a more detailed description see Rahav, Teichman, Gil, Rosenblum, & Bar-Hamburger, 1998). In the Arab communities, most of which have no maps to sample from, 22 communities were selected in four geographic regions. Within each community, a quota sample was taken defined by age and gender to represent the 18-to-40-year-old population.

The interviews were conducted with structured questionnaires, in Hebrew or Arabic, according to the respondent's language. The substance-use items in this survey have been used repeatedly in household and school-based surveys in Israel, and have shown good reliability (Barnea, Rahav, & Teichman, 1987). Anonymity and confidentiality were promised, and subjects were asked to complete the questionnaire by themselves.

The drug-use items were the Hebrew version of the items used by Johnston, O'Malley, and Bachman (2000). These items were used several times in the past (Barnea et al., 1987) and are generally accepted as the local standard. Two items dealt with alcohol consumption for nonreligious purposes: drinking during the previous 12 months and drinking during the previous 7 days. Drinking during the previous year was used as the criterion to distinguish drinkers from non-drinkers; drinking during the previous week was taken as an indicator of moderate to high drinking. For all other substances, use during the previous year was the criterion applied to determine a behavior pattern. These items were used in their dichotomized form because of the extremely skewed distributions that could bias most analyses based on categorization of the original items.

RESULTS

Table 4.1 presents the percentage of subjects reporting use of psychoactive substances. Binge drinking is presented as a percent of those drinking during the previous month. The table also presents the odds ratios, which were determined by dividing the chance of the behavior occurring among Jews divided by the chance of the behavior occurring among Arabs. The table shows that alcohol consumption is higher among the Jews, with about 64 percent consuming during the previous year as compared with 30 percent among the Arabs and 27 percent versus 15 percent consuming during the previous week. On the other side of the severity scale are the hard drugs. In this case, prevalence in the Jewish population (nearly 1 percent) is considerably lower than that in the Arab population (over 3 percent). The odds ratios indicate that the chances of a Jewish person drinking alcohol based on the frequencies used for this analyses are about two times higher than the chance for an Arab person doing the same. On the other hand, Arabs are two times more likely than Jews to use hard drugs.

Regarding the odds ratios, the highest relate to yearly alcohol consumption with considerably lower ones for weekly drinking. They are about balanced for cannabis,

Table 4.1
Percent Using Psychoactive Substances by Ethnicity

	Alcohol—Year	Alcohol—Week	Alcohol—Binge*	Cannabis—Year	Prescription—Year	Hard—Year	Any Illicit—Year
All Subjects							
Jews	64.40	27.0	39.1	4.4	2.9	0.9	6.7
Arabs	29.8	15.3	54.0	4.2	5.1	3.2	7.2
OR	2.06	1.43	0.74	1.02	0.75	0.53	0.96
p <	.001	.001	.001	.76	.001	.001	0.45
Males							
Jews	81.6	43.1	45.2	6.4	3.3	1.6	8.6
Arabs	53.2	31.5	58.8	9.0	8.7	6.2	13.5
OR	1.97	1.23	0.76	0.83	0.59	0.50	0.78
p <	.001	.03	.001	.03	.001	.001	.001
Females							
Jews	53.0	16.4	24.5	3.2	2.7	0.4	5.5
Arabs	14.0	4.6	43.6	1.1	2.6	1.2	3.1
OR	2.59	2.01	0.65	1.72	1.01	0.60	1.34
p <	.001	.001	.01	.002	.90	.01	0.01

*Binge drinking was calculated only for subjects who drank in the previous month.

and are lower for the use of pills, with hard drugs being the lowest. Apparently, the more serious, or dangerous the consumption, the higher the likelihood of Arab involvement. It is interesting to note, furthermore, that binge drinking (among those who drink) takes the pattern of the more dangerous substances, with an odds ratio of 0.75.

Among both Jews and Arabs, males tend to use substances more than females. Regarding odds ratios, a similar picture tends to emerge in terms of Jewish and Arab consumption of alcohol and illegal substances. The major difference in the odds ratios, however, seems to be that the chance of Jewish females using substances is greater than the chance of Arab females using substances. Use among males is more similar across the two groups. The major differences between the patterns of males and females are in the use of cannabis and prescription drugs. Cannabis is used by Jewish females much more often than by Arab females; Arab males use the substance more often than their Jewish counterparts.

This analysis does not take into consideration several variables that may have confounded the findings. For example, in Israel, Arab residents are overrepresented in the lower socioeconomic strata. The findings may be biased, therefore, because consumption of substances is greater, in general, among those of lower socioeconomic status. Another potentially confounding factor is religiosity. Generally speaking, the Arab population seems to be more religious than the Jewish population. Since religion tends to be a significant protective factor against substance use, the findings may be affected. In order to overcome these issues, logistic regressions were used with psychoactive substance consumption serving as a dependent variable.

Table 4.2 presents the results of these analyses. The first independent variable is the respondent's ethnic group (1 for Jews, 0 for otherwise). Three indicators of the socioeconomic status were used: educational attainment, occupational prestige level, and income. Occupations were classified according to the Central Bureau of Statistics into nine groups designating professional and academic occupation. The highest of one's own and one's spouse's occupation was considered. Income was assessed subjectively on a five-category scale, from much more to much less than the mean. Religiosity was measured by a five-category scale ranging from very religious, ultra-orthodox to non-religious, secular.

For the purposes of this description, the most important finding is the strong, significant relationship between ethnic status and substance use even in this multivariate model of analysis. The effect of being Jewish on alcohol consumption is positive, both for being a drinker (previous year) and for present, or frequent drinking (previous week). The chance of a Jewish person in Israel drinking in a specific year is 71 percent higher than that of an Arab resident, and the chance of a Jewish person drinking during the previous week is 29 percent higher than that for an Arab person. After controlling for age, sex, socioeconomic status, and religiosity, it was found that a Jewish person is 53 percent less likely to use hard drugs than an Arab person.

Table 4.2
Logistic Regression Results (Odds Ratios)

	Alcohol— Year	Alcohol— Week	Alcohol— Binge*	Cannabis— Year	Prescription— Year	Hard— Year	Any Illicit—Year
Jewish	1.71***	1.29***	0.73***	0.77***	0.70***	0.53***	0.78***
Sex	2.10***	2.04***	1.58***	1.47***	1.21**	1.98***	1.32***
Age	1.00	1.01**	1.00	1.00	1.03**	0.95**	1.01
Education	1.08***	1.00	0.92	1.00	0.87**	0.74***	0.95
Occupation—SES	0.99	1.01	1.01	0.92**	1.00	1.06	0.95
Income	0.96*	0.98	0.99	0.97	1.06	0.99	0.99
Religiosity	1.44***	1.31***	0.99	1.83***	1.28***	1.20#	1.56***

*$p < 0.05$. **$p < 0.01$. ***$p < 0.001$. #$p < 0.10$.

While our focus is on ethnic group membership, it is worth noting the strong effects of two other variables. First, gender has a strong effect, with all forms of substance use being higher for males than for females. Second, religiosity is strongly associated with use, so that the least committed to a religion (who have the highest score) are the most likely to use alcohol and drugs. Furthermore, it is worth noting that additional analyses testing for interactions did not considerably alter the findings.

The interaction of ethnicity with religiosity is rather interesting and important, and, therefore, justifies additional attention. Table 4.3 presents these interactions in detail. The first section of the table presents the percent drinking alcohol during the previous 12 months by ethnicity and religiosity. In each level of religious devoutness, Jews are more likely to drink than Arabs. Actually, drinking prevalence among the most religious category of Jews is about the same as that of the least religious among the Arabs. What is more interesting, however, is the interaction of ethnicity, religiosity, and substance use. The odds ratio between Jewish and Arab alcohol use is 1.41 among the least religious, and increases to 3.34 among the most religious. A similar but somewhat less pronounced trend (in the ratio of Jewish to Arab users) is reflected by the figures for previous-week drinking. This trend completely disappears in the examination of illicit drug use. In all religiosity levels, Jewish use of illicit drugs is lower than that of Arab use. Moreover, the interaction effect changes its nature: in the cases of hard drugs and illicit use of prescription drugs, the difference between Jews and Arabs is high for the least religious and for the highly devout. It is lower for the moderately religious. In the case of cannabis use, the difference tends to be the same, with a modest variation in terms of chance of use.

SUMMARY AND CONCLUSION

The major finding of this study is that psychoactive substance consumption differs between Jewish and Arab Israelis. Alcohol consumption is much more prevalent among the Jews, while illicit substance use is more prevalent among the Arabs. Representation of Arabs among the users changes from high underrepresentation in the case of alcohol drinking during the previous year to high overrepresentation in the case of hard drug use. The rates of cannabis use are similar for Arabs and Jews. A more thorough analysis reveals that these overall trends are rather stable when sex, age, socioeconomic status, and religious devoutness are controlled for. Differences do exist, however, among males and females and between different ethnic groups, as well as among those with various levels of religiosity.

ACKNOWLEDGMENT

The surveys that served as the source of the data for this chapter were conducted for the Anti-Drug Authority of Israel (ADAI). The authors are grateful to the ADAI

Table 4.3
Prevalence of Substance Use by Religiosity

	Religiosity		
	High	**Moderate**	**Low**
Alcohol: Past Year			
Jews	48.1	59.1	73.6
Arabs	14.4	28.4	52.3
Ratio	3.34	2.08	1.41
Alcohol: Past Week			
Jews	17.9	24.1	32.3
Arabs	7.1	14.0	28.8
Ratio	2.52	1.72	1.12
Cannabis: Past Year			
Jews	0.9	2.5	7.1
Arabs	2.1	2.8	10.2
Ratio	0.43	0.89	0.70
Medications: Past Year			
Jews	1.3	3.3	3.1
Arabs	3.1	5.0	7.8
Ratio	0.42	0.66	0.40
Hard Drugs: Past Year			
Jews	0.5	1.1	0.9
Arabs	2.6	1.7	7.2
Ratio	0.19	0.65	0.13
Any Illicit: Past Year			
Jews	1.8	5.3	9.4
Arabs	4.4	6.5	12.7
Ratio	0.41	0.82	0.74

and its chief scientist, Dr. Rachel Bar-Hamburger, for the data and the help they provided.

REFERENCES

Bales, R. F. (1946). Cultural differences in rates of alcoholism. *Quarterly Journal of Studies on Alcohol, 6,* 480–499.

Barnea, Z., Rahav, G., & Teichman, M. (1987). The reliability and consistency of self-reports on substance use in a longitudinal study. *British Journal of Addiction, 82,* 891–898.

Bilu, Y., & Witztum, E. (1997). The mental health of Jews outside and inside Israel. In I. Al-Issa, M. Tousignant, et al. (Eds.), *Ethnicity, immigration, and psychopathology.* New York: Plenum.

Engs, R., Hanson, D., & Isralowitz, R. (1988). Drinking problems among Jewish college students in the United States and Israel. *Journal of Social Psychology, 128*(3), 415–417.

Glassner, B., & Berg, B. (1980). How Jews avoid alcohol problems. *American Sociological Review, 45,* 647–664.

Johnston, L. D., O'Malley, P. M., & Bachman, J. G. (2000). *The Monitoring the Future National survey results on adolescent drug use: Overview of key findings, 1999* (NIH Publication No. 00-4690). Rockville, MD: National Institute on Drug Abuse.

Matza, D., & Sykes, G. (1961). Delinquency and subterranean values. *American Sociological Review, 26,* 712–719.

Neumark, Y., Friedlander, Y., Thomasson, H., & Ting-Kai, L. (1998). Association of the ADH2*2 allele with reduced ethanol consumption in Jewish men in Israel: A pilot study. *Journal of Studies on Alcohol, 59,* 133–139.

Rahav, G., Teichman, M., Gil, R., Rosenblum, Y., & Bar-Hamburger, R. (1998). *The use of psychoactive substances among Israeli citizens 1998: Epidemiological study 4.* Tel Aviv: Pori Institute, Tel Aviv University, Anti-Drug Authority (in Hebrew).

Room, R. (1968). Cultural contingencies of alcoholism: Variations between and within nineteenth-century urban ethnic groups in alcohol-related death rates. *Journal of Health and Social Behavior, 9,* 99–113.

Sellin, T. (1938). *Culture conflict and crime.* New York: Social Science Research Council.

Snyder, C. (1958). *Alcohol and the Jews: A cultural study of drinking and sobriety.* Glencoe, IL: Free Press.

Weiss, S., Sawa, S., Abdeen, Z., & Yanai, J. (1999). Substance abuse studies and prevention efforts among Arabs in the 1990s in Israel, Jordan and the Palestinian Authority: A literature review. *Addiction, 94,* 177–198.

5

Alcohol Use among Moslems and Druze in Israel, Jordan, and the Palestinian Authority: Theoretical Aspects and Trends

Shoshana Weiss, Ghazi H. Sawa, Ziad Abdeen, and Joseph Yanai

INTRODUCTION

Arab people in the Middle East are currently facing a process of transition: the transformation from conflict to coexistence (Hermann & Yuchtman-Yaar, 1997) and changes in their way of life (Bar, Eldar, & Yarom, 1987). The process of transition is not unique to the Moslem and Druze residents of Israel, for it characterizes most Arab societies in the whole of the Middle East. However, the process of transition among Arab people is most significant in Israel, due to the influence of the nontraditional Western Jewish society. One behavioral aspect that has been tremendously affected by the process is the alcohol consumption in the Arab sector. The Islamic and Druze religions are examples of abstinence-teaching faiths that prohibit the consumption of alcoholic beverages. However, the transition from conflict to coexistence has contributed to alcohol use and to the emergence of alcohol-related problems among the Arab people, especially in Israel.

ARAB PEOPLE IN ISRAEL: CONTRIBUTING FACTORS TO ALCOHOL USE

Transition

For decades, the influence of religion has weakened among Arab people in Israel (Hermann & Yuchtman-Yaar, 1997; Laish, 1981; Laish & Fallach, 1981), even though there are places where religious groups such as the Islamic Movement are strong. Alcohol is widely available in Israel, since Israel is a non-Moslem country.

The Islamic and Druze religions prohibit drinking and provide arguments against drinking and about its dangers, but do not provide guidelines concerning drinking or create norms about how to drink. In addition, the secular educational system does not provide a comprehensive alcohol education program (Weiss, Sawa, Abdeen, & Yanai, 1999). With the weakening of religion and the strengthening of secularization (Ramberg & Moshkovitz, 1988), religious rules tend to have little effect on actual behavior. When nonobservant people come into contact with Western norms and drinking patterns in a non-Moslem country, they do not know how to cope with alcohol. They do not see the consumption of alcohol as something that deserves special reference and learning. For many who drink, religion does not serve as a protective factor against abuse of the substance. Thus, Moslems and Druze, as members of abstinence-teaching religious groups, are likely to have a low prevalence of drinking in comparison to people who belong to prescriptive religious groups (such as Jews), but are likely to have a relatively high prevalence of excessive drinking and harm among the drinkers (Teichman, Rahav, & Barnea, 1994). In other words, the Islamic and Druze religions may be negatively precipitating alcohol-related problems among drinkers rather than preventing them, particularly in an environment where alcohol is available (Weiss, in press a).

Contact with the Jewish Sector

The Israeli Arab population is engaged in a process of transition mainly because of its close contact with the Jewish population (Ben-Dor, 1995; Hermann & Yuchtman-Yaar, 1995; Ramberg & Moshkovitz, 1988). Arab people, particularly young people, adopt "Western thinking" in many aspects of life (Smooha, 1984). Jewish secular values concerning alcohol use have been imported to a great degree from Europe and America. Moslems absorb these values as a result of employment that takes them from their villages to places of work that are Jewish owned or operated. Development of transportation networks reducing the travel time to and from work and improved methods of communications are additional factors that have brought modernization to Moslems in the region (Israeli, 1976; Laish & Fallach, 1981; Ramberg & Moshkovitz, 1988).

In addition to work-related contact, many Arab people are living in cities, which have mixed Arab-Jewish populations, and many visit the entertainment and shopping centers in the Jewish towns. The increasing proportion of high school students among the Arab people increases the flow of students to the universities (Hermann & Yuchtman-Yaar, 1997). These contacts also expose Arab people to the influence of different socialization patterns that strongly reflect Western culture (Bar et al., 1987; Ramberg & Moshkovitz, 1988). The number of Arab people who interact regularly with Jews is much higher than the number of Jews who maintain day-to-day relations with the Arab people. In a 1995 study of Arabs ($n = 483$) and Jews ($n = 1{,}221$), 86 percent of Jews reported that they had never visited Arab areas or towns, while only 20 percent of the Arab people had never visited Jewish localities (Hermann & Yuchtman-Yaar, 1995).

Among the Druze, integration into Israeli society is a common theme as evidenced, in part, by increased access to population centers of Jewish economic and employment activity (Ben-Dor, 1995). Furthermore, due to their compulsory service in the Israeli army, the Druze are placed in situations that expose them to drinking.

Modernization and the Standard of Living

In the Middle East, modernization involves a change from a traditional agricultural community to one based on technology, modern agriculture, and industry (Ben-Dor, 1995; Ramberg & Moshkovitz, 1988). During the slow process of industrialization in Arab and Druze villages, a stratum of wealthy intellectuals, industrialists, developers, and suppliers has emerged (Ramberg & Moshkovitz, 1988). Arab people throughout the region have been involved in a process of catching up with modern conditions in education, technology, and science. As a result, while there has been improvement in the economic condition of the Arab people living in Israel, their living conditions and economic status are still inferior to those of the Jewish citizens in the country (Landau, 1981). One outcome of this improved status is an increased rate of alcohol consumption. Many more Arabs than ever can afford to purchase alcoholic beverages in large quantities, and by doing so are adopting the norms of an affluent society as well as one of its symbols, which is prominently displayed through advertisements (Moore & Weiss, 1992). In addition, similar to Jews, Arabs are influenced by television programs and other communication means that reflect Western customs and values. Drinking is viewed as a symbol of "doing well" and being a "sophisticated person," a "modern citizen of the globe."

The Family

Modernization, the spread of Western culture, exposure to media, and the relocation of people from Arab villages to Jewish centers are among the factors that have reduced the importance of the extended family and the clan (hamula) (Hermann & Yuchtman-Yaar, 1997; Ramberg & Moshkovitz, 1988). Over time, the Arab family has become more nuclear, leading to a greater sense of individualization and familial disintegration. The transition in family structure has weakened the power of the father in the family by subverting his authoritative role, and with it, his ability to control problem behaviors, including those related to alcohol use. In practice, many married young Arab people from villages leave their fathers because of the shortage of land (Ramberg & Moshkovitz, 1988), migrating to other places, mainly urban, looking for employment. This creates a sense of economic independence from their fathers. These factors have resulted in a loosening of interpersonal bonds and a weakening of individuals' connection to the traditional extended family, causing isolation and confusion for many (Miller, 1977). In short, the Arab family is in transition as a result of multiple factors, and that transition is accompanied by an increase in alcohol use as a convenient and cheap way to relieve tension (Bar et al., 1987).

COEXISTENCE AND EQUALITY

The numerous stressors affecting Israeli Arabs exacerbate the use of alcohol. Among them are the complex political situation, which entails a dilemma of national and civil identity—their Palestinian nationality on the one hand and their life in Israel as a minority on the other (Hermann & Yuchtman-Yaar, 1995; Ramberg & Moshkovitz, 1988); discrimination in terms of unequal spending for the education of children and allocations to local authorities; and the lack of free and equal competition in the work force (Hermann & Yuchtman-Yaar, 1995, 1997).

These complexities, combined with the wide gap between expectations (i.e., for rapid but positive fundamental changes in policy that will impact external and domestic relations and support systems) and the reality of the strained and drawn-out peace process (Hermann & Yuchtman-Yaar, 1997), lead to feelings of inferiority, dissatisfaction, uncertainty, anger, neglect, frustration, tension, and rage among Arabs, feelings that are often associated with alcohol use.

Adjusting to change is not a simple process; traditions and response patterns in terms of addressing and coping with situations do not evolve overnight. In such an environment, change can cause confusion and ambivalence with respect to social controls that have been in put in place to protect Arab society against problems associated with alcohol use. In sum, processes of transition including social, cultural, and political problems, as well as the adaptation to Western values and culture, contribute to an understanding of why drinking and alcohol-related problems are becoming more prevalent in the Arab sector.

PALESTINIAN PEOPLE: TRANSITIONS AND ALCOHOL USE

If there is one phrase that characterizes Palestinian society, it is “in transition.” The Palestinians are going through a radical, long, and arduous process of normalization involving national consolidation, socioeconomic development, political transformation, and institution building that includes governmental mechanisms that address human needs (Hassassian, 1995; Sabella, 1995). Even prior to the peace agreements, however, Palestinians faced challenges and changes that might have had an impact on alcohol use.

The trade structure (Awartani, 1995) has been heavily dominated by links with Israel, and there has been a heavy dependence on Israel as a source of employment. The movement of Palestinians (especially young males) from the West Bank and Gaza to work inside the “green line” has given such people access to alcohol and a drinking culture in Israel. They then bring a drinking ethic back to the Palestinian territories. Palestinians have been exposed to Western culture, not only through the media and contact with Jews, but also through contacts with tourists and with the

Palestinians who have returned home from abroad. Economic development and an increase in income have made it financially feasible for many people to afford alcohol, which is relatively cheap in Israel. While a low level of industrialization exists in Gaza and the West Bank, the standard of living has changed with modernization and alcoholic beverages have become readily available and easily attainable.

Another important factor is that the social and cultural influences of the Intifada and Israeli occupation have led to the weakening of social controls over young males, possibly giving them greater opportunity and reason to use alcohol. A survey among 1,874 people in the West Bank and Gaza in 1994 (Sabella, 1995) revealed that 71 percent of the Palestinian people were not happy with life. This mood, as well as feelings of uncertainty and fears about the future may explain alcohol use.

JORDANIAN PEOPLE: TRANSITION AND ALCOHOL USE

In Jordan two main processes are affecting alcohol use: its suppression and its spread. The trend toward suppressing alcohol use seems to be associated with an emerging sector of the Jordanian society that leans toward strict Islamic values and moral codes of conduct. This sector's main political premise is religiously bound, as are its modes of expression and norms of interaction. In a way, elements of this movement are becoming characteristic of Jordanian institutions ranging from mosques and benevolent associations to schools, universities, and the parliament. The growing emergence of this religiously oriented sector of the Jordanian society, including the formidable force of preaching and precepts that relate to the teachings of Islam, can lead to the suppression of alcohol consumption.

The other trend, leading to increasing alcohol consumption and abuse, is associated with various transitions that have taken place in Jordan during the last 10 years or so including:

- The social change from the extended family to nuclear families, which gives young married couples the opportunity to use alcohol because they are no longer under the watchful eyes of their elders.
- The growing influence of media that reflects Western lifestyles and culture that tolerate and encourage the use of alcohol.
- The spread of private universities and the concomitant increase in the freedom available for young students to try alcoholic drinks that may in turn lead them to becoming social drinkers, abusers, or dependents.
- The growing trend of tourism from the Gulf region and Saudi Arabia, which leads to a growing demand for the availability and use of alcohol.
- The gradual improvement in the standard of living and a growth in the adoption of Western lifestyles, even among rural peoples such as the desert-dwelling Bedouin. There has been growth in the number of well-to-do families of prosperous businessmen, pro-establishment people, and Westernized upper-middle-class status among both secular

Moslems and Christians. This sector of the Jordanian society is not a new one. It has slowly emerged since the 1970s. Most of the upper-middle-class members tend to use alcoholic beverages and are social drinkers (while the lower-working-class members in the Jordanian society tend to be alcohol abusers). The affluent people and their lifestyle can impact all of society by sending implicit messages that alcohol use is an acceptable indulgence.

- Feelings of frustration and disappointment concerning the peace agreements with Israel, which have failed, so far, to deliver significant economic benefits. Such feelings can lead to drinking. (This factor also can contribute, however, to the growth of the religious sector, which condemns drinking.)
- The spread of illegal drug addiction that contributes to alcohol abuse.

Up to this point, the unique situation among the Arab people in the process of transition and its relation to alcohol use has been described. Now, we shall review alcohol use patterns over the last decade and projected trends.

ALCOHOL USE STUDIES IN THE MIDDLE EAST

During the 1990s, 12 epidemiological and social studies were carried out on Israeli Arabs, two on Jordanians, and two on Palestinians (see Table 5.1).

In addition, reports of Arabs receiving services in alcohol treatment centers in Israel are published every year and provide information about the socio-demographic characteristics of these people. These reports, as well as a report on hospitalized Arab alcoholics in an Israeli residential center and two Jordanian reports, appear in Table 5.2.

Israel: Alcohol Use Trends

Tables 5.1 and 5.2 reflect the various local and national studies that have been conducted in the region during the last decade. It is impossible, however, to compare the results, because they differ in methodology, samples, and other data collection factors. In spite of these difficulties, studies and reports prepared over the last decade by certain researchers provide insight into alcohol use patterns and trends. Thus, this chapter will present major examples of the incidence of alcohol use drawn from studies and reports that encompass at least three points of time, and identify the trends that took place during the last 10 years or so.

Treatment

Table 5.3 presents the number of Moslem and Druze patients in the open alcohol centers from 1993 to 1999.

The population of alcoholics throughout the world is much greater than the number of alcoholics who apply for treatment. For the most part, alcoholics deny their addiction or attempt to withdraw from their habit by themselves. For these

Table 5.1
Alcohol Studies on Arabs in the Trilateral Region

Reference	Year of Study	Topic	Population	Sample Size
Moore & Weiss, 1991, Israel	1990	Alcohol use	Youth	1,147
Weiss & Moore, 1992, Israel	1991	Perception of alcoholism	Teachers	273
Dgani, 1992; Israel	1991	Alcohol use	Youth	160
Weiss, in press b; Israel	1992	Alcohol use	Youth	156
Weiss & Moore, 1995a,b; Israel	1994	Alcohol use/reasons for abstinence	Youth	1,591
Rahav et al., 1995; Israel	1994–95	Alcohol use	Adults	954
Weiss, 1996; Israel	1995	Knowledge of alcohol & driving	Youth	825
Abu Saad, 1996; Israel	1995–96	Alcohol use	Youth	731
Weiss, 1997, in press b; Israel	1996	Alcohol use/opinions/warning labels	Youth	2,220
Abu Saad, 1998; Israel	1997	Alcohol use	Youth	312
Weiss, 1999; Israel	1997	Alcohol use/ opinions/alcohol control	Youth	799
Rahav et al., 1998; Israel	1998	Alcohol use	Adults	397
Weiss et al., 1999; Al-Farah, 1991; Jordan	1990–91	Alcoholic traits	Adults	200
Weiss et al., 1999; United Nations, 1993; Jordan	1991	Alcohol use	Adults/Youth	172
Weiss et al., 1999; Abdeen, 1997; P.A.	1996	Alcohol use	Youth	603
Abdeen & Natsheh, 1998; P.A.	1998	Alcohol use	Youth/Adults	320

Table 5.2
Reports on Arab Patients and Arabs Convicted for Drunkenness

Reference	Topic	Number of Persons
Weiss et al., 1999; Jordan	Alcoholics treated in Al-Fueis Hospital 1990–97	146
W. Sarhan, personal communication, November 1, 2000; Jordan	Alcoholics treated in Al-Rashid Hospital 1990–99	229
Weiss et al., 1999; Directorate of Public Security, 1990-2000; Jordan	Adults convicted for drunkenness 1990–99	36,364
Weiss et al., 1999; Marchevsky & Weiss, 1997; Israel	Hospitalized Arab alcoholics 1982–94	84
Weiss et al., 1999; Israel	Arab patients in open centers 1991–96	597
Weiss et al., 1999; Michaely, 1998b; Israel	Arab patients as children of alcoholics	107
Michaely, 1998a; Israel	Moslem & Druze patients in open centers 1997	123
Michaely, 1999; Israel	Moslem & Druze patients in open centers 1998	207
Michaely, 2000; Israel	Moslem & Druze patients in open centers 1999	304

Table 5.3
Moslem and Druze Patients (New Admissions) in Ambulatory Treatment

Reference	Weiss et al., 1999	Weiss et al., 1999	Weiss et al., 1999	Weiss et al., 1999	Michaely, 1998a	Michaely, 1999	Michaely, 2000
Year	1993	1994	1995	1996	1997	1998	1999
Moslems	45	46	64	114	102	180	272
Druze	8	12	11	17	21	27	32
Total	53	58	75	131	123	207	304

Table 5.4
Drinking among Arab Adolescents (15–18 Years of Age) in Northern Israel by Gender and Religion

Year	Reference	*N* of Sample	*N* of Locations	Male Christians	Male Druze	Male Moslems	Female Christians	Female Druze	Female Moslems
1994	Weiss & Moore, 1995	1,591	9	73%	43%	30%	52%	9%	12%
1996	Weiss, in press b	2,220	13	82%	50%	32%	37%	11%	13%
1997	Weiss, 1999	799	4*	67%	59%	50%	48%	19%	24%

* Four Arab locations known for a high rate of alcoholism among adults.

reasons, alcoholics seek treatment only after many years of drinking. Moreover, in a closed, traditional, and abstinent society such as those in the Moslem and Druze sectors, there are strong social pressures to conceal the problem. Consequently, the appeal for help to a professional body tends to be less frequent and occurs later in terms of the problem. Furthermore, the situation of Arab alcoholics differs from that of Jewish alcoholics because of the different role of women in the family (Bar et al., 1987).

One of the most influential factors in moving the male alcoholic to treatment is his wife, but even wives have limited influence. Women have a lower status and less influence than men in Moslem society (Ramberg & Moshkovitz, 1988), and, as in other societies, drinking in Arab society is often seen as an expression of masculinity. Because of this and the fact that Arab women often have many children to care for, most Arab women have limited impact, if any, on persuading their husbands to seek treatment (Ramberg & Moshkovitz, 1988). As for the Druze, women have the same position as men in the Druze religion, but in daily life the woman's position is also lower (Ben-Dor, 1995; Ramberg & Moshkovitz, 1988). Therefore, the number of Arab people in treatment is only a small portion of those affected (Bar et al., 1987).

The rise in the number of patients in treatment in the last decade reflects the increase in the rate of alcoholism and the number of alcohol treatment centers in the Arab sector. Because treatment centers in the Arab villages provide local treatment programs, alcoholics do not need to travel to faraway cities to get help. At the end of the twentieth century, there were four alcohol treatment centers in the Arab sector and 12 in the Jewish sector. In addition, Arab people received attention in treatment centers in major population centers including Haifa, Jerusalem, and Carmel. The numbers of Arab people in treatment are expected to increase because no educational programs are available in Arab schools in Israel (Weiss et al., 1999) and no other preventive mechanisms exist. This trend may be further exacerbated by two opposing factors. The first is an improved standard of living, which enables Arab people who "do well" to easily purchase alcoholic beverages. The second factor is unemployment. The unemployment rate among Arab people is similar or somewhat higher than the rate among Jews (Hermann & Yuchtman-Yaar, 1997), but in the Arab sector, it has national and political meaning. It stems from unequal work opportunities, one example of which is that even though the educational level of the Arab people has risen, they have not been able to convert this gain into jobs, better jobs, or occupationally appropriate advancement (Hermann & Yuchtman-Yaar, 1997). Unemployed Arabs may turn to drinking alcohol, which as mentioned earlier is relatively cheap, in order to cope with the emptiness and spare time, and the feelings of anger, uselessness, alienation, and discrimination that their situation creates.

Adult Alcohol Use

A nationwide study conducted in 1995 among 954 male Arabs (mostly Moslem), 18 to 40 years of age (Rahav, Teichman, Gil, Rosenblum, & Bar-Hamburger, 1995), revealed that 31.8 percent of the participants reported drinking alcohol in the previous year. Another study was carried out by the same group of researchers (Rahav et al., 1998) in 1998 among 397 male Arabs 18 to 40 years of age, and revealed that 36.6 percent of respondents reported drinking. An impending investigation is expected to find a higher rate due to the lack of prevention programs among Israeli Arabs, and the continuation of the transitions in the political and social conditions of the Arab citizens in the country.

Youth Alcohol Use

Table 5.4 (see page 79) shows previous-year drinking among Arab youth in the northern part of the country by religion. In the aggregate, there is an increasing trend in drinking among Moslems and Druze. A 1996 study (Weiss, in press b) also revealed that among male drinkers, 13 percent of Moslems, 15 percent of Druze, and 12 percent of Christians had consumed five drinks or more in a row. (A drink was defined as one can of beer [330 cc], half a glass of wine [100 cc], or a small glass of distilled spirits [40 cc]). Those drinking five drinks or more daily or every two or three days were 4 percent of Moslems, 3 percent of Druze, and 2 percent of Christians. These percentages were higher than the percentages reflecting heavy drinking among Jewish male drinkers. The 1994 study revealed (Weiss & Moore, 1995b) that young Moslems and Druze drink at home, perhaps in order to hide the "sin," or at restaurants, perhaps to drink "while eating," and not in pubs, which are popular among Jewish adolescents. Moslem and Druze male drinkers obtain alcohol from friends or purchase it themselves, while Christians get it from their parents at home.

These findings should be considered in light of the fact that drinking is a legitimate act for the Jewish respondents, while consumption of alcohol by Moslems and Druze is a vice that is unacceptable according to religious canons. It can be assumed, therefore, that the rate of alcohol consumption among the Arab respondents might be higher than reported. Without adequate prevention programs in the schools and community, it is expected that drinking and the problems associated with alcohol use will continue to rise among young Druze and Moslems (Weiss et al., 1999).

Jordan: Alcohol Use Trends

Alcohol abuse among Jordanians is not studied to the extent that other abused drugs are investigated; nevertheless, Tables 5.5 and 5.6 merit consideration. Table 5.5 presents (W. Sarhan, personal communication, November 1, 2000) the numbers of patients treated for alcoholism from 1990 to 1999 in Al-Rashid Hospital, the sole private psychiatric treatment facility in Jordan, which serves Jordanians and Arabs from other countries. The figures given in Table 5.5 are not indicative of the real prevalence of alcoholism in Jordan, and not all alcoholics who seek treatment are treated in Al-Rashid Hospital. Alcoholics, for the most part, seek treatment in public

Table 5.5
Numbers of Patients Treated for Alcoholism at Al-Rashid Hospital

Year	Alcoholics	Males	Females	Jordanians	Non-Jordanians
1990	1	1	-	1	-
1991	4	1	3	4	-
1992	20	19	1	16	4
1993	23	22	1	18	5
1994	15	15	-	13	2
1995	20	18	2	19	1
1996	36	35	1	30	6
1997	45	45	-	33	12
1998	38	35	3	30	8
1999	27	26	1	21	6
Total	229	217	12	185	44

centers or choose to be treated abroad in order to avoid the stigma associated with a psychiatric hospital and with alcoholism.

Table 5.6, based on the Annual Statistical Report of Crimes of the Department of Criminal Investigation, Directorate of Public Security (Directorate of Public Security, 1990–2000; Weiss et al., 1999), shows the number of Jordanians convicted for drunken disturbance from 1990 to 1999. While Table 5.5 shows increases and decreases within an overall increasing trend of the number of Jordanian alcoholic patients from 1990 to 1999, Table 5.6 shows a definite increase in the number of convicted Jordanians. The tables may suggest that alcohol use today has become a social phenomenon of considerable magnitude, while a couple of decades earlier it was not noticeable.

It is difficult to predict what will happen in the years to come. It can be assumed, however, that the trend toward increasing alcohol use and abuse will continue to grow as a result of modernization in Jordan, inadequate attention given to prevention and the problems of alcohol use in the public schools and universities, a lack of support services to families of alcoholics, and the lack of enforcement of alcohol

Table 5.6
Numbers of Jordanians Convicted for Drunken Disturbance

Year	Convictions
1990	1,310
1991	2,205
1992	2,447
1993	2,740
1994	2,885
1995	5,242
1996	3,085
1997	4,162
1998	5,754
1999	6,534
Total	36,364

regulations. On the other hand, it is possible that the growing trend will be curtailed as a result of an increase of religiosity among Jordanian people.

Palestinian Authority: Alcohol Use Trends

Research among Palestinians is in its infancy. Two studies conducted in 1996 and in 1998 in East Jerusalem and the West Bank dealt with alcohol use (Abdeen, 1997; Abdeen & Natsheh, 1998; Weiss et al., 1999). In the 1996 study (Abdeen, 1997), the subjects were 603 school children 11 to 17 years old; 86 percent were Moslem and 14 percent were Christian, and the study had an even number of males and females. Among the study subjects, 6 percent of males and 16 percent of females (11 percent of the total sample) had previously drunk an alcoholic beverage. Additionally, it was found that 2 percent of the sample reported drinking beer every day, 0.7 percent reported drinking wine daily, and 3 percent reported drinking alcoholic apple juice every day. About 35 percent of drinkers had their first drink before the age of 9, 21 percent first drank when they were 9 or 10 years old, and 23 percent first drank when they were 15 or 16 years old. About 1 percent of Moslem and 10 percent of Christian Arabs drank alcohol daily.

Table 5.7
Number of Drinks Consumed Weekly among Palestinians by Gender

No. Drinks	Males (n = 245)	Percent	Females (n = 74)	Percent
0	84	34.28	34	45.94
1–5	104	42.44	30	40.54
6–10	32	13.06	5	6.75
11–15	15	6.12	3	4.05
15+	10	4.08	2	2.70

Table 5.8
Number of Drinks Consumed Weekly among Palestinians by Age

Age Group	0 Drinks	1–5 Drinks	6–10 Drinks	11–15 Drinks	15+ Drinks
15–19 (n=67)	45 (67.16%)	18 (26.86%)	3 (4.47%)	1 (1.49%)	0
20–24 (n=61)	29 (47.54%)	24 (39.34%)	5 (8.19%)	2 (3.27%)	1 (1.63%)
25–34 (n=86)	21 (24.41%)	45 (52.32%)	10 (11.62%)	6 (6.97%)	4 (4.65%)
35–44 (n=51)	9 (17.64%)	24 (47.05%)	9 (17.64%)	5 (9.80%)	4 (7.84%)
45–54 (n=32)	8 (25.00%)	13 (40.62%)	6 (18.75%)	3 (9.37%)	2 (6.25%)
55+ (n=23)	7 (30.43%)	10 (43.47%)	4 (17.39%)	1 (4.34%)	1 (4.34%)

In the 1998 study (Abdeen & Natsheh, 1998), the subjects were 67 young people 15–19 years of age and 253 adults, 246 males and 74 females, most of whom were Moslem. This is the first study to investigate alcohol use among adults. The study focused mainly on heavy drinkers. A heavy drinker was defined as any respondent who reported drinking 15 or more drinks in the week prior to the study. Heavy drinking was found only among adults (N = 12; 5 percent). Table 5.7 presents the number of drinks per week by gender, and Table 5.8 shows number of drinks per week by age.

As far as youth are concerned, the two studies mentioned above do not offer insight regarding trends mainly because of a difference in the age groups studied (an 11-to-17-year-old group in the first study as compared to a 15-to-19-year-old group in the second). Nevertheless, the rate of drinking involvement (33 percent) provides insight into future trends of alcohol use. Due to the continuation of modernization and development in the Palestinian Authority, and the absence of alcohol control measures and of prevention programs aimed at schools or the public, the rate of alcohol use and problems associated with excessive drinking are expected to rise.

ACKNOWLEDGMENT

The authors thank Dr. Walid Sarhan, the general manager of Al-Rashid Hospital in Jordan, for his assistance in providing data and insight concerning alcohol use in Jordan.

REFERENCES

Abdeen, Z. (1997). *Substance abuse among Palestinian youth in 1996*. East Jerusalem: Al-Quds University.

Abdeen, Z., & Natsheh, W. (1998). *Palestinian health promotion survey*. East Jerusalem: Jerusalem Public Health Society.

Abu Saad, I. (1996). *Substance abuse among Bedouin Arab youth in planned and unplanned settlements in the Negev*. Beer Sheva: Ben-Gurion University (in Hebrew).

———. (1998). *The influence of settlement on substance use and abuse among nomadic populations in Israel and Kenya*. Beer Sheva: Ben-Gurion University, Center for Bedouin Studies and Development.

Al-Farah, Y. F. (1991). *Familial upbringing patterns and personality traits that discriminate between alcoholics and non alcoholics* (Master's Thesis in Arabic). Amman: University of Jordan.

Awartani, H. (1995). The psychology of peace—A Palestinian perspective. In R. Moses (Ed.), *The psychology of peace and conflict —The Israeli-Palestinian experience* (pp. 170–173). Jerusalem: Center for Public Affairs, Konrad Adenauer Foundation.

Bar, H., Eldar, P., & Yarom E. (1987). *Survey of Arab clients of the Alcoholism Treatment and Rehabilitation Service*. Jerusalem: Israel Institute of Applied Social Research.

Ben-Dor, G. (1995). *The status and problems of the Israeli Druze minority in the mid-1990s*. Jerusalem: Center for Public Affairs, Konrad Adenauer Foundation.

Dgani, A. (1992). *Drug use in Tel Aviv—Jaffa*. Tel Aviv: Geocartography Institute (in Hebrew).

Directorate of Public Security. (1990–2000). *Annual statistic reports of crime*. Amman: Department of Criminal Investigations.

Hassassian, M. S. (1995). Palestinian public opinion polls, democracy and the peace process. In R. Moses (Ed.), *The psychology of peace and conflict—The Israeli-Palestinian experience* (pp. 59–70). Jerusalem: Center for Public Affairs, Konrad Adenauer Foundation.

Hermann, T., & Yuchtman-Yaar, E. (1995). Two people apart: Israeli Jews' and Arabs' attitudes toward the peace process. In R. Moses (Ed.), *The psychology of peace and conflict—The Israeli-Palestinian Experience* (pp. 33–58). Jerusalem: Center for Public Affairs, Konrad Adenauer Foundation.

———. (Eds.) (1997). *Israeli society and the challenge of transition to co-existence*. Tel Aviv: Tel Aviv University: Tami Steinmetz Center for Peace Research.

Israeli, A. (1976). The employment revolution in the minority sector in Israel. *New Middle East, 26,* 229–231 (in Hebrew).

Laish, A. (1981). The ethnic organization of the Moslems. In A. Laish (Ed.), *The Arabs in Israel: Continuity and change* (p. 121). Jerusalem: Hebrew University of Jerusalem, Magnes (in Hebrew).

Laish, A., & Fallach, S. (1981). The religious organization of the Moslems. In A. Laish (Ed.), *The Arabs in Israel: Continuity and change* (pp. 138–139). Jerusalem: Hebrew University of Jerusalem, Magnes (in Hebrew).

Landau, I. (1981). Alienation and tensions in political behavior. In A. Laish (Ed.), *The Arabs in Israel: Continuity and change* (pp. 197–212). Jerusalem: Hebrew University of Jerusalem, Magnes (in Hebrew).

Marchevsky, S., & Weiss, S. (1997). Characteristics of hospitalized alcoholics in the residential center in Ramat Gan in 1982–1994 and their implications. *Harefuah, 132,* 586–590 (in Hebrew).

Michaely, N. (1998a). *A survey of patients in the open alcohol centers in 1997.* Ramat Gan: EFSHAR Association (in Hebrew).

———. (1998b). Children of alcoholics—the present picture. In N. Michaely & O. Naor (Eds.), *Children of alcoholics—Children at risk.* Ramat Gan: EFSHAR Association (in Hebrew).

———. (1999). *A survey of patients in the open alcohol centers in 1998.* Ramat Gan: EFSHAR Association (in Hebrew).

———. (2000). *A survey of patients in the open alcohol centers in 1999.* Ramat Gan: EFSHAR Association (in Hebrew).

Miller, L. (1977). Toward a theoretical approach to contemporary drug abuse problems. *Public Health, 19,* 429–433 (in Hebrew).

Moore, M., & Weiss, S. (1991). Alcohol drinking among Moslem and Druze adolescents in Israel in 1990. *Drug and Alcohol Dependence, 28,* 189–193.

———. (1992). Israeli Christian, Druze and Moslem adolescents' attitudes toward magazine alcohol advertisements. *International Journal of the Addictions, 27,* 735–741.

Rahav, G., Teichman, M., Gil, R., Rosenblum, Y., & Bar-Hamburger, R. (1995). *The use of psychoactive substances among Israeli citizens 1995: Epidemiological study 3.* Tel Aviv: Pori Institute, Tel Aviv University, Anti-Drug Authority (in Hebrew).

———. (1998). *The use of psychoactive substances among Israeli citizens 1998: Epidemiological study 4.* Tel Aviv: Pori Institute, Tel Aviv University, Anti-Drug Authority (in Hebrew).

Ramberg, A., & Moshkovitz, A. (1988). *The Arabs citizens of Israel.* Jerusalem: Ministry of Education, Van-Leer Institution (in Hebrew).

Sabella, B. (1995). Palestinians in the transitional period: Classical and pragmatic orientations. In R. Moses (Ed.), *The psychology of peace and conflict—The Israeli-Palestinian experience* (pp. 23–32). Jerusalem: Konrad Adenauer Foundation.

Smooha, S. (1984). *The orientation and politicization of the Arab minority in Israel,* Monograph No. 2. Haifa: Haifa University, Jewish-Arab Center for Middle East Research (in Hebrew).

Teichman, M., Rahav, G., & Barnea, Z. (1994). Alcohol consumption among non-Jewish men in Israel, *Alcologia, 6,* 201–206.

United Nations. (1993). *Impact of drug abuse among youth in the economic and social commission for Western Asia Region (ESCWA): Approaches to social reintegration.* New York: United Nations.

Weiss, S. (1996). What do Israeli Jewish and Arab adolescents know about drinking and driving? *Accident Analysis & Prevention, 28,* 765—769.

———. (1997). Israeli Arab and Jewish youth knowledge and opinion about alcohol warning-labels: Pre-intervention data. *Alcohol & Alcoholism, 32,* 251–257.

———. (1999). Attitudes of Israeli Jewish and Arab high school students toward alcohol control measures. *Journal of Drug Education, 29,* 41–52.

———. (in press a). Religious influences on drinking: Illustrations from selected groups. In A. Roche & E. Houghton (Eds.), *Learning to drink.* New York: Taylor & Francis Publishers.

———. (in press b). Review of drinking patterns of rural Arab and Jewish youth in the north of Israel. *Substance Use & Misuse.*

Weiss, S., & Moore, M. (1992). Perception of alcoholism among Jewish, Moslem and Christian teachers in Israel. *Journal of Drug Education, 22,* 253–260.

———. (1995a). How do Israeli adolescents of four religions obtain alcoholic beverages and where? *Journal of Child & Adolescent Substance Abuse, 4,* 79–87.

———. (1995b). Reasons for abstinence among Moslem, Druze and Christian adolescents in Israel. *International Journal of the Addictions, 30,* 1499–1508.

Weiss, S., Sawa, G. H., Abdeen, Z., & Yanai J. (1999). Substance abuse studies and prevention efforts among Arabs in the 90s in Israel, Jordan and the Palestinian Authority—A literature review. *Addiction, 94,* 177–198.

6

Russian-Speaking Immigrants: Factors Associated with Heroin Use

Richard Isralowitz and Sofia Borkin

IMMIGRATION AND SUBSTANCE ABUSE

At the end of the 1980s, the tightly controlled emigration policies of the former Soviet Union were liberalized, providing massive numbers of people with the opportunity to leave that part of the world. This situation allowed literally millions of people, most notably those who were Jewish, claimed to be Jewish, or were related to a Jewish person, to relocate to Western countries such as the United States, Canada, and Israel. In the case of Israel, a country that imposes an ethno-religious test of fitness for naturalization, only Jews are acceptable for automatic naturalization under Israel's law of return (Light & Isralowitz, 1997). The extent of immigration to that country was so overwhelming that government authorities could barely manage the detailed inspection of those who met acceptance criteria based on religious grounds let alone examine the mental and physical health, criminal experience, or addiction to illegal substances of the immigrants. In fact, during the one-year period of 1990–1991, the number of Russian-speaking persons who immigrated to Israel was approximately 370,000, reaching nearly the number of immigrants who had settled in the country over the entire previous 40 years (Goldscheider, 1992; Rosenbaum-Tamari & Dimian, 1991). Since the initial influx of immigrants from the former Soviet republics in 1989, the population of Israel has increased by more than 1,000,000, which represents nearly 18 percent of the current residents in the country (Isralowitz & Abu Saad, 1997; Abu Saad & Isralowitz, 1997).

The illegal drug scene in Israel, prior to the immigration that began in 1989, was about 95 percent heroin addicts of Middle East origin primarily from Morocco and

Tunisia, who prefer smoking the substance. These addicts tend to be male (about 80 percent), between the ages of 18 and 30, poorly educated (less than high school completion), and of low socioeconomic status (Isralowitz, Telias, & Abu Saad, 1994). Soon after 1990, the profile of the nation's heroin addict population changed, a change attributed to immigrants, primarily intravenous users from the former Soviet republics. Currently, it is estimated that 25 percent of the country's 25,000 addicts (Elisha, 1998) came to the country after 1989 from Russia, the Ukraine, Georgia, Azerbaijan, and the Caucasus region near the Caspian Sea, which includes numerous small republics.

The Israel Ministry of Health and the Ministry of Labor and Social Affairs, both with responsibilities for addressing the drug problem, have expressed concern about Russian-speaking addicts. Little documentation exists, however, about their psychosocial profile and patterns of substance use. This chapter reports the findings of a study conducted in 1999 and 2000 of 152 male and female Russian-speaking heroin addicts who are now citizens of Israel. The study is the first detailed examination to be conducted of Russian-speaking substance abusers in Israel.

METHODS

Sample

A purposive sample of 152 Russian-speaking addicts (i.e., immigrants mostly from Russia and the Ukraine) now living in the southern "Negev" region of Israel were interviewed. This number represents 17 percent of the estimated 875 Russian-speaking addicts from the region, which is home to about 3,500 of the country's total population of 25,000 heroin addicts. A questionnaire in Russian was distributed to the addicts while they were in the process of, or recently completed, detoxification, day treatment, or methadone maintenance for heroin addiction. The addicts were assured that their responses would be confidential. No one targeted for participation refused to provide the information requested. In fact, many reported that they were pleased someone cared about their condition and hoped that the information would be used for good purposes, including the establishment of treatment services targeted for Russian addicts only. The data collection method was discussed with officials from the Israel Ministry of Health, Substance Abuse Treatment Unit, as well as the directors of the drug treatment facilities where the information was collected.

Instrument

The instrument used in this study was adapted from research conducted by Isralowitz and colleagues (Isralowitz, Abu Saad, & Telias, 1996; Isralowitz & Peleg, 1996; Isralowitz & Troestler, 1996) for research of illegal and legal drug use in Israel and in other countries. The instrument consisted of 68 items including: (1) predisposition (e.g., sociodemographic status including gender, marital status, place of birth, year of immigration to Israel; education; military experience in Russia; religious status in terms of whether the respondent and partner, if present, is Jewish; and the impact of immigration on family relations); (2) prison and mental health experience, including their relationship to the decision to immigrate; (3) details about body tattooing; (4) physical and sexual abuse; (5) licit and illicit drug use or abuse; (6) self-esteem; and (7) familial drug use (e.g., father, mother, and sibling use of alcohol, prescription, and illegal drugs). The questionnaire was anonymous and precoded.

Validity and Reliability

From the data collected and analyzed, it appears that the questionnaire used for this study has a high degree of validity—a necessary condition for reliability (Johnston & O'Malley, 1985). Among the reasons for this conclusion are: (1) the Russian version of the questionnaire was reviewed for content purposes by Russian-speaking professionals who directly worked with the addicts; (2) the respondents to the questionnaire were highly consistent in reporting their behaviors among logically related measures of substance use; (3) it was found that self-reported substance use related to other attitudes, beliefs, and behavior (i.e., there is strong evidence for construct validity in consistent and expected ways to a number of other attitudes, beliefs, and behavior); and (4) the missing data rates for the self-reported substance use questions were only slightly higher than for the preceding nonsensitive questions.

A question that often arises regarding studies of substance use attitudes and behavior is whether prevalence and trend estimates from such research are an accurate representation of substance users who were not included in the study cohort (Casper, 1992; Johnston, O'Malley, & Bachman, 1992). It is believed, based on the clinical experience of those responsible for data collection, that there is a greater likelihood of underestimation or underreporting of certain attitudes and behavior related to substance use than overreporting. Furthermore, it is believed by the authors that the analyses provided in this chapter do characterize Russian-speaking drug addicts in Israel.

Analysis

The study results and profile projected from the findings have the potential to play an important role in policy formation as well as improving the scientific understanding of the substance abuse of Russian-speaking addicts. In addition to descriptive statistics, Chi-square analysis and ANOVA were added to examine relationships between selected background characteristics, including self-esteem and substance use. Also, multiple regression analysis was conducted on self-esteem and its relation to a range of background characteristics of the addicts.

RESULTS

Background Characteristics: Male and Female Russian-Speaking Heroin Addicts

The average age of the subjects was 31.4 years, ranging from 19 to 55 with a median of 30. Age was not a factor differentiating male and female addicts. Most of the Russian-speaking addicts were born in the Ukraine (41 percent) or Russia (37 percent). The majority of the men (51 percent) were single, compared to 23 percent of the women, and the women were more likely than men to be divorced (35 percent vs. 15 percent). (See Tables 6.1–6.3.)

The vast majority of the addicts interviewed (95 percent) came to Israel after 1990. Eighty percent reported finishing high school, trade school, or some other form of education. In terms of religious status, 64 percent of the overall sample reported to be Jewish; this was true for only 53 percent of the female respondents, an important factor in Israel since by religious law the woman passes "Jewish" status on to the child. Although most of the non-Jewish subjects had Jewish spouses, 12 percent of the addicts who were not Jewish also did not have a Jewish spouse. Regarding the effect of immigration on family relations, 50 percent of those interviewed reported that their family relationships deteriorated since coming to Israel.

Forty-four percent of the subjects reported a history of imprisonment in the former Soviet Union, and 21 percent had been in a psychiatric hospital primarily for detoxification purposes. Among those who had been in prison or a psychiatric hospital, 14 percent reported that they were released in order to immigrate to Israel. Ten percent of the respondents said that they were under criminal investigation/judicial processing at the time of their emigration, and 6 percent reported that they had an open criminal file when they left. Forty-five percent of the men and 31 percent of the women reported having tattoos.

Gender Differences

Chi-square tests revealed significant differences between male and female addicts in terms of marital status, education; experience being jailed, release from jail in order to immigrate to Israel, sexual abuse as a child, physical abuse while in an institution, father's alcohol use, mother's illicit drug use, trouble with police, fighting because of drug use, and reasons for wanting to stop drug use. These differences are listed in Tables 6.1 and 6.3.

No difference was found regarding the self-concept of male ($M = 3.46$; $SD = 0.58$) and female ($M = 3.37$; $SD = 0.72$) addicts. Additional analysis regarding self-esteem, however, has shown it to be related to a desire to quit drugs, better family relations after immigration, and experience in an institution (both prison and a mental hospital). In terms of multiple regression analysis ($R^2 = 0.316$), the best predictors of positive self-esteem were good family relations, prison experience, and personal health status.

History of Physical-Sexual Abuse

Physical abuse as a child was reported by 46 percent of the female and 37 percent of the male addicts. Sexual abuse as a child was reported by 25 percent of the women compared to 5 percent of the men. While in prison, 16 percent of the men reported being physically abused, and 12 percent said they were sexually abused. Women, however, reported fewer incidences of physical (3 percent) and sexual (10 percent) abuse while incarcerated.

Family History of Addiction

Questions about the parents of the addicts revealed that alcohol was used always or often by 38 percent of the fathers and 8 percent of the mothers, whereas illegal drugs were used by 4 percent of the fathers and 4 percent of the mothers. Excessive alcohol use was reported significantly more often for the parents of female addicts than males: 46 percent of the addicted females had alcohol-abusing fathers, compared to 31 percent of the males. Moreover, addicted females had almost three times as many alcohol-abusing mothers as did the males (14 percent vs. 5 percent).

History of Licit and Illicit Substance Use

Table 6.2 provides the average and median age of the addicts as well as *t*-test analysis of the subjects at the time of first use of cigarettes, alcohol, and illicit drugs. Table 6.3 lists the resulting problems experienced by these heroin users. The study findings reflect the typical gradient pattern of drug use. In other words, the subjects began using cigarettes first (median age = 14.0), followed by alcohol (15.0), marijuana (16.0), hashish (17.0), amphetamines (18.0), sedatives (18.5), opium (19.0), and then heroin (21.0). No significant differences were found for age of first time use or gender.

Current Substance Use

Among the respondents, who ranged from those still in various stages of outpatient treatment to those who completed treatment within the past year, 39 percent reported that they were still using heroin or opiate-type drugs, and the majority of this group (72 percent) were using such substances in combination with alcohol. Forty-four percent of the subjects claimed to be "clean" of heroin but using alcohol or other drugs such as amphetamines, benzodiazepines, marijuana, and hashish. Only 17 percent reported to be free of any licit or illicit substance use; 37 percent reported smoking 20 or more cigarettes a day.

Nearly three-quarters (73 percent) of the addicts reported that their first use of heroin was in the company of friends. Fifteen percent first used it while alone, and the rest (12 percent) first used the substance with a family member or spouse. A similar pattern of first-time use was found for alcohol, marijuana, and hashish. The

Table 6.1
Background Characteristics of Male and Female Russian-Speaking Heroin Addicts

Variable	**Male** (98; 64%)	**Female** (54; 36%)	**Total** (152; 100%)	X^2
		Percentiles		
Country of Origin				
Russia	31	48	37	
Ukraine	41	41	41	n.s.
Other	28	11	22	
Marital Status				
Single	51	23	41	
Married (no children)	8	13	10	
Married (with children)	23	23	23	13.59**
Divorced	15	35	22	
Widow/Widower	3	6	4	
Education				
< high school	23	12	20	
High school	50	42	47	
Vocational school	16	33	21	12.91*
College	11	13	12	
Religious Status (affirmative response)				
Jewish	71	53	64	n.s.

Family Relations after Immigration				
Better	9	12	10	
No change	45	32	40	n.s.
Worse	46	56	50	
Institution Experience (affirmative response)				
Prison	53	28	44	8.91**
Mental hospital	20	25	21	n.s.
Prison/Mental Hospital Release Conditioned on Immigration (affirmative response)	19	6	14	4.17*
Tattoos (affirmative response)	45	31	40	n.s.
Abused as Child				
Physically	37	46	41	n.s.
Sexually	5	25	12	11.33***
Abused in Prison/Mental Hospital				
Physically	16	3	13	4.17*
Sexually	12	10	12	n.s.
Parental Substance Use (affirmative)				
Father: alcohol use (always or often)	31	46	38	4.28*
illicit drug use (yes only)	5	4	4	n.s.
Mother: alcohol use (always or often)	5	14	8	11.94*
illicit drug use (yes only)	2	8	4	n.s.

$^{*}p \leq 0.05$. $^{**}p \leq 0.01$. $^{***}p \leq 0.001$.

Table 6.2
Male and Female Russian-Speaking Heroin Addicts: Age at First Time Drug Use–Mean (Standard Deviation), Median Age, and *t*-Test Analysis

Substance	**Male ($N = 98$)** *M* (S.D.); Median	**Female ($N = 54$)** *M* (S.D.); Median	**Average** *M* (S.D.); Median	***t*-Test; df; *p* level**
Cigarettes	14.62 (8.87); 14.00	15.02 (3.29); 15.00	14.76 (7.42); 14.00	-.31; 146; n.s.
Alcohol	16.37 (9.55); 15.00	15.51 (3.30); 15.00	16.08 (7.98); 15.00	.56; 118; n.s.
Marijuana	16.25 (4.58); 16.00	17.22 (5.20); 16.00	16.57 (4.79); 16.00	-1.00; 110; n.s.
Hashish	16.83 (3.43); 16.50	17.11 (4.52); 17.00	16.91 (3.75); 17.00	-.32; 91; n.s.
Amphetamines	19.33 (3.34); 20.50	19.14 (7.49); 16.00	19.26 (5.05); 18.00	.08; 17; n.s.
Sedatives	20.50 (5.48); 20.00	18.65 (5.06); 18.00	19.96 (5.39); 18.50	1.30; 66; n.s.
Opium	18.97 (4.17); 19.00	19.49 (5.04); 17.00	19.14 (4.45); 19.00	-.53; 93; n.s.
Heroin	21.68 (5.74); 21.00	22.43 (7.04); 22.00	21.94 (6.21); 21.00	-.65; 123; n.s.
Cocaine	23.32 (6.68); 23.00	24.31 (9.37); 20.00	23.66 (7.61); 21.00	-.42; 45; n.s.
Methadone	27.83 (6.06); 27.00	28.08 (6.66); 29.00	27.92 (6.26); 28.00	-.18; 82; n.s.

Table 6.3
Male and Female Russian-Speaking Heroin Addicts: Physical, Psychological, and Behavioral Characteristics

Variable	Male (98; 64%)	Female (54; 36%)	Total (152; 100%)	X^2
	Percentile			
Continuing Drug Use (affirmative response)				
Using heroin/opiates (with or without alcohol)	38	40	39	n.s,
Alcohol and other drug use while "clean" of heroin	43	46	44	n.s.
Clean of any illegal drug or alcohol use	19	14	17	n.s.
Physical (affirmative response = *always* or *often*)				
Feel depressed, anxious, and/or restless	46	31	41	n.s.
Feel weak with pain	41	31	38	n.s.
Have problems sleeping	31	25	29	n.s.
Behavior Related (affirmative response = *always* or *often*)				
Criticized because of drug use	16	15	16	n.s.
Lost a job because of drug use	35	43	38	n.s.
Trouble with police related to drug use	37	48	41	19.21***
Fought because of drug use	54	88	66	24.57***
Caused property damage because of drug use	50	68	56	n.s.
Attitude Related (affirmative response)				
Russian-speaking treatment personnel/program needed to address treatment	87	75	83	n.s.
Would like to quit heroin use	93	100	96	n.s.
Reasons for stopping drug use:				
fatigue	39	32	37	
regain family (children)	14	18	15	
restore health	30	45	34	36.25***
out of money	17	5	14	

$^*p \leq 0.05$. $^{**}p \leq 0.01$. $^{***}p \leq 0.001$.

vast majority of study subjects (97 percent) reported immigrating to Israel already addicted.

Impact of Substance Use

Many of the subjects reported that they "always" or "often" suffered severe negative physical and psychosocial consequences due to their drug use: 66 percent were in fights over drug use; 56 percent caused property damage because of drugs; 41 percent felt depressed, anxious, and/or restless; 41 percent had trouble with the police because of their drug behavior; 38 percent felt weak and had muscle pain; 38 percent had lost a job because of drugs; and 29 percent claimed sleeping problems. Only 16 percent reported being criticized about their drug use. Common reasons for wanting to stop drug use included "tired of drug use," "restore personal health," "regain children," and "cost."

Male Jewish and Non-Jewish Heroin Addict Comparisons

Based on percentages, Jewish addicts (78 percent) were more inclined than non-Jewish (73 percent) addicts to complete high school; also, Jewish addicts (16 percent) were more likely than non-Jewish (0 percent) addicts to have some college education. Chi-square analysis revealed no significant difference in the education pattern of Jewish and non-Jewish addicts, X^2 (5, $N = 99$) = 10.5, $p < 0.05$. (See Tables 6.4–6.6.)

The mean ages of first use of common substances, including cigarettes, alcohol, hashish, and heroin, were used to compare the Jewish and non-Jewish addicts. The mean age for first use of cigarettes for Jewish addicts was 15.35 ($SD = 10.31$) and for non-Jewish addicts, 13.00 ($SD = 3.34$), $t(98) = 1.22$, $p < 0.05$; first use of alcohol for the two respective groups, 15.81 ($SD = 4.00$) and 14.72 ($SD = 3.80$), $t(65) = 0.99$, $p < 0.05$; hashish, 16.86 ($SD = 3.46$) and 16.89 ($SD = 2.67$), $t(67) = 0.03$, $p < 0.05$; and heroin 21.54 ($SD = 6.18$) and 22.16 ($SD = 4.62$), $t(82) = 0.45$, $p < 0.05$. The age differences between Jewish and non-Jewish addicts did not differ significantly. The findings were similar for self-esteem. The mean scores (1 = low; 5 = high) of Jewish and non-Jewish addicts were, respectively, 3.48 ($SD = 0.62$) and 3.42 ($SD = 0.47$), $t(98) = 0.42$, $p < 0.05$, and were not significantly different.

Native-Born and Russian-Speaking Immigrant Female Heroin Addict Comparisons

Background characteristics (see Table 6.7). Among the female addicts surveyed, 46 percent (53) were immigrants from the former Soviet Union (i.e., the majority from Russia and the Ukraine), and 54 percent (61) were born in Israel. The findings show that 30 percent (34) were single; 9 percent (10) married without children; 18 percent (21) married with children; 38 percent (43) divorced; and 5 percent (6)

Table 6.4
Percentage Comparison of Male Jewish and Non-Jewish Russian-Speaking Heroin Addicts

Variable	Jewish (71%; 70)	Non-Jewish (29%; 29)
Marital Status		
Single	52	48
Married (no children)	11	4
Married (with children)	20	22
Divorced	12	26
Widow/Widower	5	0
Education		
< high school	21	30
High school	48	48
Vocational school	14	22
College	17	0
Family Relations after Immigration		
Better	11	5
No Change	41	59
Worse	48	36
Institution Experience (affirmative response)		
Prison	47	65
Mental Hospital	17	22
In Prison/Mental Hospital and Release Conditioned on Immigration (affirmative response)	16	14
Tattoos (affirmative response)	44	38
Abused as Child (affirmative response)		
Physically	35	46
Sexually	6	4
Abused in Prison/Mental Hospital (affirmative response)		
Physically	17	16
Sexually	11	13

widowed. Regarding education, 63 percent (72) reported finishing high school, trade school, or some other form of education; 26 percent (30) did not finish high school; and 11 percent (12) had no formal education. In terms of religious status, 78 percent of the study group reported being Jewish. Non-Jewish women constituted 47 percent of the immigrant cohort, and all of them were from the former Soviet Union. The female addicts were asked about relations with family members. Satisfactory relations were reported as follows: mother, 81 percent (92); father, 73 percent (83); brother(s), 80 percent (92); sister(s), 80 percent (91); and spouse, 84 percent (96). Regarding alcohol use among parents, 36 percent of the addicts reported that their fathers were heavy users of alcohol compared to 9 percent of their mothers. Illicit drug use among fathers was 7 percent and mothers 6 percent. (See Tables 6.8 and 6.9.)

Table 6.5
***t*-Test Score Comparison of Male Jewish and Non-Jewish Russian Drug Addicts**

Variable	Mean Score (Jewish, $n = 70$)	(Non-Jewish, $n = 29$)	t Value	df	p level
Times Jailed	2.48	1.67	1.61	44	n.s.
Total Months Jailed	34.14	30.86	0.27	37	n.s.
Times in Mental Institution	2.33	3.17	-0.52	13	n.s.
Total Months in Mental Institution	2.56	2.00	0.36	11	n.s.
Cigarettes (first use)	15.37	12.70	1.28	90	n.s.
Alcohol (first use)	16.75	15.30	0.56	73	n.s.
Marijuana (first use)	16.30	15.89	0.33	70	n.s.
Heroin/Opiates (first use)	20.74	19.23	0.73	86	n.s.
Driving Misbehavior (Drug use before or while driving) (1 = *yes*; 2 = *no*)	1.81	1.69	0.43	87	n.s.
Self-Esteem (1 = *low*; 5 = *high*)	3.48	3.38	0.71	90	n.s.

Table 6.6
Chi-Square Score Comparison of Male Jewish (*n* = 70) and Non-Jewish (*n* = 29) Drug Addicts

Variable	N	df	X^2
Married Religious Status			
Jewish Addict/Spouse Jewish	34	4	10.53*
Non-Jewish Addict/Spouse Jewish	10		
Period of Immigration and Religious Status			
1989–1993/Jewish—Non-Jewish	54	2	7.27*
1994–1998/Jewish—Non-Jewish	58		10.53*
Pattern of Heroin Use			
Jewish	52	12	21.56*
Non-Jewish	30		
Pattern of Hashish Use			
Jewish	45	9	20.23*
Non-Jewish	24		

*$p < .05$.

Regarding drug use, 29 percent said they were using heroin at the time of the interview, and the majority of these women (56 percent) were using the substance with alcohol; 30 percent of the addicts reported they were clean of heroin but were using alcohol or other drugs. The majority of study participants (86 percent; 98) reported they would like to stop using drugs; however, only 68 percent (77) believed it was possible. The main reasons for trying to stop were to regain custody of their child(ren) (57 percent; 65) and to improve their health (45 percent; 51).

In terms of institutional experience, 32 percent (37) reported being in prison, and 26 percent (30) spent time in a psychiatric hospital. Among those interviewed, 42 percent (48) reported being physically abused as a child, and 32 percent (36) reported being sexually abused.

Table 6.7
Background Characteristics of Female Immigrant and Native-Born Heroin Addicts

Variable	Immigrant ($n = 53$)	Native Born ($n = 61$)	Total ($N = 114$)	X^2
		N (%)		
Marital Status				
Single	12 (23)	22 (36)	34 (30)	
Married (no children)	7 (13)	3 (5)	10 (9)	
Married (with children)	12 (23)	9 (15)	21 (18)	n.s.
Divorced	19 (35)	24 (39)	43 (38)	
Widow/Widower	3 (6)	3 (5)	6 (5)	
Education				
< high school	6 (12)	36 (59)	42 (37)	
High school	23 (43)	16 (26)	39 (34)	35.83***
Vocational school	17 (31)	9 (15)	26 (23)	
College	7 (14)	0 (0)	7 (6)	

Satisfactory Relations (affirmative response)				
mother	41 (77)	51 (83)	92 (81)	n.s.
father	36 (67)	47 (77)	83 (73)	*n.s.*
brother(s)	47 (89)	45 (73)	92 (80)	n.s.
sisters(s)	42 (80)	49 (80)	91 (80)	n.s.
spouse	45 (85)	51 (84)	96 (84)	n.s.
Institution Experience (affirmative response)				
Prison	15 (28)	22 (36)	37 (32)	n.s.
Psychiatric institution	13 (25)	17 (28)	30 (26)	n.s.
Abused as Child (affirmative response)				
Physically	24 (45)	24 (39)	48 (42)	n.s.
Sexually	13 (25)	23 (37)	36 (32)	n.s.
Parental Substance Use (affirmative)				
Father: alcohol use (always or often)	24 (46)	14 (56)	38 (36)	23.74***
illicit drug use (yes only)	2 (4)	5 (9)	7 (7)	n.s.
Mother: alcohol use (always or often)	7 (14)	3 (5)	10 (9)	n.s.
illicit drug use (yes only)	4 (8)	2 (4)	6 (6)	n.s.

$^*p \leq 0.05$. $^{**}p \leq 0.01$. $^{***}p \leq 0.001$.

Chi-square analysis was used to determine whether a relation existed between the female addict background characteristics, attitudes, behavior, and group status. Background characteristics and attitudes that were found to differentiate the two groups were: education, immigrant women had more years of formal schooling ($p < 0.001$); father's alcohol use, immigrant women had fathers who were more inclined to drink frequently or often ($p < 0.001$); wish to stop addiction, immigrant women had a stronger desire to quit drug use ($p < 0.05$); concern about health, immigrant women were more likely to want to stop drug use in order to improve their health status ($p < 0.01$); and retention of children, immigrant women were more inclined to believe this condition is desirable ($p < 0.05$).

Licit and illicit substance use; self-esteem and other factors (see Tables 6.8 and 6.9). Generally, immigrant women began using substances at an earlier age. Closer examination revealed, however, that the only statistically significant difference was for sedatives ($p < 0.01$). While receiving treatment for addiction, immigrant women, more often than native-born women, reported they were using heroin ($p < 0.05$), heroin with alcohol ($p < 0.001$), or alcohol and other drugs while clean of heroin ($p < 0.001$). Regarding self-esteem, the two subgroups did not differ. No difference was found among immigrant and native-born addicts regarding the number of times spent in a mental institution; native-born addicts, however, were referred more often to prison ($p < 0.05$).

DISCUSSION

Russian-Speaking Addicts and Substance Abuse

Immigrant absorption and substance abuse treatment are processes of transition, and as such, certain elements tend to underscore both. Specifically, these include: (1) the development of values, beliefs, and goals that guide behavior; (2) the establishment of personal identity and self-esteem; (3) the development of interpersonal skills and relationships that can be supportive in promoting a certain type of adjustment during the transition period; and (4) the clarification of a person's goals and roles in terms of work, marriage, family, and future lifestyle (Blum & Singer, 1983).

From the perspective of drug treatment policy in Israel, a major challenge exists in terms of how best to address the needs of addicts with culturally distinct background characteristics, such as Russian-speaking people. Researchers have not provided compelling evidence that separate programs for immigrants or substance abusers from different ethnic or cultural groups are superior to mainstream efforts. Experts question the cost-effectiveness of such "special" programs and caution clinicians that they must be wary of defining any patient in relation only to ethnic- or racial-group membership, especially considering that other patient-related variables have been found to have greater implications for successful outcomes, such as addiction severity, employment stability, criminal involvement, education level, and socioeconomic status (Sullivan & Fleming, 1997). Nonetheless, clinical obser-

Table 6.8
Female Immigrant and Native-Born Heroin Addicts: Age of First Time Use of Substances, Self-Esteem, and Institution Experience

Variable	Immigrant ($n = 53$)	Native Born ($n = 61$)	ANOVA (df)
	Mean Score (S.D.)		
Age of First Use			
Cigarettes	15.1 (3.3)	14.7 (2.7)	0.45 (104) n.s.
Alcohol	15.5 (3.3)	17.6 (6.4)	-1.69 (99) n.s.
Marijuana	17.2 (5.2)	18 0 (5.4)	-0.64 (65) n.s.
Hashish	17.1 (4.5)	17.9 (6.7)	-0.48 (49) n.s.
Opiates	19.5 (5.0)	19.7 (7.2)	-0.16 (46) n.s.
Heroin	22.4 (7.0)	22.3 (7.2)	0.15 (91) n.s.
Methadone	28.0 (6.7)	27.3 (7.7)	0.80 (63) n.s.
Sedatives	18.7 (5.1)	24.9 (9.1)	-2.70 (42) **
Other Factors			
Jailed (Total Times)	1.2 (0.3)	2.3 (1.9)	-2.14 (30) *
Mental Institution (Total Times)	1.6 (0.8)	2.5 (1.9)	-1.57 (23) n.s.
Self-esteem	3.3 (0.7)	3.4 (0.6)	-1.40 (103) n.s.

*$p \leq 0.05$. **$p \leq 0.01$. ***$p \leq 0.001$.

vations have shown that treatment of special populations may be enhanced if their particular needs are considered and met (American Psychiatric Association, 1995; Institute of Medicine, 1990; Landry, 1996; Sullivan & Fleming, 1997). In the case of Russian-speaking addicts, this may mean providing help to deal with difficulties such as personal adjustment and family relations attributed to low income, inadequate housing, unemployment, and underemployment.

Table 6.9
Female Immigrant and Native-Born Heroin Addicts: Patterns of Substance Use While in Treatment and Attitudes

Variable	Immigrant ($n = 53$)	Native Born ($n = 61$)	Total ($N = 114$)	X^2
		N (%)		
Patterns of Substance Use				
Heroin Use While in Treatment	21 (40)	11 (19)	32 (29)	7.73*
Heroin Use with Alcohol While in Treatment	15 (28)	3 (5)	18 (16)	11.38**
Clean of Heroin but Using Alcohol and Other Drugs While in Treatment	23 (46)	8 (15)	31 (30)	12.42***
Attitudes				
Wish to Stop Heroin Addiction	49 (93)	49 (80)	98 (86)	4.07*
Believes Can Stop Addiction	36 (68)	41 (68)	77 (68)	n.s.
Concern about Health (main reason to stop drug use)	35 (67)	16 (27)	51 (45)	30.63**
Desire to Retain Child(ren)	39 (74)	26 (43)	65 (57)	5.28*

*$p \leq 0.05$. **$p \leq 0.01$. ***$p \leq 0.001$.

Religious Considerations

Based on select social and psychological characteristics, few distinctions exist between Jewish and non-Jewish Russian-speaking heroin addicts in Israel. In other words, it appears that, based on a limited sample, religious affiliation does not influence the attitudes and behavior of heroin addicts.

For Russian-speaking heroin addicts in Israel, religion, and the values associated with it, tends to have little, if any, meaning. The lives of Russian-speaking heroin addicts appear to be defined by social, cultural, and economic conditions and relations. Consistent with this conclusion, Engs, Hanson, Gliksman, and Smythe (1990) found that among less cohesive groups, cultural norms prevail over those of a religious nature. In the United States, where Jewish young people tend to be more acculturated with mainstream values and norms than with those of a religious nature, substance use tends to be greater than in Israel, where religious values are more prevailing (Engs, Hanson, & Isralowitz, 1988). A similar conclusion was made by Lieberman (1987), who found social drinking among assimilated Jews to be a threat to the traditional social control mechanisms that differentiate Jewish communal ritual drinking from drinking in non-Jewish communities.

According to Gorsuch (1995), studies have typically found that religiousness is associated with lower substance abuse and the negative consequences associated with such behavior because religious people have been socialized to accept anti-abuse norms, are involved with anti-abuse peers, and have a mechanism for satisfying the need for social contact and meaning in life. However, the relationship occurs only for a nurturing and supportive religiousness and not a situation where there is no religion or religion is associated with restrictive, negative, and ritualistic rules of behavior—conditions that tend to reflect most Russian-speaking addicts' relationship to Judaism in the former Soviet republics.

Details regarding the extent of non-Jewish people who entered Israel during the last 10 years or so may be of concern to religious and immigration officials among others. The fact remains, however, that up to one-third, if not more, of the Russian-speaking immigrants who entered into Israel are not Jewish. Nevertheless, they are all now citizens of Israel, and as such, they are entitled to treatment services.

Regarding treatment, the Jewish and non-Jewish addicts involved in this study reported the need for Russian-speaking treatment personnel able to provide culturally sensitive services. The world of drug addiction treatment services in Israel tends to be shaped in response to or as a result of the majority group of addicts, who are of Sephardi origin. Consequently, Russian-speaking addicts may feel, and rightly so, out of place in a treatment facility and limited in terms of their level of involvement because of language and cultural factors.

In providing support to Russian-speaking addicts, even if they had a greater degree of religious affiliation, it must be realized this is not a homogeneous group. In other words, each Russian-speaking addict has his or her unique personality and physical characteristics even if they all came from the same part of the former Soviet Union, which they did not. Too often in the provision of human services, there is a tendency to provide clients with only the services that are available. If a client does not match the service(s), there is a good chance that the individual will fall through the cracks between programs and not receive the service(s) needed. In other words, substance abuse addicts must be treated as the individuals they are. Religion has not been a factor in their lives, but religion should not be excluded as a possible means of shaping a positive, more healthy individual able to withstand the temptation of drug use.

Former Soviet Union and Israeli-Born Female Heroin Addicts

In spite of the kinds of psychological distress, for example, anxiety and hostility, and other conditions associated with being an immigrant and having to adjust to a new living environment (Ponizovsky et al., 1998), few differences exist among immigrant and native-born female heroin addicts in Israel. Health, child custody, and education are factors that differentiate the two study groups and have important implications for the needs and treatment of female addicts.

While relatively little is known about the children of heroin addicts, researchers suggest that the children of addicted parents are at greater risk for later dysfunctional behaviors (Johnson & Leff, 1999). From the present study, both immigrant and native-born female addicts, especially Russian-speaking women, report that being able to retain custody of their children is an important reason for them to try to overcome addiction. This finding and the need to prevent intergenerational drug abuse provide good reasons for providing parenting skills development as part of the treatment process of female addicts.

Another important differentiating factor found between immigrant and native-born female addicts is education. Clearly, female heroin addicts from the former Soviet Union tend to have more education, including that of a vocational nature, than their peers born in Israel. This background characteristic may open up the world of work more easily to immigrant addicts; both groups of women, however, need the ability and motivation to seek and sustain legitimate employment. One area that may provide formerly addicted women with employment is the development of gender- and culture-specific drug treatment facilities and programs.

Policy and Program Development Implications

Regarding the opportunity to emigrate, it is not too surprising that a percentage of addicts would be given release from prison conditioned on leaving the country. It seems that such action on the part of Russian prison authorities was taken not so much for humanitarian purposes but rather as a cost- and space-saving opportunity. The study results do not indicate that this policy, that is, prison release conditioned on emigration, was carried out on the level demonstrated by Fidel Castro of Cuba when people were allowed to leave that country for the United States during the Carter Administration (1977–1981).

From an epidemiological perspective, the issue of tuberculosis (TB) needs to be considered in the context of treatment. Tuberculosis is a serious issue related to immigration, substance abuse, and imprisonment. Countries with large numbers of immigrants, such as the United States and Israel, are likely to receive an increase of patients with this contagious illness. It has been reported that "the overall TB rate in New York City is . . . 21.3 per 100,000. Compare that to Bombay, where the rate is 500 per 100,000. The crisis in Russia's prisons, in turn, makes the Bombay statistics seem insignificant. If you were a diabolical terrorist and you wanted to manufacture multi-drug resistant tuberculosis, you would create an environment and a system like the one in the Russian prisons. . . . [P]risons are poorly ventilated rooms where 30 prisoners share 10 beds, sleeping in shifts. Last year 20,000 Russian prison inmates fell ill with strains of TB that resisted known medications. Many of those infected inmates were then released, and they spread the disease to 15,000 civilians" (Belkin, 1999). While reports from Israeli drug treatment physicians indicate that tuberculosis among drug users is not a problem, it must be kept in mind that the vast majority of addicts do not seek treatment. In fact, from a study of addicts in the southern region of Israel it was found that less than 20 percent find their way to detoxification and treatment programs (Isralowitz, Telias, & Tabu, 1996).

Another health-related issue worth noting is the amount of child physical and sexual abuse reported among the Russian-speaking drug addicts, especially females. Much more research needs to be done on this subject; however, the findings in terms of abuse patterns tend to be consistent with those of Dansky and colleagues (1996), Gil-Rivas, Fiorentine, and Anglin (1996), and Bernstein, Stein, and Handelsman (1998).

It has been estimated that 18 percent of heroin addicts in Israel are women. In this study's Russian-speaking cohort, however, the proportion of women is larger—in the area of 20 to 22 percent. Nevertheless, women warrant special concern because of their gender status and their relation to prostitution in order support their "habit." In a study by the U.S. National Institute on Drug Abuse (NIDA), it was found that at the end of 1994, 58,000 women were reported to be HIV infected, and 41 percent of these cases resulted from injection drug use. Indeed, women's drug and sexual risk for HIV frequently co-occur. Women's drug use often involves membership in a network of HIV-infected individuals where direct and indirect sharing of injection equipment or sexual liaisons are transacted and where the social context (e.g., shooting gallery) increases the likelihood of transmitting HIV. According to NIDA, drug-dependent women are more likely than men to engage in high-risk sex, and women who inject drugs are more likely to acquire HIV sexually than men. Violence may be an additional risk factor. This is because women with abusive partners practice more HIV risk behaviors and are less likely to seek drug treatment or disclose their HIV status to their partners than nonabused women. Women's unique HIV transmission context and behaviors, including the link between drug dependence and risky sex as well as the potential transmission to infants, have implications for the development of targeted, gender-specific and risk-related treatment (National Institute on Drug Abuse, 1995). While the proportion of HIV and female drug users is expected to vary from location to location, it is an issue that must be considered to be one of the most serious drug-related problems. Outreach activities to Russian-speaking female drug users, gender-specific treatment activities, including individual and group counseling, and relapse-prevention activities must be given priority development and service provision status.

Finally, additional research is needed, including a wider investigation of a larger cohort of Russian-speaking addicts, to confirm the results of this study as well as to build a larger base of information for policy and service decision makers. Such empirically grounded information is needed to promote prevention and treatment programs that can best control drug addiction and the crime and diseases associated with it.

REFERENCES

Abu Saad, I., & Isralowitz, R. (1997). Social cohesion and intergroup conflict in the Negev: Jewish and Arab attitudes toward the absorption of Russian immigrants. In I. Light & R. Isralowitz (Eds.), *Immigration and immigrant absorption in the United States and Israel* (pp. 95–116). Burlington, VT: Ashgate Publishing.

American Psychiatric Association. (1995). *Practice guide for treatment of patients with substance use disorders: Alcohol, cocaine, opioids.* Washington, DC: American Psychiatric Association.

Anglin, M., Caulkins, J., & Hser, Y. (1993). Prevalence estimations: Policy needs, current status, and future potential. *Journal of Drug Issues, 23,* 345–360.

Belkin, L. (1999, May 30). A brutal cure. *New York Times Magazine,* p. 36.

Bernstein, D., Stein, J., & Handelsman, L. (1998). Predicting personality pathology among adult patients with substance use disorders: Effects of childhood maltreatment. *Addictive Behavior, 23,* 855–868.

Blum, A., & Singer, M. (1983). Substance abuse and social deviance: A youth assessment framework. In R. Isralowitz & M. Singer (Eds.), *Adolescent substance abuse* (pp. 7–21). New York: Haworth Press.

Casper, R. (1992). Follow-up of nonrespondents in 1990. In C. Turner, J. Lessler, & J. Gfroerer. *Survey measurement of drug use: Methodological studies* (pp. 155–173). (U.S. Department of Health and Human Services Publication No. ADM 92-1929). Washington, DC: National Institute on Drug Abuse.

Dansky, B., Brady, K., Saladin, M., Killeen, T., Becker, S., & Roitzsch, J. (1996). Victimization and PTSD in individuals with substance abuse disorder: Gender and racial differences. *American Journal of Drug and Alcohol Abuse, 22,* 75–93.

Elisha, D. (1998). Israel Ministry of Health, Substance Abuse Treatment Unit: An overview. In R. Isralowitz, M. Afifi, E. Awwad, & G. Sussman (Eds.), *Palestinian and Israeli people against drug use: Problems, policies and programs. A cooperative effort to address the problem through communication, cooperation and coordination, Conference proceedings*. Tel Aviv: Economic Cooperation Foundation.

Engs, R., Hanson, D., Gliksman, L., & Smythe, C. (1990). Influence of religion and culture on drinking behaviours: A test of hypotheses between Canada and the United States. *British Journal of Addiction, 85,* 1475–1482.

Engs, R., Hanson, D., & Isralowitz, R. (1988). Drinking problems among Jewish college students in the United States and Israel. *Journal of Social Psychology, 128,* 415–417.

Gil-Rivas, V., Fiorentine, R., & Anglin, M. (1996). Sexual abuse, physical abuse, and posttraumatic stress disorder among women participating in outpatient drug abuse treatment. *Journal of Psychoactive Drugs, 28,* 95–102.

Goldscheider, C. (1992). Demographic transformations in Israel: Emerging themes in comparative context. In C. Goldscheider (Ed.), *Population and social change in Israel* (pp. 1–38). Boulder, CO: Westview Press.

Gorsuch, R. (1995). Religious aspects of substance abuse and recovery. *Journal of Social Issues, 51,* 65–83.

Institute of Medicine. (1990). *Broadening the base of treatment for alcohol problems.* Washington, DC: National Academy Press.

Isralowitz, R., & Abu Saad, I. (1997). Ethnic conflict and social cohesion among Israeli adolescents toward Russian immigrants. In I. Light & R. Isralowitz (Eds.), *Immigration and immigrant absorption in the United States and Israel* (pp. 82–94). Burlington, VT: Ashgate Publishing.

Isralowitz, R., Abu Saad, I., & Telias, D. (1996). Work values among heroin addicts: A status model perspective. *Journal of Offender Rehabilitation, 24,* 141–154.

Isralowitz, R., & Peleg, A. (1996). Israeli college student alcohol use: The association of background characteristics and regular drinking patterns. *Drug and Alcohol Dependence, 42,* 147–153.

Isralowitz, R., Telias, D., & Abu Saad, I. (1994). Psychological characteristics of heroin addicts and non-drug users in Israel: A status model comparison. *Journal of Social Psychology, 134,* 399–401.

Isralowitz, R., Telias, D., & Tabu, N. (1996). *Drug services in the Negev: A study of organization problems and needs, staff training and treatment issues. A report to the Negev Development Authority.* Beer Sheva: Ben-Gurion University.

Isralowitz, R. & Troestler, N. (1996). Substance use: Toward an understanding of its relation to nutrition-related attitudes and behavior among Israeli high school youth. *Journal of Adolescent Health, 19,* 184–189.

Johnson, J., & Leff, M. (1999). Children of substance abusers: Overview of research findings. *Pediatrics, 103,* 1085–1099.

Johnston, L., & O'Malley, P. (1985). Issues of validity and population coverage in student surveys of drug use. In B. Rouse, M. Kozel, & L. Richard (Eds.), *Self-report methods of estimating drug use: Meeting current challenges to validity* (pp. 31–54). Washington DC: National Institute on Drug Abuse.

Johnston, L., O'Malley, P., & Bachman, J. (1992). *Smoking, drinking, and illicit drug use among American secondary students, college students, and young adults, 1975–1991, 1&2.* (National Institutes of Health Publication No. 93-3480). Washington, DC: National Institute on Drug Abuse.

Landry, M. (1996). *Overview of addiction treatment effectiveness.* (U.S. Department of Health and Human Services Publication No. SMA 96-3081). Washington, DC: U.S. Government Printing Office.

Lieberman, L. (1987). Jewish alcoholism and the disease concept. *Journal of Psychology and Judaism, 11,* 165–180.

Light, I., & Isralowitz, R. (1997). *Immigrant entrepreneurs and immigrant absorption in the United States and Israel*. Aldershot, England: Ashgate.

National Institute on Drug Abuse. (1995, August 18). Women's HIV Risk and Protective Behaviors. (National Institutes of Health Guide, 24). Washington, DC: National Institute on Drug Abuse.

Ponizovsky, A., Ginath, Y., Durst, R., Wondimeneh, B., Safro, S., Minuchin Itzigson, M., & Ritsner, M. (1998). Psychological distress among Ethiopian and Russian Jewish immigrants to Israel: A cross-cultural study. *International Journal of Social Psychiatry, 44,* 35–45.

Rosenbaum-Tamari, J., & Dimian, N. (1991, April). *The two waves of immigration: The Soviet immigrants in the 1970's and the onset of the 1990's.* Paper presented at the annual meeting of the Israel Sociological Association, Tel Aviv.

Sullivan, E., & Fleming, M. (1997). *A guide to substance abuse for primary care clinicians.* (U.S. Department of Health and Human Services Publication No. SMA 97-3139). Washington, DC: U.S. Government Printing Office.

7

Social Change and Substance Use among Bedouin Arabs in Southern Israel*

Ismael Abu Saad

INTRODUCTION

In recent decades, substance use and abuse have increased greatly in many parts of the world, including the Middle East (Weiss, Sawa, Abdeen, & Yanai, 1999). This chapter explores the development of substance use among a traditionally nomadic and seminomadic population in the process of urbanization, the Bedouin Arabs in southern Israel. The experiences of many developed and developing countries confirm that radical social change tends to produce severe disruption of social and cultural patterns that may, in turn, be associated with a wide range of social problems, including substance abuse (Berry, Trimble, & Olmedo, 1986; Kiev, 1972; Trimble, 1996). This study, which is based on structured interviews with 312 Bedouin Arab males, investigates the phenomenon of their substance use and abuse in the context of urbanization and other changes in their broader sociopolitical environment.

GENERAL BACKGROUND

Over the past half century, with the formation of nation-states and the encroachment of modernization, Bedouin life throughout the Middle East has changed to varying degrees. Such is the case with the Bedouin Arabs, who, having lived in the Negev desert in southern Israel, are now being resettled into urban towns by the government.

*This study was funded by the Netherlands-Israel Development Research Program (NIRP). Project No. 92-2.1.

The Negev Bedouin are among the Palestinian Arabs who remained in Israel after 1948 and are currently a part of the Arab minority in Israel. They have inhabited the Negev desert since the fifth century C.E. (Maddrell, 1990), and were traditionally organized into nomadic or seminomadic tribes that lived by raising sheep and engaging in seasonal agriculture. Prior to 1948, estimates of the Bedouin Arab population in the Negev ranged from 65,000 to 90,000 (Falah, 1989; Maddrell, 1990). During the course and aftermath of the 1948 war, the vast majority of the Negev Bedouin became refugees in the surrounding Arab countries and territories (i.e., Gaza, the West Bank, Jordan, etc.), and only about 11,000 remained in the Negev (Falah, 1989; Marx, 1967). The Israeli authorities took control of most of the land in the Negev, so the Bedouin who remained in the Negev lost the freedom to move with their herds and cultivate their lands (Bailey, 1995; Lustick, 1980). The population was confined to a specially designated "Restricted Area" (seig) in the northeastern Negev, representing only 10 percent of the territory they controlled before 1948 (Falah, 1989; Lustick, 1980; Marx, 1967). Furthermore, they were placed under a military administration until 1966, as were all other Arabs in Israel, which meant that they could not return to and cultivate their lands, they were isolated from the Arab population in other parts of Israel, and they needed special permits to leave their designated sections of the Restricted Area to look for jobs, education, markets, and other opportunities (Marx, 1967). The restrictions imposed by the Israeli government represented a form of forced sedentarization, which virtually ended their nomadic and seminomadic way of life.

The Military Administration over Arabs in Israel was lifted in 1966, after which the Negev Bedouin were brought into greater contact with the broader Israeli society. The vast majority of the Bedouin became dependent on working in the Jewish sector, primarily as unskilled laborers, since they had lost their lands and traditional livelihoods (Abu Saad, 1991b).

In the late 1960s and early 1970s, the government developed plans for the resettlement of the entire Negev Bedouin population into seven urban settlements. Part of the government rationale for establishing these urban settlements was to "modernize the Bedouin" and provide them with services more efficiently, and it used the provision of services (such as running water, electricity, health clinics, and modern schools) as an incentive to attract Bedouin to the urban settlements. This settlement program has been controversial, especially given its radical departure from the Bedouin's traditional way of life. While the majority of governments in the Middle East have developed programs encouraging the Bedouin to settle, they have, for the most part, been based on some combination of agriculture and livestock raising, rather than on the urbanization of the population.

As of 1999, the Negev Bedouin population numbered approximately 120,000 of whom 50 percent lived in the planned urban settlements and 50 percent continued to live in spontaneous tribal settlements (Abu Saad, 1999a; Hayton, 1998). The unemployment rate in the planned Bedouin urban settlements is the highest in Israel. Since these settlements lack internal sources of employment other than municipal and public services, approximately 80 percent of the employed spend up to 5 days a week away from home in other parts of the country (Ben-David, 1991). Sixty-five percent of the population in these settlements live in poverty (Ghanem, 1998; Hayton, 1998).

Bedouin living in spontaneous, nonurban settlements face a different set of pressures. Since their settlements are unplanned (i.e., unauthorized and thus unrecognized), they are denied services such as paved roads, public transportation, electricity (and in many cases running water), sewage systems, rubbish disposal, telephone service, and community health facilities. These unrecognized Bedouin settlements are not geographically isolated but are rather dispersed around and between the Jewish and Bedouin urban and agricultural settlements in the Negev that are recognized and have modern infrastructure and services. Bedouin in the unrecognized settlements are denied licenses for building any permanent housing. All housing forms except for tents are considered illegal and are subject to heavy fines and demolition proceedings (Maddrell, 1990). Despite these pressures, Bedouin remain on the lands traditionally owned by them (but considered as state lands by the government) to prevent their de facto, as well as their de jure, confiscation. Most of these Bedouin depend, at least in part, on the traditional occupations of herding, agriculture, and the processing of animal products to supplement or provide their incomes, but this is also restricted by the government. Herd sizes and grazing areas are tightly controlled and a special police unit patrols and confiscates flocks found in violation of regulations. Thus, very few Bedouin can subsist entirely on their traditional sources of livelihood, and therefore they also seek out paid employment in the larger Israeli economy (Bailey, 1995; Maddrell, 1990).

In addition to the spatial and economic changes the Bedouin have undergone, the social structure of the Bedouin, within and outside the planned urban settlements, has also changed dramatically. The traditional tribal structure, norms, and values are no longer formally operative. The patriarchal family structure also has been altered, due to so many fathers working outside of the community and having little time to spend with their families. The place of children has changed in that in the traditional economy, the children played a significant role in the family's agricultural and herding activities. Bedouin youth in the urban settlements, however, no longer play this role, and the urban settlements have no cultural centers, libraries, or other places to provide them alternative, constructive activities. In addition, the Bedouin have significant exposure to Western-oriented Israeli society through visiting or working in surrounding (Jewish) commercial centers and through the media (television, radio, newspapers). These social changes have not been addressed, leaving many people lost between traditional and modern society (Abu Saad, 1997).

Formal education is essential to success in the new context of the Negev Bedouin. There are public schools throughout the Negev serving the Bedouin population, but the schools outside the urban settlements are considered temporary by the government and are housed in makeshift facilities. None of the schools in the nonurbanized sector provide education past the eighth grade, which means all Bedouin children from nonurbanized communities who want to go to high school must go to the schools in the urban settlements. The drop-out rate in the Negev Bedouin community, in general, is the highest in Israel, with an estimated 70 percent of students dropping out before completing high school (Abu Saad, 1996a, 1997). Due to the failure of the schools to retain students, as well as to the lack of structured activities in the urban settlements, children and youth have become a part of a marginal, dependent population, at risk of adopting delinquent attitudes and behaviors.

Traditionally, in this religiously homogeneous (Moslem) community, tobacco was the only substance used, and its use was virtually restricted to males. Bedouin were on drug trafficking routes through the Middle East and even worked as traffickers, but the phenomenon of substance use never developed, nor did it ever gain social acceptability (Abu Saad, 1999b). However, recent research indicates that within the context of the radical social and economic change the Bedouin are undergoing, the phenomenon of drug, alcohol, and other substance consumption has developed (Abu Saad, 1991a, 1996b). Abu Saad's study among Bedouin intermediate and secondary school students revealed that 12 percent of the students from urban settlements and 15 percent of the students from nonurban settlements smoked cigarettes; 8 percent of those from urban settlements and 4 percent of those from nonurban settlements drank alcohol; and 8 percent of those from urban settlements and 6 percent of those from nonurban settlements used illicit drugs. Twenty percent of the illicit drug users in urban settlements and 10 percent of the illicit drug users in nonurban settlements used hard drugs, such as cocaine and heroin. Although approximately 40 percent of the respondents were female, all of the substance users were male.

Research conducted in 1998 on substance use among youth in Israeli schools in general, from the seventh to twelfth grades (13–18 years old), indicated that 21 percent smoked cigarettes, 57 percent drank alcohol, 5 percent used cannabis, and 5 percent used hard drugs within the previous year. Among adults, 42 percent smoked cigarettes, 65 percent drank alcohol, 7 percent used cannabis, and 1 percent used hard drugs (Rahav, Teichman, Gil, Rosenblum, and Bar-Hamburger, 1998).

LITERATURE REVIEW

Numerous reviews of the research on the correlates of substance use and abuse have been conducted, and there is general agreement on the major predictors of substance abuse (Braucht, Brakarsh, Follinstad, & Berry, 1973; Flay, D'Avernas, Best, Kersell, & Ryan, 1983; Isralowitz & Telias, 1998; Kandel, 1982; Murry & Perry, 1985; Ong & Isralowitz, 1996). Based on the reasonable consistency among studies in the domains of variables found to predict drug use, a number of classes of variables that encompass the most important predictors have been identified (Flay & Petraitis, 1991).

One class of variables (*social environment*) deals with the structure of the economic, legal, social, cultural, and educational systems of a society as determinants of behavior. The importance of the social environment is well established in the literature. For example, in a binational comparison of Singapore and Israeli heroin users, Ong and Isralowitz (1996) found more differences than similarities, which they attributed to the prevailing social and cultural norms of the respective societies. Jones Webb, Hsiao, and Hannan (1995) found higher rates of alcohol-related problems among African American than among white males living in economically depressed U.S. neighborhoods because they were more likely to live in block groups with low family incomes, higher population densities, and easier retail access to alcohol. They also were subject to more social conditions that have been linked to increased risk for alcohol-related problems. No differences were found between these two groups when they lived in more affluent neighborhoods.

Changes in the social environment have been found to be related to the development of substance abuse patterns. The sudden change produced by the coming together of different cultural traditions, in particular, has been found to produce "acculturative stress" and to lead to massive disruption of cultural norms and values at the group level (Berry, 1980; Berry et al., 1986; Trimble, 1996) and substance abuse at the individual level. Hunter's study of Aborigines in an isolated region of Australia describes how their entry into a cash economy and the sudden widespread availability of alcohol led to the abuse of alcohol and other self-destructive behaviors primarily among the males in this population (Hunter, 1990).

Social or cultural disorganization and breakdown may lead to inadequate socialization that alters social bonding and social learning (Merton, 1957). Wilson has found that this may, in turn, lead to increased substance use and abuse, especially among the economically or politically disadvantaged (Wilson, 1987). Research on Puerto Rican youth in the United States indicates that cultural values toward substance use or abuse and loss of cultural identity play an important role in the substance use and drug dealing of these youth (Rodriguez, Recio Adrados, & De La Rosa, 1993). Similarly, American Indian youth who lose their cultural identity have been found to be more susceptible to substance use and abuse than those who do not (Oetting, 1993).

A second set of variables, *social bonding*, is involved in the way in which social organization affects substance abuse. Conventional bonds with family, peers, school, and other community groups are important, and researchers have shown that the breakdown of family bonding leads to increased probability of bonding with delinquent peers (Elliott, Huizinga, & Ageton, 1985). Brook (1993) found that nonconflictual and affectionate mutual attachment relationships between parents and children led to lower levels of drug use among African American and Puerto Rican youth. Krohn and Thornberry (1993) studied the network systems of white non-Hispanic, African American, and Puerto Rican youth and found that drug nonusers tended to have stronger family network systems than users did, and that, conversely, users tended to have more supportive and intimate relationships with their friends than did nonusers (Krohn & Thornberry, 1993). A study of drinking behavior among young Asian American adult males revealed that the only social factor consistently related to drinking behavior was having friends who used alcohol (Chi, Lubben, & Kitano, 1989). Ong and Isralowitz (1996) reported that studies conducted in Singapore found that most drug abusers did poorly in school and dropped out prematurely.

Social learning variables are a third set of variables related to opportunities for observation and modeling of a behavior: substance availability; social normative beliefs, including collective ignorance of norms; and social reinforcement. Researchers have developed the relations among these variables from psychological and sociological perspectives (Akers, 1977; Bandura, 1986). Any particular behavior is more likely to occur when it is differentially reinforced and is seen as desirable by important others. Akers (1992) views social learning theory as providing the connection between the social environment (macrolevel factors) and the behavior of individuals (microlevel factors) insofar as social learning provides the process through which the social environment has an impact on the substance use of the individual. Society, as well as particular groups and social situations, provides environments in which the social learning variables of association, definitions, reinforcement, and imitation operate. The primary groups through which the general orientations (cultural, religious, and community) toward substance use influence an individual are family, peers, and friends, but secondary groups and the media also have an impact (Akers, 1992). The importance of such secondary groups was confirmed by Weiss and colleagues (1999) in their review of substance use studies among Arabs in Israel, Jordan, and the Palestinian Authority. They concluded that secularization and the exposure to the alcohol and drug consumption patterns of Israel and of Western culture, in general (through television, tourists, etc.), resulted in unexpectedly high levels of alcohol and other drug consumption patterns among these traditional, predominantly Moslem populations.

A fourth class of variables, *knowledge, attitudes, and behavior*, deals with the intrapersonal cognitive, affective, and conative variables. These include knowledge of physiological and social consequences of use; personal beliefs regarding consequences; general values and specific evaluations of the consequences; attitudes toward substance use and related issues; behavioral intentions; trial behavior; stages of behavior (i.e., from licit to illicit substances); and established adult behavior patterns.

These four classes of variables, which encompass many of the major variables included in other broad theories, form the theoretical basis of this study.

METHODOLOGY

The current study was designed to: (1) examine the levels of substance use among the urbanized and nonurbanized Negev Bedouin and (2) test the relationships between substance use and the theoretical dimensions of social environment; social bonding; social learning; knowledge, attitudes, and behavior (KAB); and selected demographic variables.

Participants

The study sample consisted of 312 Negev Bedouin participants from within and outside the government-planned urban settlements in Israel who were interviewed in 1995–1996. Purposive sampling was used to identify and include a broadly representative geographical distribution of subjects from the urbanized and nonurbanized sectors of the population.

The sample was all male for the following reasons: (a) Bedouin girls and women live within a very tightly controlled social structure that disapproves of women using licit or illicit substances and gives them no access to substances or opportunities for engaging in substance use; (b) given the social norms, coming into a home and asking females the questions about substance use contained in the structured interview could be interpreted as an affront to the individual female, as well as to her entire (extended) family, and could have seriously jeopardized the willingness of the Bedouin community to participate in the project; and (c) previous substance-use research conducted among Bedouin high school students (of whom approximately 40 percent were female) revealed no use of either licit or illicit substances among females (Abu Saad, 1996b).

Instrumentation

A structured interview was developed, based on the theoretical model described above. This interview also obtained detailed information on substance use and general demographic characteristics.

Procedures

The data were collected through structured home interviews. Several procedures were followed to protect the anonymity and confidentiality of subjects in the study. Neither names nor other personal codes were imprinted on any interview. All subjects were assured of complete anonymity prior to being interviewed and were advised that participation in the study was voluntary.

Data Analysis

Descriptive statistics were used to report the basic distribution characteristics of the variables, and Chi-square and ANOVA were used to examine the differences between groups.

RESULTS

Demographic Data

Among the sample of respondents, 48 percent (150) lived in government-planned urban settlements, and 52 percent lived in spontaneous, nonurban settlements (162). Neither of the groups reported being very "mobile" any longer. Those living in urban settlements were significantly more likely than those living outside of urban settlements to have moved their place of residence within the last 10 years. About 10 percent (15) of the respondents living outside the urban settlements lived in tents, while 76 percent (119) lived in zinc or wood shacks, and 16 percent (22) lived in cement block or stone houses. This differed significantly from those living in urban settlements, among whom 97 percent (117) lived in cement block or stone houses and 3 percent (4) lived in zinc or wood shacks.

The mean age of the respondents was 32 (*SD* = 10); 72 percent (224) were married and 28 percent (88) were single (a few of whom were divorced or widowed). The mean number of children was 7 (*SD* = 5). Ninety-one percent (147) of those living outside urban settlements and 82 percent (123) of those living in urban settlements reported that they lived with their extended families.

The mean number of years of schooling for the sample was 10 (*SD* = 5). There were significant differences in the educational levels of those living inside and outside the urban settlements, with those living inside the settlements having higher educational levels.

Regarding employment status, 82 percent (119) of those living in urban settlements and 75 percent (109) of those living outside urban settlements reported having a paid job at the time of the interview. In terms of land ownership, respondents living outside urban settlements were significantly more likely to own more land, now and in the past, than those living inside urban settlements.

Levels of Substance Use

Among the study subjects, 64 percent (201) reported using cigarettes, 90 percent of whom reported smoking daily. The proportion of cigarette use was significantly higher among nonurbanized (74 percent, $n = 119$) than urbanized (55 percent, $n = 82$) Bedouin (see Table 7.1); 68 percent (136) of the smokers were under the age of 35. The average age at which they began smoking was 15.

Regarding alcohol use, 31 percent (46) of urbanized and 30 percent (49) of nonurbanized Bedouin reported ever using the substance, with 85 percent of the urbanized and 98 percent of the nonurbanized Bedouin reporting they had drunk alcohol in the month prior to the structured interview (see Table 7.2). Among those reporting alcohol use, 73 percent (69) were under the age of 35, and the average age at which they began to drink was 20. Beer was the most common form of alcoholic beverage used by both groups. Urbanized Bedouin used more wine and hard liquor than their nonurbanized counterparts (see Table 7.3).

Among both urbanized and nonurbanized Bedouin, 15 percent reported ever using drugs (see Table 7.2); 83 percent (39) of those who reported using drugs were below the age of 35. The average age at which they began using cannabis was 18. The average ages at which urbanized and nonurbanized respondents began using hard drugs were 23 and 26, respectively. The patterns of drug use among urbanized and nonurbanized Bedouin were quite similar, although nonurbanized respondents reported using cannabis more frequently than urbanized respondents. The urbanized respondents reported using hard drugs and other substances more often than nonurbanized respondents (see Table 7.4).

Table 7.1
Cigarette Smoking among Urban and Nonurban Bedouin

Cigarettes	Urban (*n* = 150)	Nonurban (*n* = 162)
Have you ever smoked cigarettes?		
Yes	82 (55%)	119 (74%)
No	68 (45%)	43 (27%)
Have you smoked in the last year?		
Yes	77 (51%)	114 (70%)
No	4 (3%)	5 (3%)
Not applicable	70 (47%)	43 (27%)
Have you smoked in the last month?		
Yes	75 (50%)	114 (70%)
No	1 (1%)	0
Not applicable	74 (49%)	48 (30%)
How often do you smoke?		
Every day	68 (45%)	112 (69%)
Once a week	4 (3%)	2 (1%)
Once a month	3 (2%)	0
Not applicable	75 (50%)	48 (30%)

Table 7.2
Alcohol and Drug Use among Urban and Nonurban Bedouin

Substance	Urban (*n* = 150)	Nonurban (*n* = 162)
Alcohol		
Ever used alcohol	46 (31%)	49 (30%)
Used alcohol in last year	43 (29%)	49 (30%)
Used alcohol in last month	43 (29%)	49 (30%)
Drugs		
Ever used drugs	22 (15%)	25 (15%)

Social Environment Variables

Respondents were asked to report their level of satisfaction with their community in general; the local health, education, and leadership services; and the behavior of their youth. While both urbanized and nonurbanized respondents expressed a moderate level of satisfaction with life in their community in general, they expressed dissatisfaction with the specific aspects of local health, education, and leadership services, and the behavior of youth. Nonurbanized Bedouin were sig-

Table 7.3
Frequency and Quantity of Alcohol Use by Type among Urban (n = 150) and Nonurban (n = 162) Bedouin

	Beer		Wine		Hard Liquor	
Frequency of use	Urban	Nonurban	Urban	Nonurban	Urban	Nonurban
Every day	9 (6%)	14 (9%)	2 (1%)	0 (0%)	3 (2%)	0 (0%)
Once a week	10 (7%)	25 (15%)	1 (1%)	2 (1%)	5 (3%)	7 (4%)
Once a month	15 (10%)	9 (6%)	5 (3%)	0 (0%)	9 (6%)	3 (6%)
Quantity (cans/bottles/glasses)						
>6	4 (3%)	3 (2%)	1 (1%)	0 (0%)	0 (0%)	1 (1%)
5–6	3 (2%)	9 (6%)	0 (0%)	0 (0%)	0 (0%)	0 (0%)
3–4	10 (7%)	13 (8%)	2 (1%)	2 (1%)	4 (3%)	1 (1%)
1–2	12 (8%)	20 (12%)	1 (1%)	0 (0%)	3 (2%)	4 (2%)
<1	5 (3%)	3 (2%)	4 (3%)	0 (0%)	10 (7%)	5 (3%)

Table 7.4
Illicit Drug Use Patterns and Frequency by Type among Urban (n = 150) and Nonurban (n = 162) Bedouin

	Cannabis		Hard Drugs		Other	
Drug Use Patterns	Urban	Nonurban	Urban	Nonurban	Urban	Nonurban
Used drugs in last year	18 (12%)	22 (14%)	6 (4%)	4 (2%)	6 (4%)	2 (1%)
Used drugs in last month	18 (12%)	22 (14%)	6 (4%)	4 (2%)	6 (4%)	2 (1%)
Frequency of Use						
Every day	7 (5%)	11 (7%)	3 (2%)	1 (1%)	2 (1%)	1 (1%)
Once a week	5 (3%)	7 (4%)	1 (1%)	2 (1%)	1 (1%)	0 (0%)
Once a month	6 (4%)	4 (2%)	2 (1%)	0 (0%)	3 (2%)	1 (1%)

nificantly more dissatisfied (at a level of $p < 0.05$) than urbanized Bedouin with the quality of services in their communities and the behavior of their youth.

Many differences were found between substance users and nonusers with regard to the level of satisfaction with their social environments (see Table 7.5). Nonsmokers and nondrug users were significantly more satisfied than smokers and drug users with: life in general in their communities; health services; education services; and local community leadership. The level of dissatisfaction with the behavior of youth in their communities among smokers and drug users was very similar to that of the general population of respondents. Alcohol drinkers were significantly more satisfied with the behavior of youth in their communities than nondrinkers. However, they were more dissatisfied than nondrinkers with: life in general in their communities; health services; educational services; and local community leadership.

Urban and nonurbanized substance users (by substance) were compared on these items, but no consistent pattern of differences was found in their attitudes toward their social environment. In addition to general questions about the social environment and infrastructure, those who lived in urban settlements were asked what they thought about having moved there. Overall, people did not think that the move had been a good step. They thought that it had created social and economic problems. They missed the traditional way of life, which they did not think was being preserved in the urban settlements at all, and they were dissatisfied with the quality of the municipal services they received. Substance users did not differ from nonsubstance users on these items.

Social Bonding Variables

Respondents were asked about a number of variables that indicate the strength and type of their social bonding patterns (including marital status, living with extended family, school completion, and religiosity). In addition, respondents were asked how they would react if their children skipped school, or used or began to bond with peers who used cigarettes, alcohol, or drugs. Comparisons were made between: (a) urbanized and nonurbanized respondents in general, (b) substance users and nonsubstance users by substance, and (c) urbanized and nonurbanized substance users by substance.

Both urbanized and nonurbanized respondents indicated that they would oppose having their children skip school occasionally; use cigarettes, alcohol, or drugs; or spend time with friends who engaged in these behaviors. The level of opposition expressed by nonurbanized respondents to their children skipping school occasionally, drinking hard liquor at parties, and using illicit or other drugs was significantly stronger (at a level of $p < 0.05$) than the level of opposition expressed by urbanized respondents.

Regarding the social bonding variables, the main differences existed between substance users and nonsubstance users. Cigarette smokers did not differ from nonsmokers on the variables of marital status or social structure (i.e., living with their extended family). They were, however, significantly more likely than non-

Table 7.5
Bedouin Social Change and Substance Use: Selected Significant Factors

Variable	
General Comparisons: Urban (n = 150) and Nonurban Dwellers (n = 162)	X^2; df; sig. level
Urban more likely to be married	13.80; 2;***
Urban more likely to live with extended family	6.35; 2;*
Urban more likely to have higher education	4.52; 4;***
Nonurban more likely to own land	51.44; 4;***
Nonurban more likely to be cigarette smokers	12.00; 1;***
Social Environment Comparisons: Smokers and Nonsmokers; Alcohol Users and Nonalcohol Users; Illicit Drug Users and Non-Illicit Drug Users	F score; sig. level
Nonsmokers more satisfied with life	6.22**
education services	8.85***
health services	11.32***
community leadership	7.05**
Nonalcohol users more satisfied with life	28.92***
education services	9.37***
health services	8.59***
community leadership	11.42***
Non-drug users more satisfied with life	36.21***
education services	21.76***
health services	7.88**
community leadership	24.68***
Social Bonding Comparisons:	X^2; df; sig. level
Cigarette smokers more likely to be school drop outs	18.29; 1;***
Cigarette smokers more likely to be secular	30.27; 2;***
Alcohol users more likely to be single	7.78; 1;**
Alcohol users less likely to be living with extended family	18.12; 2;***
Alcohol users less likely to be religious	35.26; 2;***
Illicit drug users more likely to be single	30.66; 1;***
Illicit drug users less likely to be living with extended family	6.43; 2;*
Illicit drug users less likely to be religious	34.67; 2;***
Illicit drug users more likely to be school drop outs	12.36; 1;***

* $p \leq 0.05$. ** $p \leq 0.01$. *** $p \leq 0.001$.

Note: Additional statistical comparison data are available by contacting Dr. Israel Abu Saad, Department of Education, Ben-Gurion University, Beer Sheva, Israel 84105.

smokers to have dropped out of school. In general, nonurbanized Bedouin were more likely than urbanized Bedouin to drop out of school; the difference in the mean number of years of schooling for nonurbanized smokers (7 years) and nonsmokers (9 years) was statistically significant.

Cigarette smokers, in general, were also significantly more likely than the general sample of nonsmoking respondents to consider themselves secular (58 percent and 26 percent, respectively). While cigarette smokers were as strongly opposed as nonsmokers to the idea of their children skipping school or using alcohol and illicit drugs, nonsmokers were more strongly opposed than smokers to the idea of their children smoking cigarettes.

Alcohol drinkers were significantly more likely than nondrinkers to be single or not married and less likely to live with their extended family. In addition, the religiosity of drinkers differed significantly from that of nondrinkers; 70 percent (65) of the drinkers considered themselves secular, as compared to 37 percent (78) of nondrinkers.

The proportion of drinkers who were school dropouts did not differ significantly from that of nondrinkers. However, when the respondents were asked how they would react if they found out their children were skipping school or using licit and illicit substances, nondrinkers were significantly more opposed than drinkers to their children skipping school occasionally, drinking alcohol, or drinking hard liquor at parties.

Regarding illicit drug users, the proportion of users who were unmarried (62 percent) was significantly higher than that of non-drug users (22 percent). Drug users were also much less likely than non-drug users to live with their extended family. The proportion of drug users who considered themselves secular was over twice that of non-drug users (87 percent and 40 percent, respectively). In addition, the proportion of drug users who dropped out of school was significantly higher than that of non-drug users (72 percent and 45 percent, respectively). Non-drug users were more strongly opposed than drug users to their children skipping school occasionally, smoking, spending time with friends who smoked cigarettes, drinking alcohol in general, drinking hard liquor at parties, and using illicit drugs or other drugs. However, drug users and nonusers were equally opposed to their children spending time with friends who used illicit drugs.

Social Learning Variables

Four subcategories of variables were examined within the category of social learning variables: (1) opportunities for observation and modeling of behavior, (2) substance availability, (3) social normative beliefs, and (4) social reinforcement.

Opportunities for observation and modeling of behavior. Among both urbanized and nonurbanized Bedouin respondents in general, 18 percent (54) thought that there was a large illicit drug problem in their community, 53 percent (162) thought there was a small illicit drug problem in their community, and 26 percent (78) said that they didn't know. Only 4 percent (11) said that they thought there was no illicit drug problem in their community at all. Urbanized respondents, however, were more likely than nonurbanized respondents to say that they knew of drug-using adults in their community. Regarding alcohol, similar proportions of urbanized and nonurbanized respondents thought that there was a small alcohol problem in their communities (56 percent and 48 percent, respectively), or did not know (28 percent and 31 percent, respectively). Urbanized respondents, however, were significantly more likely than nonurbanized respondents to say that they knew of youth in their communities who used alcohol. In terms of cigarette smoking, nonurbanized respondents were significantly more likely than urbanized respondents to say that there was a major tobacco problem in their communities, and to know of youth in their community who smoked cigarettes.

Major differences emerged when substance users were compared to nonusers. A significantly higher proportion of smokers than nonsmokers thought there was an illicit drug problem in their communities (78 percent and 58 percent, respectively). Smokers were also more likely to think that there was a considerable tobacco problem in their community than nonsmokers. In addition, smokers were significantly more likely than nonsmokers to know of youth in their communities who used illicit drugs and smoked cigarettes.

The comparison of alcohol users to nonusers revealed that drinkers were more likely to think that there was an illicit drug problem in their communities and to know of youth who used illicit drugs. They were also more likely than nondrinkers to think that there was an alcohol problem in their communities and to know of youth who drank alcohol. There were no significant differences between urbanized and nonurbanized alcohol drinkers on other questions.

Among the drug-using respondents, 96 percent said that they thought there was a drug problem in their communities, as compared to 66 percent of the nonusers, and they were significantly more likely than nonusers to know adults and youth in their communities who used drugs. They were also more likely than nonusers to think that there was a tobacco problem in their communities and to know of youth who drank alcohol and smoked cigarettes. There were no significant differences between urbanized and nonurbanized drug users on these items.

Substance availability. Regarding substance availability, 52 percent of both urbanized and nonurbanized respondents, in general, said it was possible to buy illicit drugs in their communities. Thirty percent of nonurbanized respondents said that it was not possible to buy illicit drugs in their communities, and 18 percent said that they did not know. This differed significantly from urbanized respondents, among whom 12 percent said that it was not possible to buy illicit drugs in their community, and 33 percent said that they did not know. Smokers (61 percent) were significantly more likely than nonsmokers (40 percent) to say that it was possible to buy illicit drugs in their communities; however, among smokers, urbanized respondents were significantly more likely than nonurbanized respondents to say that it was possible to buy drugs in their community. Additionally, 72 percent of the alcohol drinkers and 94 percent of the drug users said it was possible to buy illicit drugs in their communities, as compared to 45 percent of nondrinkers and 46 percent of non-drug users. There were no differences between urbanized and nonurbanized alcohol and drug users on these items.

Social normative beliefs. Nonurbanized respondents, in general, disagreed more strongly than urbanized respondents with the following statements: "Using drugs is acceptable in society" and "My community ignores drug users." In addition, the difference in their level of their disagreement with the statement, "My community tolerates drug users," was marginally significant. They did not differ with the statement, "Using drugs, even once, is very bad." However, smoking and drug-using respondents expressed significantly less agreement with this statement than did the nonsmoking and non-drug using respondents. Comparisons of urbanized and nonurbanized smokers and drinkers revealed that the nonurbanized respondents disagreed significantly more strongly (at a level of $p < 0.05$) than urbanized ones with the statement that their community ignores drug users. There were no significant differences between urbanized and nonurbanized drug users on these items.

Urbanized and nonurbanized Bedouin expressed similar beliefs that drug users were dangerous and should be treated harshly but should also be helped. Nonsmoking respondents were more likely than smokers to think that drug users were dangerous and should be treated harshly rather than helped. Nonusers of alcohol and drugs were more likely than drinkers and drug users to agree with the statements, "Using drugs is not acceptable in society," "Drug users should be treated harshly," and "Drug users are dangerous." Conversely, alcohol drinkers and drug users were more likely than nondrinkers and non-drug users to agree with the statement, "Drug users should be helped, not punished." The only differences to emerge from the comparison of urbanized and nonurbanized alcohol and drug users was that the nonurbanized respondents were less likely to have harsh attitudes toward drug users.

Social reinforcement. Substance-using respondents were asked about their experience and knowledge of the health-related effects of the substance they used. Among smokers and alcohol drinkers, urbanized respondents were significantly more likely than nonurbanized respondents to think that smoking and drinking affected one's health and to know about the health hazards of smoking and drinking. Among drug users, urbanized respondents were more likely than nonurbanized respondents to report that using drugs had affected their work, health, and lives negatively; however, the differences were not statistically significant.

The attitudes of substance users and nonusers (by substance) on these same items were also compared. Cigarette smokers were significantly more likely than nonsmokers (at a level of $p < 0.00$) to think that drug use could be an enlightening experience and that it could help people cope with pressures at work and pressures caused by social change or problems. Nonsmokers were more likely than smokers (at a level of $p < 0.00$) to think that drug use destroys family and social relationships and that drug users cannot be trusted. They were also more likely than smokers (at a level of $p < 0.05$) to think that drug use automatically leads to moral collapse, that one should not experiment with drugs even once, and that the dangers of drug use were not overplayed. There were no significant differences between urbanized and nonurbanized smokers on these items.

Alcohol drinkers were significantly more likely than nondrinkers (at a level of $p < 0.00$) to think that drug use could be an enlightening experience, that the dangers of drug use were overplayed, and that drugs could help a person cope with the pressures of work or social change or problems. Conversely, nondrinkers were more likely than drinkers (at a level of $p < 0.00$) to think that experimenting with drugs even once was bad, that drug users could not be trusted, and that drug use destroys family and social relationships, has a negative effect on a person's health, and promotes crime. Drinkers, however, were more likely than nondrinkers (at a level of $p < 0.05$) to think that it is important to be informed about the effects of drug use on a person's health. The major difference to emerge between urbanized and nonurbanized alcohol drinkers was that urbanized drinkers were more likely than nonurbanized drinkers to think that drug use destroys family and social relationships.

In looking at drug users, again the strongest pattern of differences was found between users and nonusers, rather than between urbanized and nonurbanized users. Drug users were significantly more likely than nonusers (at a level of $p < 0.00$) to think that experimenting with and using drugs could be enlightening and help one cope with work and social pressures. Nonusers were more likely than users to think that drug users can't be trusted and that drug use destroys family and social relationships, automatically leads to moral collapse, leads to crime, and has a negative effect on a person's health. Nonusers were also more likely than drug users to think that it is important to be informed about the effects of drug use on a person's health. Only two significant differences were found between urbanized and nonurbanized drug users. Urbanized users agreed with the statements, "Drug users can't be trusted," and "Drugs destroy good social relationships with family and friends," while nonurbanized drug users disagreed with these questions/statements.

CONCLUSIONS

The results of this study are consistent with research that has found that the sociocultural environment has an important effect on people's substance use attitudes, norms, and behaviors (Berry, 1980; Hunter, 1990; Jones Webb, Hsiao, & Hannan, 1995; Ong & Isralowitz, 1996; Trimble, 1996). Radical social change caused by the urbanization of Negev Bedouin Arabs is a major factor contributing to the breakdown of traditional social structures and the development of substance use and abuse patterns among male youth and young adults.

The findings reveal that a number of substances are being used in the Bedouin community. The majority of the respondents (64 percent) reported using cigarettes. A much higher proportion of the nonurbanized than the urbanized Bedouin respondents smoked; further research is needed to confirm and better understand this finding. Since tobacco is a traditionally accepted substance, its use is not necessarily associated with the breakdown of social norms and values. Smokers, however, were more likely than nonsmokers to be school dropouts, to know youth who used alcohol and drugs, and to know how to obtain these substances in their own communities. This suggests that Bedouin who smoke are more likely than nonsmokers to observe and model the behavior of other substance users as well as bond with their substance-using peers.

Nearly one-third of the respondents reported using alcohol, and 15 percent reported using illegal drugs. In both cases, the proportion was the same among urbanized and nonurbanized respondents. While rates of alcohol use among the Bedouin in the sample are lower than those in Israeli society in general, they are unexpectedly high for a traditional Moslem community. Weiss and colleagues (1999) identified a similar phenomenon in their review of substance use studies among Arabs in Israel, Jordan, and the Palestinian Authority that they attributed to secularization, exposure to the alcohol and drug consumption patterns of Israelis, and to Western culture in general (through television, tourists, etc.). The rates of cannabis and hard drug use found among the Bedouin in the sample are higher than those found among adults in Israeli society in general (Rahav, Teichman, Gil, Rosenblum, and Bar-Hamburger, 1998).

Study data show that an association exists between substance use (i.e., alcohol and illicit drugs) and the breakdown of traditional social structures. Alcohol and drug users were more likely than nonusers to be not married, not living with the extended family, and nonreligious. In addition, drug users were more likely than nonusers to have dropped out of school. Both drinkers and drug users were more likely than nonusers (regardless of their urbanization status) to believe that there were substance abuse problems in their communities and to know youth who used substances. They were more open than nonusers to experimenting with drugs and expressed less fearful and more tolerant attitudes toward drug users. They were less opposed than nonusers to the idea of their children skipping school, drinking alcohol, and using drugs. The vast majority of Bedouin substance users in the sample were under the age of 35. This suggests that substance use (particularly alcohol and illicit drugs) is a new phenomenon being introduced to a society in transition—one that is being exposed to new social values, norms, and behavioral patterns that conflict with the traditional.

In terms of substance use patterns, fewer differences than anticipated were found to exist between those from urbanized and nonurbanized settlements. The study data provide some information that may account for this outcome. The earliest pattern of substance use (cigarettes and cannabis) tends to begin between the ages of 15 and 18, when all Bedouin youth are either studying in high school in the urban settlements or, if they have dropped out of school, are most likely to be employed within the larger Jewish economic infrastructure. Three-quarters of the respondents from the nonurbanized communities reported having a paid job at the time of the interview, indicating that for most, their livelihood did not come from traditional Bedouin economic pursuits of herding and agriculture. Thus, the socioeconomic environment of most Bedouin encompasses both urbanized and nonurbanized Bedouin communities, as well as Israeli Jewish communities and work contexts.

This means that, regardless of urbanization status, Bedouin are exposed to conflicting values and behavioral norms, greater substance availability (including that of hard drugs), and different opportunities for social bonding.

A number of differences with regard to the social impact of substance use were found among urban and nonurban respondents. Nonurban respondents were more strongly opposed than urbanized respondents to considering drug use as something that could be accepted, tolerated, or ignored by the community. Also, they expressed more conservative attitudes about the behavior of their youth (vis-à-vis missing school, using drugs, and alcohol, socializing with drug and alcohol users, etc.) than their urban counterparts, and they were generally more dissatisfied with the behavior of their youth. While nonurban Bedouin have resisted the move to towns, the data show that the nonurban youth in the sample (who are either in high school in urban Bedouin settlements or dropouts working in Jewish towns or establishments) are adopting substance use behaviors negatively associated with urbanization at the same rate as youth living in the urban settlements.

A number of differences were found between urban and nonurban substance users. Urban users were more aware than nonurban users of the negative effects of substance use on their health and work. In addition, urban alcohol and drug users were more likely than nonurban users to believe that drug use destroys family and social relationships. Traditionally in Arab culture, maintenance of family and social relationships and conformity to accepted social behavior and norms were given paramount importance (Barakat, 1993). This was even more true among the Bedouin, for whom the family and tribe were the primary source of social power and protection. Nonurban respondents, in general, and drug and alcohol users, in particular, tend to be less inclined than their urbanized counterparts to believe that substance use could destroy family and social relationships. The fact that urban users thought this was indeed a possibility suggests that within the context of urbanization, substance use could cause a breakdown in social cohesion.

Overall, the respondents expressed general dissatisfaction with the social changes occurring in the Bedouin community. As documented in the literature, stress caused by radical social change can lead to the disruption of cultural norms at the group level and to substance use at the individual level. The findings of this study suggest the presence of the same phenomenon among the Bedouin respondents interviewed. The smokers, drinkers, and drug users in the sample were more likely than the nonusers to view drug use as a mechanism for coping with the pressures of social change. Furthermore, substance users (both urban and nonurban) exhibited higher levels of dissatisfaction with services and social life in their communities than nonusers did. The fact that this dissatisfaction cuts across urbanization status suggests that it is not simply related to the objective level of services, but may well be another indication that substance users have more trouble functioning or adapting to change.

REFERENCES

Abu Saad, I. (1991a, October 19). *Substance abuse among Negev Bedouin Arab youth.* Paper presented at the 2nd Annual Conference on Health Issues in the Arab Sector in Israel, Nazareth.

———. (1991b). Toward an understanding of minority education in Israel: The case of the Bedouin Arabs of the Negev. *Comparative Education, 27,* 235–242.

———. (1996a). Provision of public educational services and access to higher education among the Negev Bedouin Arabs in Israel. *Journal of Education Policy, 11,* 527–541.

———. (1996b). *Substance abuse among Negev Bedouin Arab youth in planned and unplanned settlements.* Report submitted to the Ministry of Health, Southern District: Beer Sheva (in Hebrew).

———. (1997). The education of Israel's Negev Bedouin: Background and prospects. *Israel Studies, 2,* 21–39.

———. (1999a, July 8). *Bedouin Arabs in Southern Israel.* Paper presented at the Interim Conference of RC05—Race and Ethnicity—of the International Sociological Association, Jerusalem.

———. (1999b). *The influence of settlement on substance use and abuse among nomadic populations in Israel and Kenya.* Beer Sheva: Center for Bedouin Studies and Development, Ben-Gurion University of the Negev.

Akers, R. L. (1977). *Deviant behavior: A social learning perspective.* Belmont, CA: Wadsworth.

———. (1992). *Drugs, alcohol and society: Social structure, process and policy.* Belmont, CA: Wadsworth.

Bailey, C. (1995). Dispossessed of the desert. *The Jerusalem Report,* January 26.

Bandura, A. (1986). *Social foundations of thought and action: A social cognitive theory.* Englewood Cliffs, NJ: Prentice-Hall.

Barakat, H. (1993). *The Arab world: Society, culture, and state.* Berkeley: University of California Press.

Ben-David, J. (1991). *The condition of the Negev Bedouin.* Jerusalem: Jerusalem Institute for Israel Research (in Hebrew).

Berry, F. (1980). Social and cultural change. In H. C. Triandis & R. Brislin (Eds.), *Handbook of cross-cultural psychology: Social psychology* (Vol. 5). Boston: Allyn and Bacon.

Berry, F., Trimble, J. E., & Olmedo, E. (1986). Assessment of acculturation. In W. J. Lonner & J. W. Berry (Eds.), *Field methods in cross-cultural research* (pp. 219–234). Newbury Park, CA: Sage Publications.

Braucht, G. N., Brakarsh, D., Follinstad, D., & Berry, K. L. (1973). Deviant drug use in adolescence: A review of psychological correlates. *Psychological Bulletin, 79,* 92–106.

Brook, J. S. (1993). Interactional theory: Its utility in explaining drug use behavior among African-American and Puerto Rican youth. In M. R. De La Rosa & J. L. Recio Adrados (Eds.), *Drug abuse among minority youth: Advances in research and methodology* (pp. 79–101). National Institute on Drug Abuse Research Monograph Series 130. (U.S. Department of Health and Human Services Publication No. 93-3479). Washington, DC: U.S. Government Printing Office.

Chi, I., Lubben, J. E., & Kitano, H. H. (1989). Differences in drinking behavior among three Asian-American groups. *Journal of Studies on Alcohol, 50,* 15–23.

Elliott, D. S., Huizinga, D., & Ageton, S. S. (1985). *Explaining delinquency and drug use.* Beverly Hills, CA: Sage Publications.

Falah, G. (1989). Israel state policy towards Bedouin sedentarization in the Negev. *Journal of Palestine Studies, 18,* 71–90.

Flay, B. R., D'Avernas, J. R., Best, J. A., Kersell, M. W., & Ryan, K. B. (1983). Cigarette smoking: Why young people do it and ways of preventing it. In P. J. McGrath & P. Firestone (Eds.), *Pediatric and adolescent behavioral medicine* (pp. 132–183). New York: Springer-Verlag.

Flay, B. R., & Petraitis, J. (1991). Methodological issues in drug use prevention research. In C. G. Leukefeld & W. J. Bukoski (Eds.), *Drug abuse prevention intervention research: Methodological issues* (pp. 81–109). National Institute on Drug Abuse Research Monograph 107. Washington, DC: U.S. Government Printing Office.

Ghanem, A. (1998). State and minority in Israel: The case of ethnic state and the predicament of its minority. *Ethnic and Racial Studies, 21,* 428–448.

Hayton, B. (1998). Israel: Bedouin, *Simpson's World* (Documentary Film). London: BBC.

Hunter, E. (1990). Using a socio-historical frame to analyze Aboriginal self-destructive behavior. *Australian and New Zealand Journal of Psychology, 24,* 191–198.

Isralowitz, R. E., & Telias, D. (1998). *Drug use, policy, and management.* Westport, CT: Praeger Publishers.

Jones Webb, R. L., Hsiao, C. Y., & Hannan, P. (1995). Relationships between socio-economic status and drinking problems among Black and White men. *Alcoholism: Clinical and Experimental Research, 19,* 623–627.

Kandel, D. B. (1982). Epidemiological and psychosocial perspectives on adolescent drug use. *Journal of American Academy of Clinical Psychiatry, 21,* 328–347.

Kiev, A. (1972). *Transcultural psychiatry.* New York: Free Press.

Krohn, M. D., & Thornberry, T. P. (1993). Network theory: A model for understanding drug abuse among African-American and Hispanic youth. In M. R. De La Rosa & J. L. Recio Adrados (Eds.), *Drug abuse among minority youth: Advances in research and methodology* (pp. 102–129). National Institute on Drug Abuse Research Monograph Series 130. (U.S. Department of Health and Human Services Publication No. 93-3479). Washington, DC: U.S. Government Printing Office.

Lustick, I. (1980). *Arabs in the Jewish State: Israel's control of a national minority.* Austin: University of Texas Press.

Maddrell, P. (1990). *The Bedouin of the Negev.* Minority Rights Group Report No. 81, London.

Marx, E. (1967). *The Bedouin of the Negev.* Manchester: Manchester University Press.

Merton, R. K. (1957). *Social theory and social structure.* Glencoe, IL: Free Press.

Murry, D. M., & Perry, C. L. (1985). The prevention of adolescent drug abuse: Implications of etiological, developmental, behavioral and environmental models. In C. L. Jones and R. J. Battjes (Eds.), *Etiology of drug abuse: Implications for prevention* (pp. 236–256). National Institute on Drug Abuse Research Monograph Series 56. Washington, DC: U.S. Government Printing Office.

Oetting, E. R. (1993). Orthogonal cultural identification: Theoretical links between culture identification and substance use. In M. R. De La Rosa & J. L. Recio Adrados (Eds.), *Drug abuse among minority youth: Advances in research and methodology* (pp. 32–56). National Institute on Drug Abuse Research Monograph Series 130. (U.S. Department of Health and Human Services Publication No. 93-3479). Washington, DC: U.S. Government Printing Office.

Ong, H. T., & Isralowitz, R. E. (1996). *Substance use in Singapore: Illegal drugs, inhalants and alcohol.* Singapore: Toppan Company.

Rahav, G., Teichman, M., Gil, R., Rosenblum, Y., & Bar-Hamburger, R. (1998). *The use of psychoactive substances among Israeli citizens 1998: Epidemiological study 4.* Tel Aviv: Pori Institute, Tel Aviv University, Anti-Drug Authority (in Hebrew).

Rodriguez, O., Recio Adrados, J. L., & De La Rosa, M. R. (1993). Integrating mainstream and subcultural explanations of drug use among Puerto Rican youth. In M. R. De La Rosa & J. L. Recio Adrados (Eds.), *Drug abuse among minority youth: Advances in research and methodology* (pp. 8–31). National Institute on Drug Abuse Research Monograph Series 130. (U.S. Department of Health and Human Services Publication No. 93-3479). Washington, DC: U.S. Government Printing Office.

Trimble, J. E. (1996). Acculturation, ethnic identification and the evaluation process. In A. Bayer, F. L. Brisbane, & A. Ramirez (Eds.), *Advanced methodological issues in culturally competent evaluation for substance use prevention. CSAP Cultural Competence Series 6* (pp. 13–62). (U.S. Department of Health and Human Services Publication No. SMA 96-3110). Washington, DC: U.S. Government Printing Office.

Weiss, S., Sawa, G. H., Abdeen, Z., & Yanai, J. (1999). Substance abuse studies and prevention efforts among Arabs in the 1990s in Israel, Jordan and the Palestinian Authority—A literature review. *Addiction, 94,* 177–198.

Wilson, W. J. (1987). *The truly disadvantaged: The inner city, the underclass, and public policy.* Chicago: University of Chicago Press.

PART III

Toward an Understanding of Drug Prevalence Estimation and Evaluation for Palestinian and Israeli Populations

8

Rapid Assessment and Response (RAR) to HIV and Psychoactive Substance Use: Relevance for the Eastern Mediterranean Region

Gundo Weiler, Shekhar Saxena,
Ahmad Mohit, and Andrew Ball

WHY RAPID ASSESSMENT AND RESPONSE?

Since the outbreak of Human Immunodeficiency Virus (HIV) epidemics among injecting drug users, investigating the association between substance use and HIV infection has been high on the World Health Organization's (WHO) agenda. Consequently, as early as 1989, WHO initiated a large comparative study on HIV-transmission and prevention strategies among injecting drug users in 13 cities globally (Stimson, Des Jarlais, & Ball, 1998). Notably, the study was able to identify four major features that distinguished settings where HIV epidemics were averted from those in which HIV epidemics escalated within a short period of time: (a) availability of outreach programs to drug users that were based on a trusting relationship with the provider; (b) access to sterile needles and syringes; (c) access to drug treatment and education; and (d) establishment of such comprehensive responses before the HIV-prevalence among injecting drug users exceeded 5 percent. In short, the study demonstrated that, despite all skepticism, substance users can change their behavior and thus prevent HIV infection if the appropriate interventions are in place.

What the study did not reveal, however, was how these principles are being best translated into specific local action and how resistance to the interventions can be overcome. In this sense, the study reflected a dilemma that has occurred before in other settings, namely the obtaining of general insights at the expense of their applicability. In the 1970s rural developmental experts faced a similar situation in regard to specific problems such as farming, firewood consumption, and water hygiene. Their response, namely the application of multiple qualitative methods at the local level, is now seen as the origin of rapid assessments and the inspiration for WHO to formalize rapid assessment and response (RAR) as a set of tools for generating local knowledge and structures that are indispensable for the successful translation of global experience into community action.

Since the first *Rapid Assessment and Response Guide on Injecting Drug Use* (*IDU-RAR*; World Health Organization, 1998a) was made available in draft form almost four years ago, WHO has complemented the guide with others that specifically address the association between substance use and sexual risk behavior (*SEX-RAR*; World Health Organization, 1998c) and substance use among especially vulnerable young people (*EVYP-RAR*; World Health Organization, 1998b). To date, these guides have been applied in more than 100 cities worldwide. This chapter covers all the RAR work related to HIV and substance use, with special focus on injecting drug use.

What Is RAR?

RAR is a methodology that is suitable to generate knowledge and insights that lead directly to intervention responses. RAR uses well-recognized methods that are applied in traditional social science research. There are several features of RAR, however, that distinguish it from traditional research. Where pure research ideally strives to prove hypotheses under controlled conditions, RAR intends to explore and to innovate. Where research intends to be conclusive and restrictive, RAR aims to be suggestive and creative. And, finally, where a traditional research project concludes with an analysis and reporting of research findings, RAR establishes an ongoing mechanism of assessment, response development, and evaluation. Within the rapid assessment process, these "scientific weaknesses" turn out to be a necessary precondition to reach its goals, namely to base the formulation of research, intervention, and policy priorities on a comprehensive and transparent process. Rather than being just "second-rate research," RAR can serve as an instrument to prepare for more rigorous research in specific areas, based on a process that involves a variety of key stakeholders and is no longer exclusively dominated by the scientific and funding elite. RAR's egalitarian approach is underlined by its adoption not only by research institutions but also by governments, international nongovernmental organizations (NGOs), United Nations agencies, and local NGOs.

Often RAR is applied in settings where public health problems are experienced and appropriate solutions are sought through developing new interventions or upgrading existing ones. In this regard, RAR is not principally distinguishable from many research projects that inform public health responses, even though RAR-based responses might be more numerous and might occur more immediately. The main purpose of RAR, however, is not to generate knowledge but to *prepare* for interventions. In a broad understanding, these interventions might include the initiation of immediate responses, the development of targeted research projects, and the establishment of sustainable coordinating mechanisms and policies. While the basis on which such interventions were designed may be unclear, the benefit of RAR is to increase the transparency of their development, to strengthen their scientific and situational appropriateness, and to foster active participation by affected individuals and communities.

Being neither research nor an intervention, RAR combines *components* that are found in science (data gathering, data analysis) and interventions (community mobilization, immediate response implementation). In addition, RAR includes elements that are found in strategic planning (consultations, programming) and policy development (needs and resource assessment). To this end, RAR might be more comparable to engineering rather than science, which provides a good sense of what RAR wants to achieve: to be the connecting wheel between the above-mentioned domains, which too often function independently or in isolation—if they are in place at all. In this sense, RAR does not aim to replace either of these areas, but rather to act as a complementary and catalyzing mechanism, based on a number of simple principles:

RAR uses multiple methods and data sources to depict the local extent and nature of drug use. A sound knowledge of substance use and its determinants is seen as the starting point for the development of appropriate interventions. In this, RAR emphasizes understanding the local system in which the context of drug use, risk behaviors, and adverse health consequences are closely interrelated. There is no one method, however, suitable to generate insights that will make us understand how such systems work and know the potential entry points for change. Exploring the local situation, therefore, necessitates the application of a range of different methods, each of them proving to be particularly useful with regard to specific information sources. The comprehensiveness of knowledge gained is further enhanced through the use of multiple data sources. This usually includes a review of all existing data, such as previous reports and available statistics, as well as gathering primary data from substance users, health professionals, and other community members. Such an approach resembles a jigsaw puzzle in which, over time, the RAR team connects the various pieces of information gained from different data sources and research methods to arrive at a picture of the whole system.

RAR bridges the gap between research and public health action to develop appropriate interventions. As mentioned earlier, the generation of any knowledge within the RAR process is purposefully directed toward intervention planning. To this end, it is crucial to integrate those who usually develop and implement services relevant to drug users into all stages of the rapid assessment. During the data-gathering process, the inclusion of service providers and health politicians will significantly contribute to the formulation of appropriate questions and facilitate access to a range of data sources that normally might be inaccessible. Even more important, the integration of a range of disciplines in the RAR process is the precondition for the process of translating findings into practical action. This is usually done through a consultation in which research might play a moderating role but which draws heavily on the input and ideas of those who are in daily touch with the situation, be it from the perspective of law enforcement, policy planning, or service provision.

RAR strives to build local alliances through involving the broad community. Rapid assessments in the past relied on foreign experts to conduct the work and provide recommendations. In contrast to that past approach, RAR is rooted in the local community, both in the composition of the RAR team of researchers and the involvement of other community key stakeholders in such RAR activities as regular meetings and consultations. Community involvement goes beyond providing technical advice to the RAR team to building understanding and support in the community for any recommended interventions. Experience shows that, particularly with regard to substance use issues, even a well-justified proposal might meet significant resistance from the general community or specific groups. RAR aims to anticipate this resistance and to walk the community through RAR as a learning process, which enables the community to not only understand the need for action but also actively seek solutions. Ideally, such a process generates feelings of ownership and active support for interventions that are proposed on the basis of the RAR findings.

RAR intends to facilitate rapid results and initiate sustained action. One of the starting points for developing RAR was the insight that traditional research projects often fail to deliver information about successful interventions in a timely fashion. This applies particularly to the context of HIV infection through injecting drug use, where interventions are most efficient and most needed before the HIV prevalence among injecting drug users reaches the critical 5-percent level. To this end, rapidity is central to RAR and is sought through the application of a range of methods in parallel and through inclusion of multiple data sources. For the sake of rapidity, RAR may compromise on the depth of information if it is not seen to be crucial for the development of interventions. A number of examples have shown that rapid assessment may reveal initial viable results in as little as two weeks. RAR should not be seen, however, as a one-shot exercise. Rather, it can be perceived as a start-up for an ongoing process in which situation assessment and the implementation and evaluation of responses complement each other.

How Does RAR Work?

Because its approach is flexible, each RAR will necessarily be distinct from any other RAR in terms of activities performed as well as in terms of outcomes and recommendations. Experience shows, however, that certain steps are crucial in enhancing the success of RAR. Such a standardized approach to RAR can be best described along five steps.

Step 1: Recruiting the RAR team. Rapid assessments may be initiated by a variety of interest groups, such as the government, research institutions, or service providers, or by members of the target group themselves. As a first step, usually a small number of people are sought to take responsibility for the execution of the rapid assessment and who undertake the day-to-day work. Ideally, this core RAR team should include members from a variety of professional backgrounds, including social science research, service provision, and policy planning. Such a multidisciplinary approach is desirable to enhance both the range of skills of the RAR team and the scope of entry points to the community. Thus, the RAR team will evaluate the situation from different perspectives and be able to cross-check data whenever appropriate. This procedure is essential to ensuring a high degree of validity of the research results. In addition to the representation of different professions on the RAR team, it has been proven that a mix of people from other societal backgrounds can be useful. This also refers to a balance of genders and the representation of individuals who are close to the age of the target group. A core RAR team normally consists of three to six individuals who might be supported by individuals who are specifically trained for certain purposes such as interviewing substance users in the field. It is crucial, however, that the RAR team members be given the chance to devote a significant proportion of their time throughout the rapid assessment process in order to be the driving force that keeps up the momentum behind the local effort (see Figure 8.1; Peleru, 2000).

Step 2: Building community alliances. A rapid assessment is unlikely to achieve its aim unless it receives broad community support. It is crucial, therefore, to include all those members into the assessment process who have the potential to support or to obstruct the RAR process and follow-up. Often, an exercise in mapping power in the community will reveal insights into who these potential allies might be. Some of the most frequently mentioned people with regard to assessments on psychoactive substance use include health authorities, law enforcement agencies and police, religious leaders, members of the media, and, of course, users themselves. The objective of community involvement in RAR is to make these key stakeholders part of the process from the outset rather than to confront them with the findings after the conclusion of RAR. Many sites found the establishment of community advisory boards a practical and feasible way to ensure community involvement. Again, it is important to make these boards active participants in the RAR process and not to

Figure 8.1
Case Example: RAR in Romania

In 1999 the Romanian Institute of Health Services Management initiated a rapid assessment on injecting drug use. The composition of a multidisciplinary RAR team allowed for using a range of methods and access points to a variety of data sources, including:

Secondary data from police, customs, prisons, drug treatment centers, emergency rooms, school health inspectorates, and ministries.

Primary data collection through observation, focus groups, key informant interviews, and application of estimation techniques.

Figure 8.2
Case Example: RAR in India

In 1998, a consortium of governmental and nongovernmental organizations (NGOs) in Madras, South India, conducted an RAR on injecting drug use. Prior to the assessment being conducted, a community advisory board of 20 members was established, involving representatives from the police, the community council, the youth federation, Narcotics Anonymous, women's groups, scheduled casts, and prominent Moslem, Hindu, and Christian citizens. The board was entirely responsible for the evolution and implementation of RAR.

In addition, RAR results were disseminated during a two-day advocacy meeting with more than 60 participants.

Both activities contributed to the endorsement of an RAR-based action plan by senior government officials, leading NGOs, drug treatment professionals, and users.

merely inform them on the proceedings and results. Tasks of the advisory board might encompass steering and supporting the assessment phase, active participation in the process of translating findings into responses and, most notably, establishing a climate that enables interventions to be implemented thereafter. With regard to the latter, it has been demonstrated that community ownership plays a crucial role. To enhance such ownership, some sites found it beneficial to assign official responsibility for the entire rapid assessment to the board, with the RAR team merely being its executing arm (see Figure 8.2; Kumar et al., 2000).

Step 3: Mapping key areas of assessment. Once an RAR team has been formed and community support established, information gathering will commence. The challenge is to embrace factors that contribute to the onset of adverse social and health consequences among drug users as well as factors that potentially protect individuals from the development of such adverse consequences. In reality, these factors are likely to be interwoven and constitute a complex system that is determined by components at the individual level, the community level, and the national level. Even though interventions initiated at a later date might specifically target one of these components, developing an understanding of the whole seems imperative in order to assess the intervention's potential benefits. Recognizing that such a whole is difficult to grasp, RAR proposes to focus the assessment on four main areas. First, the *context assessment* aims to determine the local mix of social, religious, and cultural characteristics that encourage or discourage drug use and possible interventions (see Context Assessment case example: Siri & Inchaurraga, 2000). A characteristic example for this assessment area is the legal and organizational framework under which substance users are addressed. Second, the *drug use and risk behaviors assessment* aims to describe the nature, scope, and trends of drug use in the local context and to identify behaviors that put drug users at risk. Classical examples embrace the exact description of drug consumption patterns, including

Figure 8.3
Case Example: Context Assessment

In Rosario, Argentina, it was found that a particular law can be used to punish any institution that publishes information on safer methods of using drugs. This *context finding* was seen as an important hurdle in the process of ameliorating existing educational material.

needle-sharing practices (also see Risk Behavior Assessment case example: C. Fitch, personal communication, 1997). Third, the *health consequences assessment* seeks to determine the nature and extent of adverse social and health consequences of psychoactive substance use. Obviously, in many settings, this assessment focuses on a description of the spread of blood-borne diseases, including HIV and hepatitis. Fourth, a *thorough intervention assessment* will depict the existing range of prevention and treatment interventions for drug users and explore the potential for future improvements. This part of the assessment process prepares the grounds for proposed RAR-based ameliorations later on (see Figures 8.3 and 8.4).

Step 4: Translating findings into action. Proposing interventions that are both effective and acceptable to the community is the primary objective of the rapid assessment. The success of this stage will depend heavily on how the previous steps were implemented, as all of them play a decisive role in the intervention development process: the interdisciplinary RAR team as the driving force that moderates a consultation among key community stakeholders; the advisory body as the main resource for intervention entry points and political support; and a comprehensive knowledge of the situation as a basis for discussions about possible interventions. The notion of "intervention" in this understanding refers to a broad spectrum of activities that might be seen as suitable to ameliorate the current situation. Such activities are not only restricted to the establishment of potentially cost-intensive new services, but might also include the refinement of existing services and policies. Even the initiation of further, traditional research might be part of the RAR recommendations. Usually, such recommendations are summarized in an action

Figure 8.4
Case Example: Risk Behavior Assessment

In Odessa, Ukraine, drug production included a testing system in which one drug user assesses the quality of the drug solution through filling his syringe from a common container and injecting the drug. In the distribution process, 50 percent of all drugs were sold in prefilled syringes. Drug consumption itself proved to often include group settings with a high prevalence of sharing patterns. All three findings were seen to represent important risks factors for transmission of blood-borne diseases through injecting drug use.

Figure 8.5
Case Example: RAR in the Russian Federation

In September 1997, Médecins Sans Frontières-Holland started a training program in the Russian Federation that eventually resulted in rapid assessments being completed in 28 cities by local professionals.

The results revealed a wealth of insights in similarities and differences in local problems and resources. Consequently, each of the resulting action plans included a different combination of interventions, tailored toward what was needed and feasible in the community.

As a result of the RAR, harm reduction programs were established in 14 cities, each of them embracing a unique mix of mass media campaigns, vaccination, and/or outreach work to drug users and sex workers, various drug treatment services, HIV and STI testing, and establishment of prison programs.

plan. Experience shows that the action plan has to be based on a skillfully moderated debate among the various participating groups and individuals. In order to support this process, RAR proposes a number of steps that for each key finding explores general responses and the relevance, effectiveness, and feasibility of possible specific interventions, as well as possible obstacles to the intervention. Such a discussion is likely to result in a mix of proposed interventions that takes maximum advantage of existing local capacities (see Figure 8.5; Burrows et al., 2000).

Step 5: Sustaining the difference. Usually rapid assessments will not only result in locally specific action plans but will also create a powerful momentum of community awareness and involvement. This momentum is, in itself, an important outcome of the RAR, and sustaining it should be given high priority. For instance, some sites succeeded in keeping the advisory board functioning as an ongoing forum for information exchange and coordination. The advisory board can also serve as a platform for fundraising, overseeing the implementation of interventions, and, eventually, playing an important role in their evaluation. Ideally, such sustained involvement will result in an ongoing process in which regular reassessments of the situation are accompanied by continuous refinement of existing interventions, which again will be subject to evaluation (see Figure 8.6; Sutherland, 1999).

Examples of Rapid Assessment and Response Initiatives in the Region

The use of RAR methods in the Eastern Mediterranean region of WHO are still at an initial level. Some initiatives, however, have been launched. These are briefly described here.

A summary of the results of two *Rapid Assessment and Response Studies* recently done in Egypt and Iran and a limited study performed in Pakistan are

Figure 8.6
Case Example: RAR Canada

In Canada the national health authorities commissioned a rapid assessment on drug use in 1998. Findings of this RAR were incorporated in the national drug strategy. This included the development of a set of indicators for drug use and adverse social and health consequences based on the assessment findings. In addition, it was decided to periodically reassess the situation.

presented here. A part of this material was presented to the "Intercountry Consultation on Development of Guidelines for Demand Reduction in Substance Abuse with Special Emphasis on Injecting Drug Use" held by the WHO Eastern Mediterranean Regional Office (EMRO) in November 1999 in Beirut, Lebanon.

Egypt

The Rapid Assessment Study in Egypt took place between 1998 and 1999 under the auspices of the Ministry of Health and United Nations International Drug Control Programme (UNDCP.) The primary purpose of this study was to provide original data collected from the drug users to complement the existing survey and research material, particularly data from the National Research on Addiction. To this end, a National Scientific Committee was convened to oversee and guide the project.

Five study sites were identified to provide a geographically and socioeconomically representative sample. A cross-sectional survey was conducted at each site using a semistructured interview schedule. Respondents were recruited and interviewed at a number of treatment centers, as well from the community (cafes, schools, streets, etc.). A total of 696 interviews were conducted. The sites and samples were Cairo, 177; Gharbiah, 144; Ismailiah, 140; Qena, 125; and South Sinai, 110.

Although differences were noted among the research sites, common features of substance use were the widespread use of bango (cannabis herb) and alcoholic beverages. Use of psychotropic substances and heroin injecting were more common in the large urban centers. In general, 17 percent of the subjects interviewed reported injecting as their main route of drug use. One-third of the injecting drug users reported sharing injecting equipment with friends, and 13 percent reported sharing such equipment with strangers. Nearly two-thirds of the injection users reported "always sterilizing injecting equipment" if reusing it, although 16 percent reported no sterilization. Thirty percent of the sample had adequate knowledge about the various ways of transmitting HIV, but knowledge on hepatitis was less thorough.

Analysis of the data confirmed the findings of the National Research on Addiction regarding the vulnerability of 15-to-20-year-olds in terms of initiation of drug use. Consistently, "friends," "curiosity," and "invitation/gift" were given as reasons for first drug use. Peer pressure was strongly correlated with drug use in this age group.

Concerns regarding health, family, and finance were given as reasons for stopping drug use, and informal help was often sought from family members. Opportunity for access to treatment was not evenly distributed throughout the country.

Islamic Republic of Iran

The Rapid Situation Assessment (RSA) of Drug Abuse in Iran was performed in 1998–1999 and involved the Prevention Department of the Iranian Welfare Organization and the UNDCP. Consistent with other assessment efforts, data and information were collected from multiple sources and multiple categories of key informants. In this study, drug users, members of their families, and other key informants were interviewed. Due to a number of difficulties in recruiting drug users by traditional random sampling methods, the sampling was done by using innovative methods in each site. All the newcomers attending the treatment centers during the study period were included in the assessment. Drug users in prisons were recruited if they were new inmates who were registered 30 days prior to the start of the study. Drug abusers in the street were selected by using a snowball sampling strategy that included ex-drug-using key informants who were members of the research team. The study was limited in terms of not revealing drug use prevalence, being restricted to urban settings, and not having a representative sample of drug users. The information collected, however, revealed the clearest picture of substance use in the country. Selected results regarding injecting drug use from this study included:

Injecting drug use. Almost 22 percent of the subjects interviewed had a history of ever having injected drugs. The mean age of injecting drug users in the sample was 31.7, and the mean age for starting to inject was 26.3. About half of the injecting drug users reported injecting two to three times a day. Almost always, an intravenous route was used. About half of the sample reported having shared syringes and needles. Sharing of needles was reported by 70 percent of the drug injectors recruited from the streets. Pharmacies were the most common source of syringes and needles. Key informants in the prison system believed that, in spite of strong security and control measures, drug injecting took place inside the prisons, albeit infrequently. Used and handmade needles (also known as pumps) and droppers were used to inject in the prisons.

In light of the fact that injecting has not been the favorite route of drug use in Iran, these findings point to a new trend that needs to be taken seriously. Many of the key informants who were interviewed have also pointed out that injecting drug use seems to be rapidly growing. The findings of the study in the area of sexual behavior of the drug-using respondents make this issue even more important. About one-third of the married respondents reported having had sexual intercourse outside of marriage. This figure was about 50 percent for the divorced or separated respondents and over 70 percent for unmarried respondents. The rates for condom use at the time of last sexual intercourse was reported to be 32 percent for the single and only 20 percent for the divorced or separated respondents. Together, these findings show the potential dangers involved with injecting drug use and the transmission of HIV. The problem of such transmission was evident in 1996–1997 with the prison outbreaks of HIV/AIDS.

Pakistan

The total number of people who are afflicted with substance use disorders in Pakistan is estimated to be around three million. The traditional routes of taking drugs have been inhaling heroin on foil (chasing the dragon) and smoking. Currently, there are indications of a serious increase in injecting drug use The issue has become even more serious since the official publication of a combined UNDCP and UNAIDS report in December 1999: "Baseline Study of the Relationship between Injecting Drug Use, HIV and Hepatitis C among Male Injecting Drug Users in Lahore."

The baseline study of injecting drug users in Lahore, undertaken in January and February 1999, revealed an alarmingly high rate of infection by hepatitis C virus (HCV) among the study population. The study results suggest the potential for an even greater public health challenge in the form of an epidemic of HIV once the virus enters this highly vulnerable population. In addition, there is the possibility of a more generalized HIV epidemic as a result of secondary transmission through sexual activity. The study results will have important implications for the formulation of Pakistan's strategies regarding illicit drug use, especially among injecting drug users, and for the development of plans for programs of HIV/AIDS awareness and prevention.

There is very little documentation of the extent and nature of the injecting drug use problem in Pakistan. Anecdotal evidence suggests that injecting is on the rise, and findings from this study suggest that injecting drug use is becoming increasingly popular in the early stages of drug dependency among drug users in Pakistan. Drug treatment services are limited, and such services that are available are often not easily accessible to injecting drug users.

Of the 200 study respondents, 178 (89 percent) tested positive for HCV, and no respondent tested positive for HIV. This extremely high HCV infection rate combined with high rates of acknowledged needle sharing (64 percent) and very limited awareness of proper needle sterilization procedures indicate that there is a considerable danger for transmission of blood-borne infections in this population.

The study results dispel the notion that drug dependents are sexually inactive, since just over half of the respondents reported involvement in sexual activity of varying types and frequencies within the previous year. In addition, nearly one-half (48.5 percent) of the study respondents reported having had sex with commercial sex workers. These findings indicate the danger for secondary transmission to the general population through sexual activity.

Finally, the study suggests that a shift from smoking or sniffing heroin to injection of polydrug "cocktails" is rapidly occurring. Forty-nine percent of the respondents had switched to injecting from smoking or other oral drug use within the previous year. The drug cocktails being injected by the study respondents are composed of combinations of legal prescription drugs (easily available over the counter without prescription) and illegal drugs. Research in other parts of Asia indicates that diffusion of new patterns of drug use, and shifts from opiate smoking to drug injecting in particular, may be an important contributing factor to rapid increases in HIV infection levels among injecting drug users. The possibility that a shift in drug use is currently occurring in Pakistan may be an important early warning sign necessitating a call to action.

Judging from experiences of greater work in this region, not only will a better understanding of the situation in the region result from the use of RAR, but the RAR methodology will itself get richer and more effective. The unique sociocultural environment of this region poses a lot of challenges as well as offers solutions.

CONCLUSION

Experience with the use of RAR shows that it is useful where drug use is emerging and is subject to rapid change. This finding is particularly important in terms of monitoring the extent of blood-borne diseases such as HIV in the community of psychoactive substance users and being able to respond to the spread of the use and abuse of other harmful substances through appropriate intervention policies and programs.

During a regional consultation for the development of guidelines for demand reduction organized by the WHO Eastern Mediterranean Regional Office held in November 1999, governmental representatives uniformly expressed concern about the recent introduction of HIV into this part of the world (World Health Organization, 1998d). While still in an early low-level epidemic stage, the spread of HIV among drug injectors poses a serious threat to the health and welfare of the region. This is only one reason, but an important one, to use Rapid Assessment and Response in response to psychoactive substance use in the Eastern Mediterranean region.

REFERENCES

Burrows, D., Trautmann, F., Frost, L., Bijl, M., Sarankov, Y., Sarang, A., & Chernenko, O. (2000). Processes and outcome of training on rapid assessment and response methods on injecting drug use and related HIV infection in the Russian Federation. *International Journal of Drug Policy, 11,* 151–167.

Kumar, M. S., Mudaliar, S., Thyagarajan, S. P., Kumar, S., Selvanayagam, A., & Daniels, D. (2000). Rapid assessment and response to injecting drug use in Madras, South India. *International Journal of Drug Policy, 11,* 83–98.

Peleru, G. (2000). Injecting drug use in Romania. *International Journal of Drug Policy, 11,* 145–150.

Siri, P., & Inchaurraga S. (2000). "First Steps": Using rapid assessment and response methods to develop research, intervention and advocacy capacity for addressing drug use in Rosario City, Argentina. *International Journal of Drug Policy, 11,* 125–132.

Stimson, G. V., Des Jarlais, D. C., & Ball A. (Eds.). (1998). *Drug injecting and HIV infection.* London: Taylor and Francis.

Sutherland, D. (1999). *Results of a rapid assessment and response in Canada.* Oral report to the World Health Organization, Geneva, Switzerland.

World Health Organization. (1998a). *Rapid assessment and response guide for injecting drug use (IDU-RAR).* Draft for Field Testing, Geneva, Switzerland.

———. (1998b). *Rapid assessment and response guide for substance use among especially vulnerable young people (EVYP-RAR).* Draft for Field Testing, Geneva, Switzerland.

———. (1998c). *Rapid assessment and response guide for substance use and sexual risk behaviour (SEX-RAR).* Draft for Field Testing, Geneva, Switzerland.

———, Regional Office for the Eastern Mediterranean. (1998d). *Draft report on the intercountry consultation for the development of guidelines for demand reduction in substance abuse with special emphasis on injecting drug use.* Alexandria, Egypt.

9

Middle East Drug Use Watch (MEDUW): A Trilateral System to Measure the Type and Extent of Psychoactive Substance Use in Palestinian and Israeli Communities

Richard Rawson, Albert Hasson, Richard Isralowitz, and Mohammed Afifi

INTRODUCTION

Drug abuse is a worldwide problem that has damaged the health, social institutions, and political stability of many countries. Drug abuse, like many other health and social problems, is not static. Different drug problems emerge in different places at different times and produce a complex and sometimes unpredictable set of problems. For example, in the United States, cocaine had been viewed for decades as an interesting but generally unimportant drug of abuse. However, in the 1980s, the greater availability of cocaine resulting from increased coca production in South America combined with the development of smokable forms of cocaine (i.e., "crack") produced a national emergency. Similarly, in the past decade in the western and rural areas of the United States, methamphetamine production and use have devastated small rural towns, creating health care and law enforcement problems in epidemic proportions.

The rapid emergence of new, powerfully disruptive, and dangerous drug abuse problems is not limited to the United States. For example, health and law enforcement reports indicate that methamphetamine-related problems are very significant and increasing in the Philippines and other areas in Southeast Asia. Similarly, there are numerous reports that in many areas of the former Soviet Union and in India, heroin use is rapidly escalating. Furthermore, World Health Organization (WHO) reports (M. Monteiro, personal communication) indicate that for the first time there is significant evidence of substantial amounts of heroin use in developing countries, including many African nations. In all of these situations, drug abuse is a concern in its own right; however, there are many who are equally or more concerned about the associated sequellae of drug use. There is extensive evidence that illicit drug use is a major contributor to crime. Drug trafficking and the property crime associated with the acquisition of drugs often can overload and corrupt law enforcement and judicial systems. Of equal concern are the health care concerns from HIV, hepatitis, and TB transmission, which in some parts of the world are primarily associated with injection drug use and prostitution related to drug acquisition. Clearly, drug abuse and its associated problems are of great importance to the health and social stability of all world communities.

SUBSTANCE USE IN THE MIDDLE EAST

There is reason to believe that the societies of the Middle East are not immune to the problems of substance use and abuse. In fact, data collected during the 1990s suggest that drug and alcohol use has increased throughout the area (Rahav, Teichman, Gil, Rosenblum, & Bar-Hamburger, 1995,1998; Teichman, Rahav, & Barnea, 1994). A recent review article catalogued what is known about the nature and extent of substance use among the people of the many diverse cultures and religions of the Middle East (Weiss, Sawa, Abdeen, & Yanai, 1999). Particular attention is given to creating a compendium of the studies that have been conducted on the topic of substance abuse published in the 1990s. Included in the review is a description of the traditions and religious positions toward the use of substances among Moslems, Christians, Jews, and the Druze. Similarly, the article contains reports that focus on the geographical areas of Jordan, Israel, and the areas of the Palestinian Authority (West Bank communities and Gaza). Many of the studies draw on relatively small samples of individuals who are selected from convenience samples or from larger samples of individuals who have participated in large-scale surveys.

The Weiss and colleagues (Weiss et al., 1999) article provides an extraordinarily thorough compilation of the substance abuse research that has been reported from the Israeli, Palestinian, and Jordanian communities during the past decade. Based on the information presented in these reports, it has been found that substance users differ substantially among these communities. It appears that there are higher rates of alcohol use among Israeli youth than among Arab youth. The rates of drug use among Arab youth living in Israel appear higher than for youth living in Palestinian or Jordanian communities. Within the Moslem populations, the drug use of the Jordanians appears to be more widespread, but the drug use among the Palestinians appears to frequently involve multiple drugs. Of particular interest was the observation that even though there are religious prohibitions against substance use by Moslems, there was a perception from the compiled reports that the use of substances among young Arabs was accelerating at a much higher rate than among Jewish youth. If increased rates of substance use accompany the changes in the Palestinian society that are likely to accompany the emerging Palestinian State, there could be severe negative sequellae. Increased rates of substance use by Palestinian youth could greatly increase the crime and health care costs that accompany substance use problems. Furthermore, the damage to social and religious norms resulting from substance abuse problems can lead to a backlash of anger and animosity toward the presumed "cause" of the emergent problem. As is true in much of the world, the "cause" of substance abuse problems is viewed as members of "the other" cultural group of that area. In the case of these cultures, it is not difficult to imagine the substance abuse problem of both Israelis and Palestinians being causally attributed to the opposite group. In fact, this has already occurred.

As noted by Weiss and colleagues (Weiss et al., 1999), many of the reports used data collected by a wide variety of survey strategies, many of which were methodologically flawed. The impressions distilled from these reports clearly suggest that there are substance abuse problems in this part of the world, and they appear to be growing. The potential for substance abuse-related issues to create serious problems for the policymakers and leaders in the Middle East is quite real and profound. However, at the present time it is impossible to accurately gauge the extent of the problem. Surveys done with school children are exquisitely sensitive to the social taboos of the situation. In a culture where substance use is religiously prohibited and a source of family shame, it is very possible that the substance use of participants is significantly underreported. Conversely, surveys of treatment seeking or treatment participants frequently overestimate the frequency and amounts of substances used. Thus we do not yet know the extent of substance use in these Middle East communities. A major recommendation from Weiss and colleagues' (Weiss et al., 1999) review was to establish a process for accurately measuring drug trends and to include the leaders and communities involved in that process.

Why is it important to have data on the nature and extent of substance abuse in Palestinian and Israeli communities? There is a wealth of data to support the contention that psychoactive substance use (alcohol, tobacco, and illicit drugs) plays a major role in the public health, criminal justice, and political agendas of many of the world's nations. Although there is wide geographical and cultural variation in the nature and extent of substance use and abuse, no society is completely free from the problems of drugs and alcohol. There is consensus that if the types and amounts of substances being used are known and if it is known by whom and where substances are being used, health care, educational, social service, and criminal justice resources can be more effectively allocated. Within the complex, interconnected societies that exist under the Israeli government and the Palestinian Authority, the development of a system for identifying and monitoring the psychoactive substance use trends could provide a wealth of valuable information.

Currently, in Israel, drug treatment admission data suggest that the immigration of large numbers of Russians during recent years is associated with an increase in the heroin problem (J. Gleser, personal communication). Anecdotal reports from methadone clinics in Beer Sheva and other parts of Israel suggest that many of the new immigrants arrive in Israel with severe addictions to opiates and that there is great concern about the rates of HIV and hepatitis among this group of injection drug users. Palestinian health officials describe what they believe are increasing rates of alcohol, cannabis, and heroin use among the youth of the West Bank, but there are no data to clearly assess this situation (V. Fasheh, personal communication). Similarly, in the more shielded and conservative society in Gaza, there are anecdotal reports of major increases in what were previously very low rates of alcohol use among the youth of the cities and the large refugee camps (M. Afifi, personal communication).

Accurate information on this issue could be used by Israeli and Palestinian policymakers to plan a response to the substance use problems of the region. Public health officials would have a vastly better understanding of what groups of individuals were using what types of substances in which communities. In those circumstances in which drugs were being used by injection, infectious disease agencies could be involved. In those cases where youth are involved, prevention efforts could be intensified and made relevant to the substances used (e.g., heroin prevention efforts have little impact on alcohol use levels). In areas where the availability of drugs appears to be extreme, law enforcement efforts could be intensified. In short, the policymakers from both the Palestinian and Israeli governments would be more capable of making effective responses if they had good data.

At this time, there is inadequate information to accurately assess the type or extent of illicit drug use and drug-related health problems (e.g., HIV, hepatitis) in Israeli or Palestinian communities. Without such data it is difficult to effectively target treatment and prevention efforts and appropriately allocate resources for these efforts. Cost figures related to the drug problem in the Middle East are limited. One point is clear, however: massive amounts of money are being spent by government, communities, businesses, schools, and private individuals to address drug use. Even with these expenditures, the area lacks an adequate response to the drug problem. One prime reason for this is the absence of detailed information regarding the nature and extent of drug abuse. Such information is essential for policy and program development drug prevention and treatment.

SENSITIVITY OF DRUG USE INFORMATION

Information about drug abuse is a potentially volatile commodity. While it is necessary to the development of good health care systems and the allocation of criminal justice resources, it can also be ammunition for acrimonious political agendas. In the United States, there has been tremendous controversy and racial acrimony regarding theories that the U.S. government supplied cocaine to some major metropolitan areas (populated predominantly by African Americans and where cocaine or crack use rates were disproportionately high) to fund illegal support for the U.S.-supported Nicaraguan rebels. This accusation became an inflammatory and socially divisive issue that was the basis for significant social turmoil. One well-established principle is that "the other" sector of the community is responsible for any drug problems. In African American communities, the drug problem is generally seen as a function of the white- or Hispanic-controlled drug trafficking organizations. In predominantly Caucasian communities, drug use is generally attributed to ethnic minority communities.

As mentioned earlier, there is clear evidence that the belief that drug problems result from "the other" is a factor in Israeli and Palestinian opinion. In drug abuse training workshops and other activities (see Chapter 2), this sentiment was frequently expressed. Palestinians were heard to say that the more affluent Israeli communities were the source of the illicit drugs and if it were not for the availability of drugs from these communities, there would be no drug problem. Conversely, Israeli participants voiced opinions that much of the drug trafficking in their communities came via the day workers from Gaza and the West Bank who delivered drugs as they went back and forth to work. Also expressed by some Israelis was the opinion that the Bedouin were a major source of the illicit drug supply. This attribution of the drug problem as coming from "over there, from those people" is not unique to the factions in the Middle East, but certainly is clearly present in this region.

The sensitivity and potential volatility of data on substance use trends strongly suggest that any method for collecting this information should be carefully constructed to ensure the accuracy of the information and the appropriate use of the information. The methodologies for establishing such data collection systems are relatively new, but there are established models developed in the United States.

GENESIS OF THE MIDDLE EAST DRUG USE WATCH (MEDUW)

The idea for this initiative did not result from a hypothetical discussion among a group of academic social scientists; rather, the proposal is an outgrowth of a vigorous trilateral program of work. Over the past four years, there has been an extensive set of workshops, training sessions, and meetings discussing the need for Palestinians and Israelis to take a more active role in their communities and societies in addressing the problems associated with drug use. The array of drug abuse activities and the cooperative efforts of senior Israeli and Palestinian leaders and U.S. colleagues have been impressive.

People-to-People Initiative

Palestinian and Israeli "people-to-people" workshops were held in Beer Sheva in 1997 and Bethlehem in 1998 under the sponsorship of the U.S. Information Agency in cooperation with the Palestine Council of Health, the Child Health & Community Research Association (Gaza), Ben-Gurion University, and the Economic Cooperation Foundation (ECF). These workshops exposed the need to assess the nature and extent of the Palestinian and Israeli drug problem. Such information is needed to help Palestinians and Israelis tailor more efficient and effective drug prevention and treatment efforts.

In November 1997, the senior author (Rawson), a drug abuse research expert from the United States, was invited to lead substance abuse needs assessment training efforts in Israel and the Palestinian territories. This project included community training sessions conducted in Beer Sheva, Bethlehem, and Ramallah with Palestinian and Israeli health professionals (coordinated by the Economic Cooperation Foundation [ECF] and Ben-Gurion University, with sponsorship by the United States Information Agency [USIA]). The initial training was followed by a series of trainings involving the Palestine Health Council, the Israeli Ministries of Health and Foreign Affairs, representatives from Israeli and Palestinian Police and Judicial agencies, Ben-Gurion University, and the ECF.

In October 1998, Dr. Rawson returned to conduct a five-day intensive training at Al-Quds University at the Abu Dis Campus and a two-day training in Beer Sheva. Thirty-five senior health officials attended the Al-Quds workshops from the Palestinian Health Council from the West Bank and Gaza Communities as well as senior members of the Israeli health community. In Beer Sheva, over 50 Israeli and Palestinian participants attended the two-day training, including the senior PCH health officials and the director of the Israeli Ministry of Health's Department for the Treatment of Substance Abuse. The closing ceremony of the training session in Al-Quds was attended by Dr. Fati Arafat, representing the Palestinian Red Crescent Society, Haim Divon, deputy director general of the Israeli Ministry of Foreign Affairs, Dr. Sarri Nusseibeh, the president of Al-Quds University, and Ron Pundik, Ph.D., director of the ECF.

Project RADAR

Along with the training programs, three substance abuse resource centers have been established for health care and education professionals in the Israeli, West Bank, and Gaza communities. These centers, called Project RADAR (Regional Alcohol and Drug Abuse Resource) stations, organized with the cooperation and support of the U.S. SAMHSA (Substance Abuse Mental Health Services Administration), have compiled extensive libraries of state-of-the-art substance abuse educational materials (books, pamphlets, posters, and videotapes, as well as substance abuse prevention and treatment protocols). These materials include a collection of very recent documents developed by NIDA (National Institute on Drug Abuse) that represent the "best practice protocols," and all have a very solid scientific base. These RADAR stations represent initial "outposts" for increasing substance abuse awareness in these communities.

Middle East Regional Cooperation (MERC) Program Application Meeting

From May 9 to 13, 1999, a meeting in Los Angeles of three Israelis and three Palestinians and a group of U.S. scientists was held to plan the MERC application, a proposal to the U.S. State Department to conduct a program of trilateral substance abuse research among Israelis and Palestinians. The Israeli and Palestinian teams, which included the principal investigators of this application, met for four days in Los Angeles to discuss the scope and content of this application. A number of senior substance abuse researchers from UCLA (R. Rawson, M. D. Anglin, W. Ling) participated in these meetings and the design of the projects. The participants spent the majority of the four-day visit in meetings, trainings, dinners, and visits to local universities, all in a collegial and productive manner. This visit to the United States was funded by a donation from the board of directors of Friends Research Institute, the applicant organization for this proposal, as a contribution to support the effort. Clearly, the team that submitted this application has a very successful and productive track record of working together, and the principal investigators and the applicant organization have made substantive efforts to demonstrate their commitment to this project.

Building a Leadership Team

Even more impressive than the specific activities was the positive change in the nature of the interpersonal interactions between participants from the two groups. While the initial 1997 meetings were characterized by some awkward, suspicious, and, at times, abrasive interactions, during the 1998 and 1999 meetings and activities, the communication between the members of the two groups was open, helpful, and oriented toward joint efforts to address substance abuse problems throughout the area. Future cooperative projects are in the planning stages, and in the Palestinian communities, concrete plans have been established to create treatment, prevention, and training capabilities. The activities of this project will be an important next step in the development of a cooperative system of substance abuse services in this area of the world. There is clear evidence that the leaders of the communities want these services and that a cooperative Palestinian-Israeli effort has been established as a foundation for the project.

GOALS OF MEDUW

This project is importing two methodologies for estimating substance use prevalence to the communities of Israel and the Palestinian Authority: the Community Epidemiology Workgroup (CEWG) approach and the Arrestee Drug Abuse Monitoring (ADAM) program. The CEWG methodology has been developed by NIDA over the past 10 years as the most comprehensive manner in which to estimate the multiple domains of impact of different types of substance use problems. This approach has only recently been formalized into a manual for exportation and replication (NIDA, 1998). The ADAM approach has been used by the National Institute on Justice (NIJ) since 1987. The data from ADAM originally were used only by law enforcement officials but now are used together with other data to provide multiple windows on the problem. In 1998, an ADAM international program was initiated and has been instituted in three countries outside the United

States. The initiative described in this article will establish a Palestinian-Israeli ADAM program, to be affiliated with the International ADAM project.

The Trilateral Steering Committee for MEDUW

Establishment of an active and involved steering committee is an essential element for the success of this project. Throughout the four years of trilateral substance abuse training activities in Israel and Palestinian communities, there has been a very active and productive alliance of Palestinians, Israelis, and U.S. participants. Many individuals who have been responsible for the success of the previous activities (including the application's principal investigators) will be invited to participate in the steering committee. This committee must comprise members who have: (a) respect and trust of their constituent groups; (b) knowledge of the key community individuals and institutions that can gain access to needed data sources; (c) willingness to work as part of a cooperative Israeli-Palestinian team that will produce balanced, accurate reports; and (d) attendance at two to three meetings per year.

The steering committee will be made up of approximately 12 representatives (six Israeli and six Palestinian) of the following Israeli and Palestinian groups: substance abuse treatment and/or prevention; health care/public health; law enforcement/criminal justice; educational system/university; governmental/political official; and behavioral scientist/researcher. In addition, three U.S. members will provide technical support. It is expected that the individuals on the steering committee will be senior professionals who have extensive high-level contacts so that the project may call on them to assist in gaining access and approval for project activities.

The steering committee will be responsible for overseeing the project. They will be asked to: (1) assist with the specific design of the CEWG component of the project; (2) help with selecting the research staff; (3) help identify and recruit CEWG group members in the four communities; (4) review and approve the ADAM methodology; (5) assist in gaining access to jails for ADAM data collection; (6) assist with overcoming regulatory barriers; (7) assist with the production of the project reports; and (8) review, approve, and assist in presenting project reports to policymakers. All members of the steering committee will be asked to serve a two-year term and then remain on in an advisory capacity.

The NIDA-Sponsored CEWG Network

The National Institute on Drug Abuse (NIDA) currently funds approximately 85 percent of the world's research on drug abuse (NIDA, 1998). Along with an extensive array of treatment research and basic science research on substance abuse-related issues, NIDA sponsors and organizes the most extensive, multidimensional substance use monitoring system in the world. The centerpiece of this system is the Community Epidemiological Work Group (CEWG) network. The CEWG has been in place for more than 20 years. During this time it has developed a set of methodologies and measures that possess empirically established validity and reliability. The CEWG provides U.S. policymakers with data on topics such as: which drugs are available in what geographical areas of the United States; the purity of the drugs being used; the characteristics of the users of different types of drugs (e.g., ages, gender, ethnicity, rural, or urban); where the drugs come from; which types of drugs are increasingly being used; and how various drugs are associated with different health and criminal justice problems.

This epidemiological data collection system has been documented in two recent monographs by NIDA (NIDA, 1996, 1997). The data collected in this system are the source for thousands of policy reports for federal, state, and community health care system planners, school and drug prevention program organizers, law enforcement officials, judicial officials, and legislators. The data from this system have very substantial budgetary significance. They are used to guide the allocation of resources for everything from agencies as diverse as the Department of Health and Human Services, the Justice Department, the Defense Department, and the Department of Education. The essential methodologies for establishment of a system to collect such data in a country, region, or municipality are described in a virtual "how to" manual just published by NIDA. This volume, *Assessing Drug Abuse within and across Communities* (NIDA, 1998), provides the blueprint for the plan of research described in this proposal. The CEWG program has gained solid credibility through the well-established application of scientific methods and a process that includes a broad and inclusive set of stakeholders. The principles used to create this system of data collection and to gain acceptance for the findings are the principles upon which the MEDUW program is based.

What Is the CEWG Network?

The CEWG Network is a multiagency work group concept with a public health orientation that studies the spread, growth, or development of drug abuse and related problems. The goal of the network is elimination or reduction of drug abuse and its related consequences. To achieve this goal, network members access existing information from multiple sources, including drug abuse treatment agencies, public health offices, law enforcement agencies, hospital emergency departments, medical examiner and coroners' offices, and local school and household surveys. Members meet periodically to review, compare, and draw conclusions from the data. The data are reported in a standardized format to facilitate their review and comparative analyses. Qualitative studies may be conducted to help members understand the findings from existing data sets.

The primary objectives of the network members are to: (1) identify drug abuse patterns in defined geographic areas; (2) identify changes in drug abuse patterns over defined time periods to establish trends; (3) detect emerging substances of abuse; and (4) communicate and disseminate the information to appropriate community agencies and organizations so it can be used in developing policies, practices, prevention strategies, and research studies.

Network members are individuals who are in a position to contribute and assess information about drug use in specific geographic areas. They may represent agencies and organizations that have some responsibility for addressing drug abuse problems or that benefit directly from acquiring information about drug abuse. Researchers and other individuals who have special knowledge about a particular issue or drug-abusing population also may participate. Regularly scheduled network meetings provide a forum for members to share, review, and analyze information on the epidemiology of drug abuse (NIDA, 1998).

How Will the Middle East CEWG Network Be Organized?

The early stages of organizing the network are critical because they set the stage for what the monitoring network will be, how it will function, and how it will be perceived by participants and others. Two interrelated objectives need to be kept in mind: obtaining knowledge about drug abuse, and developing and strengthening the work group. Four principles will be observed in building the Middle East CEWG: (1) Start small and be selective in inviting individuals to attend. It is easy to add individuals once the needs and sources have been identified and to change individuals based on strengths and interests of the members. (2) Have clear, attainable objectives for the meeting. Avoid trying to overachieve at the beginning. (3) Establish the agenda in coordination with other participants so they feel invested from the beginning. (4) Give each participant a role to play and a contribution to make.

The first meeting will be organized to accomplish several objectives: (1) Identify known and potential sources of data and information. Selected participants will be asked to describe particular data sets and to prepare data from sources to which they have access. (2) Review the types of data sources (indicators) accessed by other epidemiologic networks to determine if they might be obtainable. If they are, determine what steps should be taken to identify agencies and individuals that can provide access to each of these sources. (3) Assign participants to follow up (after meetings) and, if appropriate, make contacts to find out what types of data are available, how the data can be made available, and who is most knowledgeable about the data and the data sources. (4) Determine how information from the meetings should be recorded, reported, and disseminated, including to whom it should be sent. (5) Identify current and potential sources of support for organizing and conducting the meeting, and producing and disseminating reports from the meeting (NIDA, 1998).

Within the activities of the CEWG meetings, consideration will be given to evaluation of six areas: (1) demographic characteristics, employment history, and legal history; (2) alcohol and drug-use history; (3) medical history and medical consequences of substance abuse; (4) psychiatric diagnosis; (5) family functioning;

and (6) social adjustment and social supports. Whether or not a data collection instrument responds to each of these areas, it is important that the instrumentation be developed (or selected) on the basis of the following criteria: the degree to which reliability has been established; the adequacy of findings regarding validity and psychometric properties of the instrument; its record of use in substance-abusing populations and availability of comparison data with an indication of feasibility of use with these subject groups; and efficiency and ease of administration.

THE NIJ-SPONSORED ADAM MONITORING PROGRAM

The National Institute of Justice's Arrestee Drug Abuse Monitoring (ADAM) program tracks trends in the prevalence and types of drug use among booked arrestees in urban areas. The data play an important role in assembling the picture of drug abuse in the U.S. arrestee population and have been a central component in the study of the links between drug use and crime. ADAM is the only national drug data program that utilizes drug testing. The data provided by the ADAM program allow policymakers and analysts to view developing trends, potentially permitting earlier intervention against problems. The ADAM program currently operates in 35 sites in the United States.

The International Arrestee Drug Abuse Monitoring (I-ADAM) program is envisioned as a research partnership among policymakers across the world. The goal of I-ADAM is to develop a standardized international drug surveillance system that will provide researchers the ability to compare the prevalence of drug use among arrestees in different nations and allow researchers to assess the consequences of drug abuse within and across national boundaries.

What I-ADAM Offers to the MEDUW Project

The incorporation of an ADAM methodology will allow the MEDUW project to build a future involvement with I-ADAM. This will help the long-term viability of the project in the following ways:

1. I-ADAM is one of only a few international drug prevalence measures and the only international surveillance system for arrestee drug use rates. I-ADAM's development is important because the existing drug surveillance systems across the globe are in many cases not compatible. Therefore, post-hoc comparisons across countries (with independently designed systems) are very difficult. I-ADAM has been designed from its inception to be a standardized international surveillance system (similar instruments, sampling, training, and other protocols).
2. I-ADAM also explores other issues related to drug use across national borders. I-ADAM can be used to estimate the relationship between drugs and crime, sources of illegal income for arrestees, drug dependency, use of substance abuse treatment, age of onset of drug use, drug market dynamics, and a select number of public health-related

topics. I-ADAM is a flexible platform that can be modified to address topics of local interest (e.g., domestic violence) and international interest (e.g., organized crime).

3. I-ADAM can be useful as a tool to coordinate drug-control policies and resources. Identification of similar drug problems across national borders provides a standard basis for nations to coordinate drug-control policies and resources, resulting in improved multilateral cooperation. Identification of a growing substance abuse problem in a country's arrestee population can help forecast a potential hot spot for international drug trafficking.

Requirements for Middle East I-ADAM Sites

At each of the Middle East I-ADAM data collection sites, trained interviewers (who are not law enforcement officials or staff members of the lock-up facility) will conduct private, individual interviews with adult male and female booked arrestees regarding their use of substances and will collect urine specimens from each of them. Study participants will be asked to volunteer, and the data will be kept confidential and anonymous. Data collection from juveniles is optional. Each I-ADAM site will provide the interview staff with access to arrestees within 48 hours of arrest (any longer and the drug test might not be valid). The MEDUW Steering Committee, in collaboration with the National Institute of Justice, will determine which drugs to test for and how many drugs to include in the drug test panel. At least five common drugs (marijuana, cocaine, opiates, amphetamines, benzodiazepines) will be tested for by all sites. The National Institute of Justice has developed a core I-ADAM survey instrument, in consultation with the other I-ADAM sites, and the agreed-upon core survey will be implemented by all I-ADAM sites. At a later point, common addenda surveys will be developed for special topical areas (e.g., weapons). Each international site will submit their data to I-ADAM to form an international database of core standardized data elements. Each international site will have adequate time to analyze their own data for national purposes prior to submission of their data to I-ADAM.

U.S.-Arab-Israeli Cooperation in Building MEDUW

Successful U.S.-Arab-Israeli cooperation is one of the most critical issues in the creation of MEDUW. The benefit of conducting this project across the Israeli-Palestinian communities is that the interconnectedness of these societies is likely to remain complex and intertwined for the foreseeable future. It is the belief of the organizers of MEDUW that a joint effort that emphasizes cooperation and comparable methods of data collection, common protocols for data interpretation, and participation of U.S. scientists has a better chance for producing a positive impact. The combined efforts of the staffs and the personnel participating in the meetings and training events can help to produce a cooperative response to a common enemy, substance abuse, rather than produce separate unilateral efforts, which are more likely to result in parochial responses that emphasize the blaming of "the other group."

It is clear that the MEDUW project, if successful, has the potential to increase cooperation around the issue of substance abuse in the Middle East. Furthermore, the design of the project planning, training, implementation, and report preparation and dissemination will involve interaction between Palestinians and Israelis at all stages and at all levels. First, this project would not be worth doing without the participation of both Middle East partners, and it would not be possible to do without the participation of all three partners. Project activities will bring together leaders from the Israeli and Palestinian governmental agencies in the steering committees, as well as community members, as local CEWG representative groups are established that will include civic leaders, educators, health care representatives, substance abuse professionals, and law enforcement personnel. The CEWG members from all communities will be trained together. Israeli and Palestinian research staff will be trained to conduct research, test urine samples, and enter data together.

As the project progresses, Palestinian and Israeli investigators, along with U.S. scientists who will provide technical support, will gather for multiple planning, training, and report-writing sessions. The reports that result from the project will be presented to Palestinian and Israeli agency leaders together. The success of the project will be entirely dependent on the integration of the project activities and the cooperative problem-solving that will be required.

The extent of the multilevel trilateral cooperation required to conduct this project is very ambitious. The reason for believing that MEDUW will be successful is that the organizers and their colleagues have already conducted an impressive array of collaborative efforts. The future of the system will be determined by the participants of the project, together with ongoing input and cooperation from the U.S. agencies, the National Institute on Drug Abuse (NIDA) and the National Institute of Justice. While the U.S. agencies and scientists will continue to play a role in the project, as they do in other international ADAM and CEWG training activities, the growth and maturation of the system will be dependent on an ongoing collaborative effort of the Israeli and Palestinian participants.

RELEVANCE TO THE MIDDLE EAST PEACE PROCESS

The MEDUW project has a systematic plan for developing a balanced, consensus-based organizational structure for planning the CEWG network and a specific plan of work for establishing I-ADAM. The project will create the expertise to effectively conduct the work, build the community infrastructure to collect the data, and ensure a thorough review process prior to information dissemination. Clearly, it would be desirable to see the CEWG process expand to other communities in Palestine and Israel and to neighboring countries, including Jordan and Lebanon. It would also be desirable to have this network form the basis for a Middle East Regional CEWG Network. In addition, the data collection for the ADAM component of the project will be designed with the intent to merge it into the I-ADAM system run by the National Institute of Justice.

The current situation—unilateral data collection by the Israelis and no data collection by the Palestinians—has the potential for creating friction and exacerbating tensions between the two groups. The nature of psychoactive substance use in these Jewish and Moslem societies has all of the implications and ramifications concerning public health and criminal justice seen in more secular societies. However, in these societies, with the powerful influences of religious and very conservative factions, substance use also can be viewed as an indicator of societal change and, for many, cultural deterioration. Information on drug use trends can be used as indicators to inflame passions about how political and cultural changes are influencing the youth and the future of cultures. As noted earlier, there is an almost universal trend by societies to blame their problems with psychoactive substance use on "the other." By providing accurate information to a trilateral steering committee, responses to the project findings should reduce the tension, friction, and blaming. In addition, the activities of the project itself should bring together senior health care, criminal justice, and other policymakers from both sides to work on a common system to measure and address this problem.

REFERENCES

National Institute on Drug Abuse (NIDA). (1996). *Problems of drug dependence 1995.* Proceedings of the 58th Annual Scientific Meeting of the College on Problems of Drug Dependence. (NIDA Research Monograph Series No. 174). Rockville, MD: NIDA.

———. (1997). *Problems of drug dependence 1996.* Proceedings of the 59th Annual Scientific Meeting of the College on Problems of Drug Dependence. (NIDA Research Monograph Series No. 175). Rockville, MD: NIDA.

———. (1998). *Assessing drug abuse within and across communities: Community epidemiology surveillance networks on drug abuse.* (National Institutes of Health Publication No. 98-3614). Rockville, MD: NIDA. Retrieved July 17, 2000, from the World Wide Web: http://www.nida.nih.gov/DEPR/Assessing/Guideindex.html.

Rahav, G., Teichman, M., Gil, R., Rosenblum, Y., & Bar-Hamburger, R. (1995). *The use of psychoactive substances among Israeli citizens 1995: Epidemiological study 3.* Tel Aviv: Pori Institute, Tel Aviv University, Anti-Drug Authority (in Hebrew).

———. (1998). *The use of psychoactive substances among Israeli citizens 1998: Epidemiological study 4.* Tel Aviv: Pori Institute, Tel Aviv University, Anti-Drug Authority (in Hebrew).

Teichman, M., Rahav, G., & Barnea, Z. (1994). Alcohol consumption among non-Jewish men in Israel. *Alcologia, 6,* 201–206.

Weiss, S., Sawa, G. H., Abdeen, Z., & Yanai, J. (1999). Substance abuse studies and prevention efforts among Arabs in the 1990s in Israel, Jordan and the Palestinian Authority—A literature review. *Addiction, 94,* 177–198.

10

Is There a Need for an International Screening Test? The Middle East as a Case in Point

Thomas F. Babor

INTRODUCTION

In 1982, the World Health Organization (WHO) initiated a program to develop an international screening test for hazardous and harmful alcohol use (Saunders, Aasland, Babor, de la Fuente, & Grant, 1993). The program led to the creation of the Alcohol Use Disorders Identification Test (AUDIT), which has not only been found to be reliable and valid in numerous evaluation studies (Allen, Litten, Fertig, & Babor, 1997), but also has been used widely in primary care and other health settings throughout the world as part of screening and brief intervention programs (Higgins-Biddle, Babor, Mullahy, Daniels, & McRee, 1997). The success of AUDIT raises the question of whether a similar international screening test could be developed to detect drug abuse. Before an ambitious development program is initiated, it is important to consider the prerequisites for a public health approach to screening for drug abuse on an international level.

At least four conditions should be met before recommending screening procedures for routine application: (1) the target condition should have sufficient conceptual clarity to permit reliable measurement; (2) the natural history of the disorder should be fairly well understood, along with risk factors and populations at risk; (3) the test used for screening should be reliable, valid, inexpensive, easy to administer, and acceptable to both treatment providers and the target population; and (4) appropriate treatments (or brief interventions) should exist so that persons identified can be managed effectively (Babor & Kadden, 1985).

These issues are explored in the remainder of this chapter. The first section introduces major concepts of psychoactive substance use disorders, as well as the definitions of screening and related terms. The next section describes epidemiological data so as to provide a basis for evaluating existing screening instruments and the need for a new screening test. Finally, the chapter discusses the extent to which the basic requirements of a public health approach to early identification of substance use disorders have been satisfied, and what steps should be taken next. All of these considerations have meaning to Israelis, and, in particular, Palestinians, as they move forward in terms of defining and responding to the drug abuse problem in the Middle East.

DEFINITIONS AND CONCEPTUAL ISSUES

Screening is a preliminary procedure used to gather information about the likelihood that an individual has a particular disease or condition, or is at risk for such. The screening process determines who is eligible for further assessment, which could result in a formal diagnosis and treatment. When screening results in a formal diagnosis, it is called *case finding*. When screening identifies persons at risk, it is called *screening for risk factors*. The importance of this distinction lies in the timing of screening and the type of intervention that follows screening.

In the field of substance abuse, *early identification* means that screening is initiated before the onset of severe dependence or serious substance-related problems. Its purpose is to prevent substance-related disabilities in persons at risk. It may be followed by educational and motivational interventions designed to minimize harm and dissuade the substance user from further use. Opportunistic screening or case findings take place when there is a strong suspicion that the person already has a drug-related health condition. Treatment is designed to prevent the progression of harm.

Drug-related problems comprise a broad spectrum of social, medical, and psychological disabilities that affect a significant proportion of the adult and adolescent population in many countries (United Nations International Drug Control Programme [UNDCP], 1997). The most visible group of people affected are those who have developed a syndrome of drug dependence and who are commonly referred to as addicts. A less prominent but far more numerous group consists of those people who use psychoactive substances but who are not seriously dependent on drugs. These individuals have been variously termed hazardous users, drug abusers, and recreational drug users. These two "worlds" of drug problems, one characterized by intermittent drug use and the occasional acute consequences of intoxication, the other by severe dependence and the consequences of chronic substance use, may require different approaches to screening, diagnosis, and clinical management.

A World Health Organization memorandum (Edwards, Arif, & Hodgson, 1981) uses the term *hazardous use* to refer to that level of substance misuse that, should it persist, is likely to result in harm. In contrast, *harmful drug use* is defined as drug use that has already resulted in adverse mental or physical effects. The aim of this terminology is to provide clinicians and researchers with guidelines for the identification of individuals at risk who may not meet the criteria for dependence on a psychoactive substance. One implication of these conceptual developments is that hazardous and harmful use should be the prime targets of early intervention and secondary prevention programs, respectively. This is based on the assumption that such programs are less costly and preclude the need for subsequent treatment of drug dependence.

Epidemiology and Prevalence

The usefulness of an international drug screening test will undoubtedly be determined by the prevalence of drug use and drug-related problems in different parts of the world. According to the UNDCP (1997), illicit drug consumption has increased throughout the world in recent years, as estimated from emergency room visits, drug-related mortality reports, and arrests of drug users. Any discussion of drug epidemiology is complicated by the wide variety of licit and illicit substances that are classed as psychoactive agents. These agents include naturally produced drugs, whose use is deeply rooted in many cultures, such as coca leaves in the Andean Highlands, and manufactured substances, such as codeine and crack cocaine. Conditions such as rapid social change and urbanization have created epidemics of substance use in countries such as Brazil and Peru. In Mexico, the majority of urban drug users are young and poor, and use inhalants, solvents, and marijuana. A similar situation exists in many of the sub-Saharan countries of Africa, with several countries (e.g., Nigeria) recently reporting an increase in cocaine addiction. Heroin addiction has become a significant problem in Pakistan, where production and trafficking are major features of the underground economy. A special pattern of substance misuse, the inhalation of volatile substances such as gasoline, plastic cement, shoe dye, and industrial glue, is associated with social deviance, poverty, homelessness, and delinquency in many developing countries. Khat is an important cash crop in East African countries and is used at all levels of society to produce mild euphoria. The use of these substances throughout the world is virtually impossible to estimate accurately, but morbidity and mortality statistics suggest that the problems of substance misuse are not limited to the developed countries (Des Jarlais, Eisenberg, Good, & Kleinman, 1995).

Based on unofficial UNDCP (1997) estimates, the annual global prevalence rate of illicit drug consumption is in the range of 3 to 4 percent of the world population, which is far below the estimated consumption of the two primarily legal substances, alcohol (50%) and tobacco (20%). The plant-based drug with the most widespread use internationally is cannabis (marijuana and hashish), with an estimated 141.2 million people who use the substance at least once per year. Even though the use of heroin (and other opiate-type substances) and cocaine is less prevalent worldwide (estimated at 8.0 and 13.3 million annual users, respectively), these drugs have a far more serious public health impact because of their effect on emergency room visits, HIV infection, and mortality. In recent years, the most dramatic increase in drug abuse has involved synthetic drugs, especially amphetamine-like substances (Des Jarlais et al., 1995; UNDCP, 1997).

Regional, national, and international school surveys conducted since the 1970s have consistently shown that the initiation of substance use rises dramatically during early adolescence (Des Jarlais et al., 1995; Kalant, Corrigall, & Smart, 1997; UNDCP, 1997). Students often report that they began to use inhalants and alcohol before other drugs. Marijuana use begins later, followed by prescription drug abuse and cocaine (Adler & Kandel, 1981). Substance use varies considerably based on socioeconomic status, gender, ethnic group membership, and whether one resides in an urban or rural area.

School surveys conducted in many countries have documented the consequences of using various substances. Two general types of consequences can be distinguished. The first, short-term consequences, are associated with the effects of acute intoxication and include medical emergencies, acute panic reactions, and changes in interpersonal behavior. In addition to these direct consequences of drug or alcohol intoxication, there are often secondary consequences of intoxication such as arrests and accidents. The second type of consequence is the long-term effect of chronic ingestion of psychoactive substances. Long-term consequences include impaired psychosocial development, physical health problems, as well as interference with important developmental tasks such as academic performance, career choice, peer socialization, and identity formation (Newcomb & Bentler, 1988). Another consequence of substance abuse is the establishment of habitual behaviors (e.g., smoking, alcohol use) that increase the risk of chronic health conditions such as lung cancer and cardiovascular disease. Regular use of one psychoactive substance may also increase the risk of using other substances and is closely associated with the development of pharmacological dependence.

A wide variety of etiological factors and environmental correlates increase the likelihood that psychoactive substances will be used and that problems will result. Among the characteristics of youth at high risk for substance abuse are childhood hyperactivity, attention deficit disorder, conduct problems, self-derogation, low self-esteem, shyness, aggressiveness, and emotional distress (Coombs, Fawzy, & Gerber, 1986; Huba, Newcomb, & Bentler, 1988; Kaplan, 1985; Tarter, McBride, Buonpane, & Schneider, 1977). Children whose parents are alcoholic are at increased risk of alcohol and drug abuse, as are adolescents whose parents smoke cigarettes (Barnes, 1984). Other correlates of substance abuse include inadequate family bonding, negative attitudes toward school, poor school performance, tolerance of deviance, rejection of traditional values, and low social conformity (Barnes, 1984; Jessor, Chase, & Donovan, 1980; Newcomb & Bentler, 1988). Deviant attitudes and antisocial behavior are among the most consistent predictors of substance abuse by adolescents (Newcomb & Bentler, 1988). A frequently observed feature of adolescent problem drinking and other drug use is the development of school adjustment problems, low academic achievement, and termination of schooling in favor of early entry into the workforce (Kandel, Davies, Karus, & Yamaguchi, 1986; Newcomb & Bentler, 1988).

This brief overview suggests that the development of any screening test on an international level must take into account the diverse nature of psychoactive substances and of the users themselves. Nevertheless, much has been learned in recent years about the natural history of substance abuse, including its etiology, risk factors, patterns, and consequences. These findings have provided a sound empirical basis for the design of screening tests.

Screening Tests

Another prerequisite for a public health approach to screening is the availability of one or more screening tests that can be used with various population groups in a variety of settings. In the following sections, the current status of two major screening procedures are reviewed: self-report screening tests and biological screening methods.

Self-Report Screening Tests

A number of different approaches have been developed to screen for drug abuse using self-report procedures. Given the different needs and substance-use patterns of adults and adolescents, screening tests have generally been designed and validated for one or the other of these two populations.

Screening tests for adults. Two types of screening tests have been developed for adults. The first, exemplified by the Drug Abuse Screening Test (DAST; Skinner, 1982), consists of direct questions about substance use and related problems. The second, illustrated by the MacAndrew Alcoholism Scale (MacAndrew, 1965), consists of indirect questions that measure personality traits associated with substance misuse. The DAST was originally designed as a 28-item self-report scale that yields a quantitative index of the range of problems associated with drug abuse. The item content was modeled after the Michigan Alcoholism Screening Test (Selzer, 1971). Following an initial validation study, the number of items was reduced to 20, and further revisions yielded a highly reliable 10-item scale.

The Substance Abuse Screening Instrument (SASI) is a 15-item test designed to identify persons in the U.S. criminal justice system who need further assessment and possible referral to treatment (Inciardi, 1994). Questions are phrased in a yes/no format and focus on the occurrence of alcohol and drug-related problems during the course of the individual's lifetime. No information is available on the reliability or validity of this test.

In contrast to screening tests that ask about substance use and related problems directly, a number of tests have been developed to measure nonspecific correlates or risk factors that suggest an actual or potential substance use disorder. For example, the original Minnesota Multiphasic Personality Inventory included a scale designed to detect alcohol and other drug problems in adults and adolescents. Called the MacAndrew Alcoholism Scale (MAC; MacAndrew, 1965), it was developed using samples of adults and adopted for use with adolescents with relatively few changes. The MAC scale has become a standard measure of alcohol and drug problems in both research and applied settings, in spite of some criticisms (Gottesman & Prescott, 1989). The MAC scale was primarily developed to differentiate male alcoholics from male nonalcoholic psychiatric patients in an outpatient setting. The literature, however, has indicated that the MAC scale may not be as efficient or valid a discriminator of substance abusers as previously believed (Gottesman & Prescott, 1989; Preng & Clopton, 1986).

The MMPI-2, which is the first major revision of the MMPI, included a slight revision of the MAC (MAC-R; Butcher, Dahlstrom, Graharn, Tellegen, & Kaemmer, 1989) as well as two new scales to assess alcohol and drug problems. The Addiction Acknowledgment Scale (AAS) was developed to assess an adult's willingness to acknowledge the presence of problems with alcohol or other drugs. Like the MAC-R, the Addiction Potential Scale (APS) was developed to differentiate individuals with a potential for developing alcohol or other drug problems. Whereas APS has no items with content addressing substance use directly, AAS is a collection of direct items that assess open acknowledgment of problems with drugs (Greene, Weed, Butcher, Arredondo, & Davis, 1992). Both AAS and APS have performed well in validation research.

Another potential drug abuse screening test is contained in the Millon Clinical Multiaxial Inventory (MCMI-III; Millon, 1994), a 175-item diagnostic test. The 14-item Drug Dependence Scale reflects drug abuse history and impulse control. Although the test is brief, questions have been raised about the validity and clinical utility of this scale (Bryer, Martines, & Dignan, 1990).

A variation on the use of direct screening items focusing on specific substances is the use of conjoint screening questions, which inquire simultaneously about alcohol and drug use. One such instrument is the CAGE screening test, which has been adapted to include drugs (CAGE-AID). A study of a convenience sample of primary care patients found that the CAGE-AID was more sensitive but less specific for substance use disorders than the CAGE (Brown & Rounds, 1995).

Screening tests for adolescents. Until recently there have been few adolescent-specific screening instruments designed to assess the need for further diagnostic evaluation. Recognizing the need for a comprehensive screening instrument, the U.S. National Institute on Drug Abuse (NIDA) developed the Problem-Oriented Screening Instrument for Teenagers (POSIT; Rahdert, 1991). This 139-item screening questionnaire is designed as the first stage in a sequential assessment system intended to improve the evaluation and referral of substance-involved youth. The POSIT indicates whether a problem may exist in any one of 10 functional areas: substance use/abuse, mental health status, physical health status, aggressive behavior/delinquency, social skills, family relations, educational status, vocational status, peer relations, and leisure and recreation. Following screening, a more comprehensive diagnostic assessment can be given in those areas where the POSIT indicates a problem may exist. Due to its relatively recent development, little work has been done to establish the psychometric properties for the POSIT. McLaney, Del Boca, and Babor (1994) found that the test had good reliability and validity in adolescents referred to an assessment service for evaluation of substance use problems, but the findings highlighted the need for further research on screening tests designed specifically for substance-involved youth.

A related instrument is the Drug Use Screening Inventory (DUSI; Tarter & Hegedus, 1991), a 159-item self-administered questionnaire designed to evaluate problems in health, psychiatric functioning, and psychosocial adjustment. The questions concern 10 life areas or domains, including substance use, social skills, family relations, schoolwork, peer relations, leisure, and recreation. The DUSI scores produce a profile of relative severity across the 10 domains that is used for treatment planning. Reliability and validity of the DUSI are good (Kirisci, Mezzich, & Tarter, 1995).

In contrast to the comprehensive, multidimensional screening that is included in the POSIT and DUSI, a number of shorter instruments have been developed to screen specifically for substance use. The Personal Experience Screening Questionnaire (PESQ) is a 38-item self-report instrument that focuses primarily on substance use and problems. Validation research suggests that this test has acceptable reliability and validity in the detection of individuals with various histories of substance use (Winters, 1992).

The Substance Abuse Subtle Screening Inventory (SASSI; Miller, 1997) is a 78-item self-report instrument that classifies adults and adolescents as chemically dependent. The initial item content of the SASSI was derived from the item set of the MMPI. It is designed to prevent faking and focuses on early stages of substance use. Svanum and McGrew (1995) studied U.S. university students who completed the SASSI and five direct screening questions concerning the consequences of alcohol and drug use. Although the SASSI did not accurately identify substance use disorders, the five direct screening questions were modestly useful, and it was suggested that there are advantages to directness when screening for substance use disorders. These findings are in agreement with the failure of other MMPI-based trait measures to identify substance abuse (Gottesman & Prescott, 1989; Svanum & Ehrmann, 1993).

The Drug and Alcohol Problem (DAP) Quick Screen (Klitzner, Schwarz, Gruenewald, & Blasinsky, 1987) was developed for use by pediatricians. The 42 items focus on substance use and related behaviors. Validity data have been reported using a 30-item revision (Schwartz & Wirtz, 1990).

Biological Screening Methods

Biological screening methods can serve as a preliminary screening procedure or to supplement information gathered through the use of a self-report screening tool and other sources. Drug screening through such methods as urinalysis, hair testing, and saliva tests, when performed by someone with proper training, is often the quickest, most accurate way to detect recent drug use. A review by Wolff and colleagues (1999) describes the advantages and disadvantages of these screening tests.

Currently, urine is the preferred biological fluid for the analysis of drugs of abuse. The advantage of urine is that it is generally available in sufficient quantities and the drugs or their metabolites tend to be present in relatively high concentrations. A recent innovation has been the introduction of self-contained urine testing kits. These tests offer advantages in simplicity, ease of performance, and rapid access to test results, but potential drawbacks include the subjective nature of these qualitative assays and in some instances the lack of a positive control. Other limitations of urine screening include their inability to detect the route of drug administration as well as quantity, frequency, or time of drug ingestion. They can only indicate drug use over the previous few days, and there is a risk of false positives by passive drug exposure or ingestion of foodstuffs.

The usefulness of salivary drug concentrations has been criticized in regard to many compounds because of the variability of the saliva-to-plasma concentration ratio. However, tetrahydrocannabinoid is sequestered into the buccal cavity during smoking and can be detected in this way to indicate recent use. The collection of saliva for drug analysis has other advantages: it can be carried out by untrained personnel; collection is rapid, non-invasive, and relatively easy; and no contact with biological fluids is required.

Blood is the most useful biological fluid for identifying drugs for quantitative analyses, but it is probably the least favorable procedure for drug testing. There are many problems that have to be overcome: collection requires trained personnel; there is a risk of needle-stick injury and HIV and Hepatitis B/C transmission; and blood collection is invasive and may be problematic in intravenous users. Human scalp hair testing for substances that are misused is a relatively new biological form of drug screening. However, it is still a developing technology and there are many unresolved problems. The obvious advantage of hair testing is that this technique offers the potential for examination over a much greater time than is commonly obtained with urine and blood analysis.

Evaluation of Currently Available Screening Tests

A number of important features of biological and self-report screening instruments should be taken into account in the design of a drug abuse screening program, the selection of a screening test, or the development of a new test, particularly for international applications. These features include:

- Test-retest reliability (i.e., Are the results similar across time, conditions, and types of administration?)
- Construct validity (i.e., correlation with other methods or instruments attempting to measure the same construct [e.g., problem severity])
- Ability to predict criterion measures (for example, future substance abuse)
- Availability of normative data for age, race, gender, and different types of populations and settings

- Cost and efficiency
- Cross-national validation and generalizability (i.e., Is there evidence that the test is equally valid and reliable in different cultures?)
- Susceptibility to response bias (i.e., whether a test can be deliberately faked or distorted by more subtle influences, such as the need to present oneself in a socially desirable way)

Using these criteria, the available self-report screening tests have a number of limitations from an international perspective. First, most tests have been developed and validated in the United States, with little evidence that they are sensitive or specific in other cultures. Second, many of these tests have not been subject to extensive validation research, and several have not been evaluated favorably. Third, most of the adult screening tests have been designed for case finding, not to identify risk factors. These tests typically avoid direct questions about specific drugs, focusing instead on the experience of problems associated with any drug use in the past. Such an approach may be more susceptible to response bias. Fourth, subtle or disguised screening tests do not appear to be sufficiently sensitive or specific to identify active cases, although they may be useful in screening for risk factors. Finally, comprehensive or multidimensional screening tests like the DUSI and POSIT have advantages of identifying both "caseness" and risk factors, but they take much more time to administer and score.

Similar problems exist with respect to biological screening methods (Wolff et al., 1999). Drugs may be detected in any body fluid or tissue but there are many practical limitations. The problems of handling body fluids and the need for scrupulous hygienic procedures and safety standards are major limitations. The choice of body fluid is influenced by the pharmacokinetics of the drugs being tested for. Blood gives the most accurate measurement of a drug currently active in the system and is commonly used for therapeutic monitoring. Urine provides a broader time frame with less quantitative accuracy, and hair provides a substantially longer time frame. Cost, invasiveness, lack of sensitivity, and other problems limit the usefulness of biological measures as a sole approach to screening.

In discussing self-report screening tests and biological indicators of drug use, it is important to consider specific settings where screening can be conducted. Outside the treatment system, drug screening has occurred in health care settings, such as primary care and emergency departments, the workplace (as part of broader employee assistance programs), and in the correctional system. In all settings, the detection of drug use should be linked to backup treatment and intervention strategies and should be aimed at increasing the safety of the environment or the health of the population. Other settings where screening for drug use is likely to be feasible and useful are schools, hospital services (especially obstetrics, neonatal, and psychiatry), and drug treatment services (to monitor withdrawal symptoms and treatment compliance).

As indicated by the WHO Collaborative Study on Psychological Problems in General Health Care (Ustun & Sartorius, 1995), mental disorders are frequently encountered in primary care in many countries, with the three most common conditions being major depressive episode, generalized anxiety disorder, and alcohol-related problems. Although drug abuse was not a condition included in the collaborative research protocol, the study showed that it is feasible to identify and diagnose a variety of psychosocial problems in primary health care, and that physicians, nurses, and other health workers are in a unique position to detect substance abuse at its early stages.

THE MIDDLE EAST: A CASE STUDY

The Middle East is a region of multiple identities that are defined by religion, culture, language, and history. Because of its diversity and complexity, the Middle East is an ideal area to illustrate the need for an international screening test in terms of prevalence estimation, case finding, early identification, and needs assessment.

The Middle East, particularly the region including Israel and Palestine (i.e., under Palestinian Authority control), is as culturally diverse as any part of the world in that it comprises Moslems, Druze, Jews, and Christians. For this reason, the Middle East provides a major challenge to the design of any international screening test. Moslems and Druze both belong to cultures that traditionally condemn the use of alcoholic beverages. These groups live in close proximity to Christians and Jews, who have more open attitudes toward alcohol. All religious and ethnic groups in the area have experienced a rising incidence of drug use, with heroin and cannabis prevalent among Jews (including those with diverse ethnic and cultural backgrounds, such as those from the former Soviet Union and Mediterranean region countries), Christians, and Moslems, and with alcohol use now being observed among young Arabs (Weiss, Sawa, Abdeen, & Yanai, 1999). Under these circumstances, a self-report screening test and its constituent concepts would need to be translated into Arabic and Hebrew. The test also would have to be discriminating with respect to the type of substance used, and be sensitive to the social and religious connotations of various substances. The lack of epidemiological research in the Palestinian Territories (i.e., the West Bank and Gaza) means that drug and alcohol use detected by opportunistic screening could not be compared easily with population estimates. Nevertheless, school surveys, criminal justice statistics, and informal observations suggest the need for more systematic data gathering in primary care, school, and clinical facilities in order to monitor trends, detect heavy users, and identify persons at risk (Weiss et al., 1999). The direct translation of instruments developed for more culturally homogeneous societies is probably inadvisable. Any screening procedure would need to rely on a combination of direct self-report measures, biochemical tests, clinical observations, and the measurement of risk factors that are not specific to substance use. Although the existing array of screening tests provides useful insights into all of these requirements, none of them seem to be capable of addressing the needs of cultural heterogeneity in a time of rapid social change, which is precisely the condition under which substance use is likely to flourish.

CONCLUSION: IS THERE A NEED FOR AN INTERNATIONAL SCREENING TEST?

Although self-report measures have been developed for both adolescents and adults, they have not been evaluated for use outside Canada and the United States, and often have not been developed within an organized conceptual and practical framework, as was the case with AUDIT (Saunders et al., 1993), an alcohol screening test. A critical review of current drug abuse screening techniques (U.S. Preventive Services Task Force, 1998) concluded that there is insufficient evidence to recommend for or against routine screening using currently available, standardized self-report questionnaires or biologic assays. This conclusion was based on findings suggesting that self-report tests may be, at times, inaccurate, and biological tests may be insensitive. Nevertheless, the U.S. Preventive Health Services Task Force (1998) suggested that questions about drug use should be included when health professionals are taking a history from adolescents and adults, based on the prevalence of drug abuse and the seriousness of its consequences. Given the evidence reviewed in this chapter as well as the Task Force conclusions, it appears that there is a need for an international screening test for drug abuse that is reliable, valid, flexible, comprehensive, inexpensive, and consistent with an enlightened public health approach to the early identification and management of substance use disorders.

Reliability (consistency) and *validity* (accuracy) are the sine qua non of a good screening test, but these essential criteria vary with the population screened, the nature of the test, and the person responsible for screening. Any program seeking to develop a new screening test should evaluate its reliability and validity not only in relation to external criteria, but also in relation to existing screening tests.

Validity and reliability are likely to be affected by the confidentiality of the information provided during screening. Confidentiality is especially important with regard to revealing information about adolescents to parents or guardians, interagency communication, and long-term record keeping (including the issue of who has access to the information). Privacy and confidentiality are likely to affect response bias (Babor, Brown, & Del Boca, 1990), which is the distortion of self-report information because of defensiveness, perceived threat, or memory impairment.

To supplement and corroborate the information gathered with the self-report screening instrument, data should be collected from interviewer observations, family members, and other sources. These sources include people working within the juvenile justice, child welfare, or school system; clergy; peers; family (including siblings and nontraditional family members); and the health care system. Getting information from various people using different methods (e.g., self-report and biological measures) will help the assessor to guard against developing an incorrect picture based on the person's denial, misrepresentation, or minimization of the situation, and can often serve as a way to motivate the respondent to provide more accurate information. Biological tests can be a useful adjunct to screening for drug abuse, but they need to be part of a more comprehensive screening program.

Flexibility is an important characteristic to the extent that there are many different settings, populations, screening agents, and purposes that a screening test is needed for. Ideally, an international screening test should be adaptable to different cultures, different substances, different patterns of substance use, different languages, different settings, and different purposes, such as case finding as well as screening for risk factors.

Comprehensiveness refers to the ability of a test to detect clinically meaningful forms of drug abuse as well as the risk of abuse. It also refers to the primary methods of detection, which are self-report, collateral informant, biological, and physical examination procedures. Expense is an important consideration, given the lack of resources to support drug abuse screening in many countries and the low priority given to drug abuse as a major public health problem.

Finally, there is a need for a screening test to be developed within the context of an enlightened public health approach to early intervention. Such a context includes a clear conceptual understanding of the epidemiology of drug abuse, the nature of the condition or conditions in need of detection (e.g., premorbid risk factors, hazardous use, harmful use, or dependence), the natural histories of these conditions, and the availability of appropriate interventions to manage the persons who screen positive.

The previous review suggests that progress has been made in all of these areas. Several conditions (e.g., harmful use and dependence) that could be the target of screening and a number of risk factors have been identified that may lead to early identification. Although the natural history of these conditions varies with the dependence liability of the substance, a variety of methods have been developed to specify the type of substance and stage of progression between initial use and severe dependence. A large number of screening tests have been developed, but as yet there is no consensus about the best procedure to use with either adolescents or adults. Further work is therefore needed to develop and validate accurate screening instruments, especially instruments suitable for use in primary care in areas of the world such as the Middle East, where drug abuse is prevalent but difficult to detect.

Although the major focus of the present review is on screening, it is important to view screening in the context of effective treatment and other types of intervention. If intervention does not exist or is not feasible, then screening is not useful. The term *intervention* includes any effort made to correct a problematic condition or behavior. Among the least expensive interventions are conversations between a substance user and a concerned physician, teacher, parent, or friend. Although there is good evidence of the effectiveness of brief interventions with cigarette smokers and drinkers (U.S. Preventive Services Task Force, 1998), the use of early intervention approaches with drug users has not been studied except in the case of cannabis (Stephens, Roffman, & Simpson, 1994). The most common interventions are treatment efforts that may take place in outpatient, partial hospital, or residential settings (including correctional facilities).

Given the difficulties of designing a screening test, and the wide spectrum of possible target conditions (e.g., risk, vulnerability, use, intoxication, dependence, problems), it is clear that the purpose of a screening test first needs to be stated before it can be properly evaluated against a performance criterion, and that a multipurpose screening test may be needed to cover a minimum number of important domains. Separate tests may have to be developed for adolescents and adults, with flexible procedures to gain essential and ancillary information. Finally, the test has to be adaptable to different populations defined by age, gender, language, and culture, and it needs to be acceptable to health professionals so that they will use it appropriately. Despite these challenges, the need for an international screening test is clear in light of its potential value for public health and clinical practice.

ACKNOWLEDGMENT

The writing of this chapter was supported in part from funds provided by the World Health Organization, Project on Identification and Management of Psychoactive Substance Problems in Primary Health Care Settings. The author would like to thank Drs. Maristela Monteiro, Robert Ali, Michael Farrell, Richard E. Isralowitz, and John Marsden for their helpful contributions to the initial drafts of this chapter.

REFERENCES

Adler, I., & Kandel, D. B. (1981). Cross-cultural perspectives on developmental stages in adolescent drug use. *Journal of Studies on Alcohol, 42,* 701–715.

Allen, J. P., Litten, R. Z., Fertig, J. B., & Babor, T. F. (1997). A review of research on the Alcohol Use Disorders Identification Test (AUDIT). *Alcoholism: Clinical and Experimental Research, 21,* 613–619.

Babor, T. F., Brown, J., & Del Boca, F. K. (1990). Validity of self-reports in applied research on addictive behaviors: Fact or fiction? *Behavioral Assessment, 12,* 5–31.

Babor, T. F., & Kadden, R. (1985). Screening for alcohol problems: Conceptual issues and practical considerations. In N. Chang & H. M. Chao (Eds.), *Early identification of alcohol abuse* (pp. 1–30). National Institute on Alcohol Abuse and Alcoholism Research Monograph 17 (U.S. Department of Health and Human Services Publication No. ADM 85-1258). Washington, DC: U.S. Government Printing Office.

Barnes, G. M. (1984). Adolescent alcohol abuse and other problem behaviors: Their relationships and common parental influences. *Journal of Youth and Adolescence, 13,* 329–348.

Brown, R. L., & Rounds, L. A. (1995). Conjoint screening questionnaires for alcohol and other drug abuse: Criterion validity in a primary care practice. *Wisconsin Medical Journal, 94,* 135–140.

Bryer, J. B., Martines, K. A., & Dignan, M. A. (1990). Millon Clinical Multiaxial Inventory alcohol and drug abuse scale and the identification of substance-abuse patients. *Psychological Assessment, 2,* 438–441.

Butcher, J. N., Dahlstrom, W. G., Graharn, J. R., Tellegen, A., & Kaemmer, B. (1989). *MMPI-2: Manual for administration and scoring.* Minneapolis: University of Minnesota Press.

Coombs, R. H., Fawzy, F. I., & Gerber, B. E. (1986). Patterns of cigarette, alcohol, and other drug use among children and adolescents: A longitudinal study. *International Journal of the Addictions, 21,* 897–913.

Des Jarlais, R., Eisenberg, L., Good, B., & Kleinman, A. (1995). *World mental health. Problems and priorities in low-income countries.* Oxford, United Kingdom: Oxford University Press.

Edwards, G., Arif, A., & Hodgson, R. (1981). Nomenclature and classification of drug- and alcohol-related problems: A WHO memorandum. *Bulletin of the World Health Organization, 59,* 225–242.

Gottesman, I. I., & Prescott, C. A. (1989). Abuses of the MacAndrew MMPI Alcoholism Scale: A critical review. *Clinical Psychology Review, 9,* 223–242.

Greene, R. L., Weed, N. C., Butcher, J. N., Arredondo, R. & Davis, H. G. (1992). A cross-validation of MMPI-2 substance abuse scales. *Journal of Personality Assessment, 58,* 405–410.

Higgins-Biddle, J. C., Babor, T. F., Mullahy, J., Daniels, J., & McRee, B. (1997). Alcohol screening and brief interventions: Where research meets practice. *Connecticut Medicine, 61,* 565–575.

Huba, G. J., Newcomb, M. D., & Bentler, P. M. (1988). Adverse drug experiences and drug use behaviors. A one-year longitudinal study of adolescents. *Journal of Pediatric Psychology, 11,* 203–219.

Inciardi, J. A. (1994). *Screening and assessment for alcohol and other drug abuse among adults in the criminal justice system.* Treatment Improvement Protocol (TIP) Series. (U.S. Department of Health and Human Services Publication No. SMA 94-2075). Rockville, MD: U.S. Department of Health and Human Services.

Jessor, R., Chase, J. A., & Donovan, J. E. (1980). Psychosocial correlates of marijuana use and problem drinking in a national sample of adolescents. *American Journal of Public Health, 70,* 604–613.

Kalant, H., Corrigall, W., & Smart, R. (1997). *Cannabis: A health perspective and research agenda.* Geneva: World Health Organization.

Kandel, D. B., Davies, M., Karus, D., & Yamaguchi, K. (1986). The consequences in young adulthood of adolescent drug involvement. *Archives of General Psychiatry, 43,* 746–754.

Kaplan, H. B. (1985). Testing a general theory of drug abuse and other deviant adaptations. *Journal of Drug Issues, 15,* 477–492.

Kirisci, L., Mezzich, A., & Tarter, R. (1995). Norms and sensitivity of the adolescent version of the Drug Use Screening Inventory. *Addictive Behaviors, 20,* 149–157.

Klitzner, M., Schwartz, R. H., Gruenewald, P., & Blasinsky, M. (1987). Screening for risk factors for adolescent alcohol and drug use. *American Journal of Diseases of Childhood, 141,* 45–49.

MacAndrew, C. (1965). The differentiation of male alcoholic outpatients from non-alcoholic psychiatric outpatients by means of the MMPI. *Quarterly Journal of Studies on Alcohol, 26,* 238–246.

McLaney, M. A., Del Boca, F. K., & Babor, T. F. (1994). A validation study of the Problem-Oriented Screening Instrument for Teenagers (POSIT). *Journal of Mental Health, 3,* 363–376.

Miller, F. G. (1997). SASSI: application and assessment for substance-related problems. *Journal of Substance Misuse, 2,* 163–166.

Millon, T. (1994). *Millon Clinical Multiaxial Inventory manual.* Minneapolis, MN: National Computer Systems, Inc.

Newcomb, M. D., & Bentler, P. M. (1988). *Consequences of adolescent drug use*. Newbury Park, CA: Sage Publications.

Preng, K. W., & Clopton, J. R. (1986). The MacAndrew Scale: Clinical application and theoretical issues. *Journal of Studies on Alcohol, 47,* 228–236.

Rahdert, E. R. (Ed.) (1991). *The Adolescent Assessment/referral System manual.* (U.S. Department of Health and Human Services Publication No. ADM 91-1735). Rockville, MD: National Institute on Drug Abuse.

Saunders, J. B., Aasland, O. G., Babor, T. F., de la Fuente, J. R., & Grant, M. (1993). Development of the Alcohol Use Disorders Identification Test (AUDIT): WHO collaborative project on early detection of persons with harmful alcohol consumption. II. *Addiction, 88,* 791–804.

Schwartz, R. H., & Wirtz, P. W. (1990). Potential substance abuse: Detection among adolescent patients: Using the Drug and Alcohol Problem (DAP) Quick Screen, a 30-item questionnaire. *Clinical Pediatrics, 29,* 38–43.

Selzer, M. L. (1971). The Michigan Alcoholism Screening Test: The quest for a new diagnostic instrument. *American Journal of Psychiatry, 127,* 1653–1656.

Skinner, H. A. (1982). The Drug Abuse Screening Test. *Addictive Behaviors, 7,* 363–371.

Stephens, R. S., Roffman, R. A., & Simpson, E. E. (1994). Treating adult marijuana dependence: A test of the Relapse Prevention Model. *Journal of Consulting and Clinical Psychology, 62,* 92–99.

Svanum, S., & Ehrmann, L. C. (1993). The validity of the MMPI in identifying alcoholics in a university setting. *Journal of Studies on Alcohol, 54,* 722–729.

Svanum, S., & McGrew, J. (1995). Prospective screening of substance dependence: The advantages of directness. *Addictive Behaviors, 20,* 205–213.

Tarter, R., & Hegedus, A. (1991). The Drug Use Screening Inventory: Its applications in the evaluation and treatment of alcohol and drug abuse. *Alcohol, Health and Research World, 15,* 65–75.

Tarter, R., McBride, H., Buonpane, N., & Schneider, D. (1977). Differentiation of alcoholics according to childhood history of minimal brain dysfunction, family history, and drinking pattern. *Archives of General Psychiatry, 34,* 761–768.

United Nations International Drug Control Programme (UNDCP). (1997). *World drug report*. New York: Oxford University Press.

U.S. Preventive Services Task Force. (1998). *Guide to clinical preventive services* (2nd ed.). Washington, DC: U.S. Department of Health and Human Services.

Ustun, T. B., & Sartorius, N. (1995). *Mental illness in general health care. An international study.* London: John Wiley & Sons.

Weiss, S., Sawa, G. H., Abdeen, Z., & Yanai, J. (1999). Substance abuse studies and prevention efforts among Arabs in the 1990s in Israel, Jordan and the Palestinian Authority—A literature review. *Addiction, 94,* 177–198.

Winters, K. C. (1992). Development of an adolescent alcohol and other drug abuse screening scale: Personal Experience Screening Questionnaire. *Addictive Behaviors, 17,* 479–490.

Wolff, K., Farrell, M., Marsden, J., Monteiro, M., Ali, R., Welch, S., & Strang, J. (1999). A review of biological indicators of illicit drug use, practical considerations and clinical usefulness. *Addiction, 94,* 1279–1298.

PART IV

Perspectives of Drug Services: Needs and Intervention Strategies

11

Patterns, Policies, and Treatment Strategies of Substance Abuse in Israel: Past and Present

David Elisha, Jorge Gleser, and Michael Reiter

INTRODUCTION

Since the establishment of Israel in 1948, the country has experienced significant political and social changes as well as a rapid cultural transformation. These events may be attributed primarily to the fact that Israel has absorbed millions of immigrants during its brief history and to the consequences of military conflicts with neighboring countries. This chapter begins with a review of the highlights of these events in order to provide a framework for understanding the substance abuse problem in the country over time.

Israel's population numbered 600,000 in its first year of statehood (1948), and it has grown tenfold up to the year 2000. During the 1950s and early 1960s, a large influx of refugees, hailing from Europe (fleeing the Holocaust), North Africa, and the Middle East, flooded the fledgling state. Israel was largely successful in absorbing the vast majority of these immigrants, who subsequently contributed to the enormous task of building the country. Many of these immigrants, however, experienced cultural shock as well as serious social and economic problems as a result of relocation. The result was the emergence of distressed neighborhoods in urban centers and rapidly established development towns. These neighborhoods, characterized by economic stagnation and social ills typically associated with anomie and disintegration, became centers of high rates of school dropouts and juvenile delinquency, unemployment, criminality, and an emerging culture of substance abuse. To this day, these distressed communities have remained stagnant and with substance abuse problems affecting a significant number of people.

The Six-Day War in 1967, during which time Israel occupied Gaza, the West Bank, and the Golan Heights, marked an important milestone for the country in terms of social and cultural implications. Israel moved further away from the pioneering and socialist spirit that characterized its formative years and toward a liberal, materialistic society. This change, among others, was accompanied by an increase in the recreational use of alcoholic beverages and drugs including hallucinogens imported from the United States and Western Europe. Two additional factors contributed to an increase in substance abuse. One was the changes in borders, which brought with it social and political problems resulting from the occupation of Arab populations. The changed borders also created greater opportunities for smugglers to import large quantities of cannabis and high-grade heroin into the country. The second factor was the influx of American and European young volunteers who came to Israel in the wake of the 1967 war and often brought with them a culture of drug use.

New waves of immigrants reached Israel again in the late 1970s and subsequently throughout the 1990s, mostly from the former Soviet Union. The vast majority of these new immigrants were well adjusted and productive, but a small minority came to Israel with problems such as delinquency, mental illness, chronic alcoholism, and addiction to opioids, typically taken intravenously. Although small in absolute numbers, the newly arrived drug addicts and alcoholics created a strain on the substance abuse treatment centers, necessitating an expansion of the existing services as well as changes in policies and intervention strategies.

The following review is divided into three periods, each reflecting unique patterns of substance abuse and the national response to that abuse. An attempt is made to identify, in each period, the patterns of substance abuse, the prevailing community attitudes toward the problem, governmental response, treatment approaches, and the status of the service system (see Table 11.1).

THE FORMATIVE YEARS AND COMING OF AGE (1948–1969)

Reports in major professional journals on rates of substance abuse and on treatment interventions in Israel began to appear only in the early 1970s. A review of these publications reveals that no surveys were conducted during the preceding two decades. It is possible, however, to draw a general picture of the patterns of abuse, existing service systems, and treatment practices prevalent during this period (1948–1969).

The perception shared by medical and other professionals was that substance abuse in Israel during the first 20 years of the state's existence was only a minor problem that involved primarily individuals from the lower class and the criminal underworld. There were no reliable data regarding the extent of substance abuse, but a few figures were reported that reflected the small magnitude of alcohol abuse during that period. For example, it has been reported that from 1949 to 1963, there were only 70 alcohol-related admissions to inpatient medical facilities (Kersilovsky

& Yaglom, 1977). Another report indicated that in 1966 alone, there were 76 alcohol-related new admissions (Falik, 1977). While this finding suggested an increase in the rate of alcohol abuse compared with the previous years, it still reflected a phenomenon of limited scope.

The extent of drug abuse during this period is not known because no reliable findings are available. Anecdotal reports indicated that the number of opioid abusers was around 500, that between 1966 and 1968 the number of drug-related arrests doubled, and that in 1967 the number of drug-related admissions to psychiatric hospitals increased significantly (Reiter, 1977).

The prevalent drugs of abuse were hashish, opium, heroin, and barbiturates (Miller, 1971). Individuals came to the attention of the authorities when they clashed with the law, when they came to demand drugs from medical staff in primary care clinics, or when they appeared in hospital emergency rooms suffering from medical crises caused by overdose, withdrawal, or other drug-related problems.

Although various governmental agencies, primarily the Ministry of Health and the Ministry of Labor and Social Affairs, were ostensibly responsible for dealing with substance abusers, there was no national policy regarding their treatment or management. With the absence of specialized treatment centers, substance abusers were usually referred to psychiatric units, which either rejected them or reluctantly admitted them and then managed them with major tranquilizers or antidepressant medications, after which they underwent detoxification. The use of psychiatric units for the management of alcoholics and of opioid addicts was based on the assumption that substance abuse was a result of "bad" or "flawed" character; with the absence of specialized treatment units, admission to psychiatric hospitals was a forced choice. Few, if any, of the medical or paramedical staff in psychiatric facilities, however, had any specialized training in handling or treating substance abusers. Moreover, those who did attempt to apply current treatment methods viewed substance abusers in classic psychodynamic terms.

Over time, it became apparent that attempts to apply psychodynamic principles to the treatment of substance abusers in Israel generally failed, as did efforts to integrate substance abusers into the milieu treatment programs in psychiatric units. Substance abusers, on their part, resented being forced to stay in the stigmatized psychiatric units, to mix with the "insane" and be prescribed antipsychotic or antidepressant medication. On the other hand, the staff and psychiatric patients objected to the presence in the psychiatric units of, in their view, morally flawed and violence-prone individuals with criminal records. The encounter between the mentally ill and substance abusers in psychiatric units often resulted in aggressive and occasionally violent incidences, especially when such incidences involved opioid addicts. There were numerous reports of opioid addicts threatening staff while trying to obtain benzodiazepines and other drugs or preying on vulnerable female patients sexually or otherwise harassing them. As things evolved, the treatment of substance abusers in psychiatric units was reduced to medically

Table 11.1
Chronology of Substance Abuse-Related Events in Israel

Year	Service System	Ministerial & Inter-ministerial Initiatives	Legislation	Other Events and Milestones
1936			British mandate: Dangerous Drugs Ordinance	
1961			Israel ratifies the International Convention on Dangerous Drugs	
1968	Murder of regional pharmacist in Acre by a drug addict			
1970		1st Inter-ministerial Committee on Substance Abuse		1st International Congress on Cannabis Abuse held in Israel
1972				2nd International Conference on Drug Abuse held in Israel; 1st survey on drug abuse among youth
1973			Israel ratifies revised dangerous drugs ordinance	Ministry of Health committee recommends establishing ambulatory drug treatment centers in three major cities
1975	First ambulatory drug treatment center opens in Jaffa and includes methadone treatment	The Ministry of Health establishes a special coordinator for substance abuse		Uncontrolled survey estimates there are 2,400 drug addicts in Israel
1976	An ambulatory drug treatment center opens in Jerusalem			
1977	Ambulatory drug treatment centers open in Haifa, Beer Sheva and Ramleh/Lod; Al-Sam, the 1st NGO in the field of drug abuse, begins to operate offering prevention and treatment programs in major cities	A special police commission reports a significant increase in drug-related crimes and in the use of drugs among high-school students		
1978		A ministers' committee recommends comprehensive program to combat substance abuse including enforcement, prevention, and treatment programs		
1982	First and only inpatient specialized detoxification unit for alcohol established by NGO with government funding			
1984	Medicate (a private clinic) begins dispensing methadone prescriptions			
1987	5,000 opioid addicts throughout the country receive methadone via private clinics			
1988	First inpatient detoxification unit opens in Jaffa by Ministry of Health		The Anti-drug Authority of Israel bill is enacted	

Year	Service System	Ministerial & Inter-ministerial Initiatives	Legislation	Other Events and Milestones
1989	Ministry of Labour and Social Affairs begins a national program of In Home Detoxification with freelance physicians	The Anti-drug Authority of Israel (ADAI) is established and assigned to the Prime Minister's Office	The Knesset (Israeli parliament) establishes a special committee on substance abuse	
1990	First inpatient detox unit in an Arab town is opened by an NGO with government funding	Corrections Dept. establishes an ongoing forum on substance abuse		
1991	The Ministry of Health prohibits dispensing of methadone in private clinics. Dispensing can only occur in special government-run methadone maintenance centers. Four such centers are opened in major urban areas—the number of methadone patients drops dramatically	The Ministry of Health establishes the Department for the Treatment of Substance Abuse		The 5th International Congress of Drug Abuse held in Israel
1992	The Correction Dept. begins a new and comprehensive policy to combat substance abuse in jails Mobile methadone maintenance Unit begins operating in Northern Israel	First course for immigrant physicians in substance abuse is completed. The physicians become involved with in-home detoxification, a joint program of the Ministries of Health and Labour and Social Affairs		
1993	First medical center affiliated methadone treatment center established at Ichilov Hospital in Tel Aviv		The law regulating institutions treating drug abusers is enacted [Institutions for Drug Users (Supervision and Treatment) Law, 5753-1993]	
1994	First ambulatory centers opened in Arab towns: Nazareth and Um El-Faham			
1995		Second course for immigrant physicians in substance abuse is completed		
1996	Ministry of Labour and Social Affairs discontinues in-home detoxification program; Ministry of Health expands ambulatory services including ambulatory detox.			
1998	Mobile Methadone maintenance unit begins operating in Southern Israel			
1999				The Israeli chapter of the International Society of Addiction Medicine is established
2000	Buprenorphine is introduced for opiate detoxification and maintenance			The 1st International Scientific Conference of the International Society of Addiction Medicine is held in Israel

supervised detoxification, after which they were discharged with no provisions for aftercare or for rehabilitation.

The introduction of the Methadone Maintenance Treatment (MMT) model in the United States in 1964 offered a new way of treating and managing opioid addicts. Israel was not late in applying this method, albeit in a rather rudimentary fashion that relied mostly on the psychopharmacological component with few provisions for psychosocial treatment. In 1967, the Ministry of Health hastily set up in Acre, a mixed Arab-Jewish town in the Western Galilee, a small ambulatory unit where opioid addicts were provided with methadone (Erdriech, 1977). The program was run through the District Health Office and had minimal medical and paramedical staff, who were charged mainly with screening applicants and dispensing the methadone. Although the number of registered addicts was small (30), soon the District Health Office became a focal point for local opioid addicts who saw it as a source for a government-supplied daily fix. This arrangement rapidly deteriorated, fostering aggressive acting out and violent threats that culminated in 1968 in the murder of the District Health Office's regional pharmacist. This traumatic event led to the opening of a methadone maintenance clinic in the local medical center. The clinic offered greater medical supervision but no psychosocial treatment or rehabilitation training. Lacking an appropriate therapeutic environment with treatment objectives or clearly defined boundaries, the clinic became a staging ground for opioid addicts who disrupted the daily life and operation of the medical center with their demands, threats, and manipulations. It was not until 1975 that an attempt was made to set up a therapeutic Methadone Maintenance Treatment Center in Acre, replacing the hastily organized clinic.

ACTING FOR CHANGE: THE INTER-MINISTERIAL COMMITTEES (1970–1988)

The early 1970s saw the beginning of a national initiative to combat substance abuse, especially opioid addiction. Beginning in 1970, a number of committees were assigned the task of studying the substance abuse problem and recommending steps to improve and expand treatment efforts. At the same time, official and unofficial estimates of the number of substance abusers were periodically reported.

According to data reported by the Ministry of Health, the number of opioid addicts in 1970 was estimated to be 450 (Miller, 1977). Among them, 180 were receiving treatment. The first known survey was published in 1971 (Miller, 1971). This survey, however, was aimed at hashish use among youth and did not contain any information about opioid abuse among the underclass. The survey followed the First International Congress on Cannabis Abuse held in Jerusalem. It reflected the growing concern among educators and parents at that time about the increasing use of recreational drugs among youth in Israel, a phenomenon that was regarded as part of the trend of Westernization taking place within Israeli society. The survey revealed that 5 percent of Israeli youth used hashish at one time or another. This finding raised fears that drug abuse was not a problem limited to the economically disadvantaged and criminals. As for opioid addicts, by 1975 their number was estimated at 2,400, indicating a sharp rise in the population and suggesting a problem of major proportions.

The figures for alcohol abuse were rising too but still reflected a problem of rather limited scope. The number of alcohol-related new admissions to psychiatric hospitals in 1974 was 108, rising to 144 a year later (Miller, 1977). These figures indicated to the authorities that they needed to respond to alcoholism, they had to give priority to the rapid expansion of opioid abuse.[1]

Developments in the area of community psychiatry contributed to new initiatives in the treatment of opioid and barbiturate addicts. During the period 1971–1972, the first Community Mental Health Center (CMHC) was established in Jaffa, a mixed Jewish-Arab section of Tel Aviv. A specialized treatment program for abusers was developed by one of the authors (M. Reiter), then the chief psychologist of the CMHC and one of the pioneering figures in the field of drug abuse in Israel. The program included screening of candidates, supervised referrals to inpatient psychiatric units for detoxification, and follow-up treatment in the CMHC. The follow-up treatment involved primarily group therapy, specially tailored for this patient population.

In 1974, a fact-finding mission headed by Dr. Jerome Jaffe, a substance abuse specialist in the United States, arrived in Israel to study the problem of substance abuse and to make recommendations to the Ministry of Health. The main conclusions of Jaffe's team were as follows: (1) the Ministry of Health should take primary responsibility for promoting and overseeing treatment of substance abusers; (2) as part of its overall responsibility, the Ministry of Health should develop methadone maintenance treatment centers and make methadone available to opioid addicts throughout the country; and (3) in order to be better prepared to carry out these initiatives, the Ministry of Health should establish the position of a National Coordinator of Drug Abuse Services.

The recommendations of the Jaffe mission served as a catalyst for a shift in the Ministry of Health's perception of its national role in dealing with substance abuse. All of the mission's recommendations were gradually adopted. The first to be implemented was appointment of a National Coordinator for Drug Abuse Services in 1975. Shortly thereafter, the ministry opened the first comprehensive Methadone Maintenance Treatment Center (MMTC) in Jaffa. This center grew out of the drug treatment program developed by Dr. Reiter in the CMHC. This pioneering program in Jaffa constituted the foundation for future MMTCs in Israel. The Jaffa MMTC offered a psychosocial treatment program along with psychopharmacological therapy. Attempts were made to engage clients in a specially tailored model of individual and group psychotherapy and in a carefully designed behavioral program, as well as daily on-site methadone intake and routine urine testing. By 1977, four additional ambulatory centers were opened in major cities across the country, some of them including methadone maintenance treatment as well.

In 1975, other inter-ministerial committee recommendations were implemented. Greater involvement of other ministries, notably Labor and Social Affairs, in the struggle against substance abuse was encouraged. Responding to these calls, the Ministry of Labor and Social Affairs opened two ambulatory alcohol treatment centers. This was the first major attempt to treat alcoholics through specialized programs and with trained staff. As staff of these centers gained experience, they began to engage in prevention and health-education activities in schools and other public institutions.

In 1982, the first residential center for alcoholics (25 beds) was opened by a nongovernmental organization, the Israel Association for the Prevention of Alcoholism (IAPA). Funds were obtained from the Ministry of Health, on a per-diem basis, in support of the treatment program, and the Ministry of Labor and Social Affairs covered expenses for rent and upkeep. Located in the middle of the country, the center admitted alcoholics from all locations. The treatment program of the residential center included thorough medical evaluation and treatment, specially tailored individual and group psychotherapy, and a milieu program incorporating Alcoholics Anonymous and 12-step principles. The establishment of the residential treatment center for alcoholics offered, for the first time, an alternative in the community to medical or psychiatric hospitalization. Encouraged by this initiative, the Ministry of Labor and Social Affairs increased the number of Ambulatory Alcohol Centers and thus assured continuity of care and follow-up treatment for alcoholics (Weiss, 1995).

Meanwhile, a problem of major public health consequence was developing throughout the country arising from the Ministry of Health's unofficial methadone policy and from the way local authorities handled opioid addicts. The introduction of methadone as an agonist for the treatment of opiate addiction was not supported with an adequate number of methadone centers able to accommodate the growing number of addicts seeking the substance. In response, a group of private physicians opened a clinic for opiate addicts with the sole purpose of prescribing methadone, taking advantage of the fact that there were no explicit laws or guidelines regulating its therapeutic use. The unsupervised operation of the private methadone clinic gave rise to an increasing number of registered methadone patients, who through diversion created a thriving illicit trade in methadone throughout the country. By 1988, the number of registered methadone recipients was 5,000, and the illicit trade in methadone continued to flourish so that by 1990 the number of methadone recipients reached 8,000.

During this time, a public debate over the use (and abuse) of methadone began. The use of the substance was perceived by the lay public and many professionals, including those of the medical community, as a practice that encourages drug addiction among individuals who are morally flawed and weak willed. According to this view, methadone centers enabled and encouraged government-sanctioned opioid abuse. On the other hand, those advocating the therapeutic use of methadone supported the position that opioid addicts suffered from a disease (defined years later as a disease of the brain) and that methadone maintenance is the treatment of choice for the problem. As it turned out, the unscrupulous practices of the private clinic that was doling out methadone prescriptions to thousands of individuals, some of whom were not even opioid addicts, damaged the case of those advocating methadone maintenance as a sound medical treatment. The debate continued for many years without reaching a satisfactory resolution.

While the debate over the use of methadone was going on, opioid addicts, their families, and advocacy groups pressured the Ministry of Health and other governmental agencies to make available other treatment opportunities in Israel. In fact, in the mid-1970s, contacts were made by Ministry of Health officials with representatives of Odyssey House and Phoenix House from the United States about the prospects of opening drug treatment and rehabilitation centers in Israel. These contacts failed to yield results, and the public in Israel was drawn to news about the alleged effectiveness of therapeutic communities (TCs) in Europe, especially those associated with the "Patriarch" organization. Opioid addicts and their families pressed local authorities to cover travel and treatment expenses for scores of opioid addicts who were admitted to TCs run by the Patriarch or other TCs in Europe. At the same time, public pressure was mounting for the authorities to take vigorous steps toward developing a service system that could provide drug-free treatment and rehabilitation opportunities for drug addicts in Israel.

Two examples illustrate the kind of community initiatives, characteristic of the period, taken to cope with the growing pressure of opioid addicts and their families. In Kadima, a semirural community, following the threat of an opioid addict to commit suicide, local authorities joined efforts with the police and health and welfare agencies to establish a unique program of detoxification, using a designated apartment in the community, combined with provisions for aftercare and rehabilitation. This initiative created a coalition that led successful efforts to rid the community of drug dealers and to invest in drug treatment programs for local opioid addicts. The other way of coping with the problem of opioid abuse, chosen by enterprising mayors, was to offer addicts free rent provided they agree to move out of town.

In 1985, the Mann Commission, appointed by the Knesset (i.e., the Israeli Parliament) was assigned the task of studying the drug abuse problem in Israel. The commission submitted its recommendations in 1986, calling for the expansion of the service system by increasing the number of methadone centers, opening residential drug treatment centers, and establishing therapeutic communities in Israel. The committee also proposed the establishment of an inter-ministerial antidrug authority.

The first Residential Drug Treatment Center for opioid detoxification was established by the Ministry of Health in 1988. It was, in fact, an extension of the methadone maintenance center in Jaffa that, since its inception in 1975, proved to be quite successful. Admission of opioid addicts to psychiatric or medical hospitals for detoxification gradually stopped and the era of specialized residential treatment of opioid addicts began. During that same year, the first therapeutic community was established in Israel. It was the culmination of lobbying and planning efforts of a group of professionals and members of volunteer organizations (among them, Al-Sam). Seed money was raised by Ms. Aviva Nagar, wife of a Ministry of Foreign Affairs official, who persuaded the Ministries of Health and of Labor and Social Affairs to work together to fund the project. The Beit Aviva TC, named after Ms. Nagar, who died shortly before its opening, is located in a semirural area between Jerusalem and Tel Aviv. It admitted its first residents in early 1988. Its first director, Eitan Sela, exploited the receptive attitude of government officials and succeeded in bringing together a number of ministries to work together to open the second TC in Israel (Ilanot) during that same year.

The opening in 1988, by the Ministry of Health, of the Jaffa residential detoxification program drew a large number of opioid addicts from all over the country who were seeking drug-free treatment. Having only a limited capacity (16 beds), the program could not meet the growing demand, which resulted in a substantial waiting list—six months.

During this time, the Ministry of Labor and Social Affairs was called on to become more involved with the management and treatment of opioid addicts. A number of municipal welfare offices opened, with guidance from the Department for the Treatment of Drug Addicts (Ministry of Labor and Social Affairs), that were specialized "drug treatment units" for screening, referral, and follow-up of opioid addicts. Because of the long waiting list for residential detoxification, staff of these drug treatment units considered becoming more involved in the detoxification of opioid addicts. An innovative approach, "Home Detoxification," was conceived and first tried in 1990 by staff of the Lod drug treatment unit. The method, run by social workers with the collaboration of freelance physicians, was based on a number of guiding principles, including: careful screening of applicants; a detoxification process that takes place in the client's home under conditions of curfew; strict supervision, monitoring, and active involvement of significant others throughout the detoxification process; and assured follow-up psychosocial treatment. Soon the method was employed in an increasing number of municipal drug treatment units and became an important part of the treatment response to opioid addicts in Israel.

A landmark event that was to change Israel's way of dealing with drug abuse took place toward the end of 1988. After years of inter-ministerial committee work, the Anti-Drug Authority of Israel Bill was enacted, turning the Mann Commission's recommendations (1986) into legislation. The bill called for the establishment of the Anti-Drug Authority of Israel, which was to be a statutory agency assigned the task of planning, coordinating, and overseeing all activities in Israel connected to the war against drug abuse. Various reasons dictated the exclusion of alcoholism from the authority's areas of responsibility, the major one being the legal status of alcohol use. This controversial decision has had long-ranging effects on Israel's overall strategy to combat substance abuse. It created a split, in most matters pertaining to policy, funding, and service systems, between alcoholism and drug abuse services and prevented the formation of a unified effort to combat substance abuse in Israel.

THE ERA OF THE ANTI-DRUG AUTHORITY OF ISRAEL (1989–1999)

In 1989, the Anti-Drug Authority of Israel (ADAI) began operation within the Prime Minister's Office. During the initial stage of its efforts, it brought together ministries and NGOs involved with substance abuse through joint committees and it addressed a number of pressing needs through policy decisions, prevention and treatment initiatives, and research. The Knesset took note of this development and established its own "Committee for the War against the Affliction of Drug Abuse." Unlike the ADAI, the Knesset's committee took responsibility for addressing both drug abuse and alcoholism.

One of the first major initiatives of the ADAI was to commission a comprehensive national survey of substance abuse in Israel in 1989 (Rahav, Teichman, Gil, Rosenblum, & Bar-Hamburger, 1990). This survey was subsequently repeated in the years 1992, 1995, and 1998 (Rahav et al., 1992–1998). The 1989 household survey was the first major attempt to assess rates of substance use and abuse in Israel, applying state-of-the-art survey methods and data collection instruments.[2] A major limitation of the household survey, however, is that it does not contain findings about chronic opioid addicts. Various estimates made during the 1990s ranged between the conservative figure of 10,000 (the number of opioid abusers known to authorities) and 20,000. It is estimated that 10 to 20 percent of chronic opioid abusers in Israel are women. An examination of rates of drug abuse from the subsequent household surveys suggests a small (and statistically insignificant) decline in adult drug abuse and a steady, though small, increase in drug abuse among youth, with a worrisome decrease in age of first use.

In terms of alcohol use, the survey relates to general consumption but does not provide insight into alcohol abuse or alcoholism. Estimates reported in the 1990s of alcohol abusers and chronic alcoholics show that there are between 30,000 and 50,000 in the country. The recent steep rise in the number of Israelis who suffer from alcohol abuse or addiction is generally attributed to the large influx of immigrants from the former Soviet Union. These immigrants, unlike other immigrant groups, came from cultures characterized by heavy recreational use of alcohol and by a significant alcoholism problem.

With support from the ADAI's joint committees, a number of far-reaching initiatives were taken. For example, in 1990 the Corrections Department began formulating a new rehabilitation policy and established a special "Forum for Substance Abuse." Two years later, the Corrections Department began implementing a comprehensive plan to combat substance abuse in prisons that included the introduction of innovative treatment and rehabilitation programs stressing drug-free environments within the prison. Later, an entire prison was organized around the principle of a drug-free environment and active involvement of all inmates in a drug rehabilitation treatment program.

In 1990, the Ministry of Health abolished the position of the National Coordinator for Drug Services and established instead the Department for Detoxification from Drugs and Alcohol. Later, following the initiative of one of the authors (J. Gleser), the department was designated as the Department for the Treatment of Substance Abuse and the scope of its responsibilities expanded. Encouraged by the ADAI, the department issued a decree prohibiting the prescription and sale of methadone outside of government-run methadone maintenance treatment centers (MMTC). The new regulation effectively stopped the supply of methadone by the private sector. This drastic measure created an immediate crisis for thousands of opioid addicts throughout the country. Not being able to obtain methadone through private practitioners, opioid addicts were forced to turn to one of the five government-run MMTCs, three of which were hastily opened just in time for this policy change. During the 12 months following the introduction of the new policy, the Ministry of Health managed the crisis and was able, for the most part, to successfully refer hundreds of methadone users to one of its MMTCs. Hundreds of others turned to private or public centers for detoxification. Many others continued with their abuse of heroin as well as acquiring an addiction to benzodiazepine and amphetamine. The illicit street trade for methadone was substantially reduced, and methadone gradually gained its place as a legitimate therapeutic agent for opioid addiction. By 1992, close to 900 individuals were receiving methadone maintenance treatment in the government-run MMTCs. In retrospect, this policy shift had mixed results; the control of methadone increased the problem of benzodiazepine and amphetamine abuse. A distressing indication of the problem came in 1991 and 1992, when health authorities were alerted to the fact that Israel was the country with the highest consumption of Fenitylin in the world and among the first in the consumption of Rohypnol. It took years of rigorous and determined efforts, involving the Department for the Treatment of Substance Abuse, the district pharmacists, and the Medical Board at the Ministry of Health, to reverse this trend.

Opioid and benzodiazepine addiction was another growing problem that required attention from the Anti-Drug Authority and government officials. One proposed initiative, combining medical knowledge, funding support, and vision, came from Miriam Adelson, M.D., an Israeli internist who served as a research fellow with Dr. Mary Jeane Kreek at the Rockefeller University. Dr. Adelson espoused the view that opioid addiction is a chronic disease that needs to be treated pharmacologically. Also, she believed that harm reduction is the most appropriate and promising strategy to deal with opioid addiction and the accompanying threat of Human Immunodeficiency Virus (HIV). Her response to this problem, therefore, was to establish a state-of-the-art methadone center affiliated with a major medical hospital, Ichilov in Tel Aviv. The center was to combine research with comprehensive medical and psychosocial treatment for opioid addicts in a setting free of the stigma commonly associated with methadone distribution facilities. In 1993, the center was opened and, to date, it remains the only one in Israel affiliated with a major medical hospital. The Ichilov Methadone Maintenance Center is now supported jointly by the Adelson Foundation, the Ministry of Health, and Tel Aviv municipality.

The early 1990s were challenging years for the Ministry of Health. Waves of immigrants from the former USSR reached Israel during that time, including many skilled technicians, engineers, physicians, and other professionals in need of employment. One of the creative initiatives that was suggested to alleviate the problem of unemployed immigrant physicians was to offer retraining opportunities in addiction medicine and then to integrate the graduates in the expanding substance abuse service system.

In a special project planned and coordinated by the "Treatment and Rehabilitation" committee of the ADAI, The Ministry of Health, through the newly established Department for the Treatment of Substance Abuse, ran a six-month course for 25 immigrant physicians. In 1992, nearly all of the graduates were placed in government-paid positions, employed either by the Ministry of Health or by the Department of Corrections. Those employed by the Ministry of Health were placed in one of the MMTCs or ambulatory centers or they replaced the freelance physicians working for the Ministry of Labor and Social Affairs in the special In-Home Detoxification Project. The integration of Ministry of Health immigrant physicians into the In-Home Detoxification Project was prompted by the death of a heroin addict during In-Home detoxification performed by a freelance physician working for Tel Aviv's municipal drug treatment unit. This event served as one of the catalysts that prompted the Ministry of Health to assume greater responsibility for the treatment of substance abusers. It should be noted that critics of the Ministry of Health's policies were claiming that the ministry had previously shunned its responsibility by not allocating sufficient funds and human resources to improve and expand services in keeping with the rapidly growing needs. In response, the Ministry of Health reluctantly accepted the ADAI's position that it should take full responsibility for all medical aspects of the treatment of substance abusers, including physical detoxification. In the wake of these policy decisions, the Ministry of Labor and Social Affairs agreed to phase out its In-Home Detoxification Project and focus instead on developing rehabilitation services.

An additional 25 immigrant physicians completed the Ministry of Health's retraining course three years later in 1995, and most of the graduates were able to obtain gainful employment in the field of substance abuse. The initiative to integrate immigrant physicians (from the former USSR) into the field of addiction medicine turned out to be a double blessing. As it was, the large wave of immigrants brought with it not only many professionals and medical personnel but also a sizable group of drug abusers and alcoholics or individuals at high risk of becoming alcoholic because of culture shock, stress related to absorption into a new culture, and homelessness. The availability of many Russian-speaking physicians, specially trained in addiction medicine, made coping with the influx of new cases of drug and alcohol abuse easier. In addition, the need for special training programs for physicians in substance abuse served as a catalyst for formulating policy guidelines and criteria for qualifying physicians as addiction specialists.

The year 1993 saw a major achievement in the regulation of the now proliferating market of for-profit and not-for-profit detoxification centers for heroin addicts.

After a lengthy collaborative process involving the Ministry of Health and the Ministry of Labor and Social Affairs, spearheaded by the ADAI, a bill was finally made into law (Institutions for Drug Users [Supervision and Treatment] Law, 5753-1993). This was a landmark law that established the basis for licensing and overseeing drug detoxification and rehabilitation services, which in the past were all too often run by unscrupulous profit-seeking entrepreneurs of questionable credentials.

The topic of opioid addiction received considerable media coverage in 1994. An innovative method described as a revolutionary approach, "Ultra Rapid Opioid Detoxification" (UROD), was reported by the mass media in the country. The method, introduced by CITA Medical Group, was based on clinical research conducted in Europe by Loimer and colleagues (Loimer et al., 1989) and later by Legarda and Gossaop (1994). The UROD approach uses two closely related opioid antagonists, Naloxone and Naltrexone. The detoxification process lasts only a few hours and occurs while the patient is under anesthesia. The procedure is rather painless and the success rate of the physical detoxification process itself is essentially 100 percent. Detoxification is routinely followed by Naltrexone treatment for relapse prevention and by psychosocial treatment. The introduction of this new medical procedure for opioid detoxification required the Ministry of Health to act expeditiously to study the procedure, determine whether or not to authorize its use, and formulate clinical guidelines. Spearheaded by the Department for the Treatment of Substance Abuse, and with the collaboration of expert anesthetists, the ministry reached a policy decision regarding UROD in late 1995. The policy was based on the following principles: (1) UROD was determined to be a safe procedure for the detoxification of opioid-dependent individuals provided that it is performed according to the special clinical guidelines issued by the ministry; and (2) UROD must be followed by long-term psychosocial treatment. With the absence of evidence supporting the cost effectiveness of the new procedure, the ministry initially decided not to include UROD in the government-run service system. Later, when findings suggested that this expensive method is less cost effective than the conventional methods, the Ministry of Health resolved to refrain from providing funds for public use of UROD but allowed its regulated use in authorized private clinics (Lowenthal, in press).

For a few years UROD was regarded by opioid addicts and their families as a magical procedure for detoxification. Over time, however, its popularity in Israel waned as the limitations of the method became evident. With the number of UROD seekers dwindling, the method finally attained the status of yet another alternative for opioid detoxification that requires both medical and psychosocial follow-up.

The period between 1992 and 2000 saw a significant expansion of services to address substance abuse. The Israeli Association for the Prevention of Alcoholism placed addiction specialists in ambulatory alcohol centers across the country and supervised their work; the number of beds was increased in the only residential treatment center for detoxification from alcohol; the number of MMTCs was increased from six to eight, and the number of those maintained on methadone reached 1,600; and two mobile methadone units were operating in rural areas in the northern and southern parts of the country.

The Ministry of Labor and Social Affairs, for its part, had significantly increased the number of local offices offering post-detoxification rehabilitation and day treatment and took charge of the eight existing public therapeutic communities. This last step was of special significance as it marked the resolution of a long-standing conflict within the ADAI and between the ADAI and the ministries. The conflict centered on the claim of many critics of the ADAI that it needed to confine itself to activities related to coordination and initiation of projects and refrain from running or even supervising services. By transferring the responsibility for the TCs from the ADAI to the Ministry of Labor and Social Affairs, this controversy was put to rest by limiting the ADAI to its mandated role as an inter-ministerial coordinating authority.

The Present: Year 2000

Israel's efforts to combat drug abuse have been guided, for the past 10 years, by a coordinating governmental agency, the Anti-Drug Authority of Israel (ADAI). The ADAI brings together representatives from the general public, NGOs, and government ministries dealing with drug abuse. These representatives formulate policies and establish strategic objectives and goals. Owing to the activities of the ADAI, Israel now has extensive prevention and health education programs, basic and applied research projects, specialized programs for the training and continuing education of medical and paramedical staff, coordinated law-enforcement policy, and a fairly comprehensive service system addressing drug addiction through ambulatory and residential treatment settings, continuity of care, and rehabilitation.

The Ministry of Labor and Social Affairs is charged with licensing and overseeing all drug treatment and rehabilitation services that are not medical in nature. The ministry lists the following drug-related services: 100 ambulatory units, operating through municipal welfare offices that provide screening, evaluation, and psychosocial treatment to drug addicts and their family members; 20 treatment groups for children of drug addicts; 25 programs for adolescents suffering from drug abuse or addiction; 16 day treatment programs; eight technology training programs to prepare addicts for work; and the operation and/or supervision of eight therapeutic communities. In the field of alcoholism, the Ministry of Labor and Social Affairs operates a network of ambulatory centers for alcoholics that includes health education, screening and diagnosis, medical detoxification (provided by medical personnel funded and supervised by the Ministry of Health), and follow-up outpatient treatment.

The Ministry of Education develops and implements prevention programs, targeting drug and alcohol abuse among primary and high school students. The programs are offered through publications and workshops for both students and educators and through long-term "life skills" programs.

The Ministry of Health, through the Department for the Treatment of Substance Abuse, is charged with establishing and enforcing policies, laws, and regulations in all matters pertaining to the medical aspects of substance abuse. During the 1990s, the department expanded and consolidated its various regulatory activities regarding the prescribing of controlled drugs, licensing of drug treatment programs, and the accrediting of physicians in the field of substance abuse. The department also maintains overall professional and budgetary responsibility for the rather extensive service system, spread over the entire country, that includes: seven ambulatory drug treatment centers; medical services for alcoholics in nine ambulatory centers run by the Ministry of Labor and Social Affairs; eight Methadone Maintenance Treatment Centers with two special mobile units in rural areas; six residential treatment centers for opioid addicts; and one residential center for alcoholics. A special residential program for older adolescents was opened in Jerusalem in 1999, constituting an important addition to the existing services. The opening of this service was in response to the growing problem of heroin abuse among youth. The department is also responsible professionally for two inpatient units in psychiatric hospitals for individuals suffering from a dual diagnosis of mental illness and substance abuse.

The pinnacle of activities marking the year 2000 were preparations to host the First International Scientific Conference of the International Society of Addiction Medicine (ISAM) in Jerusalem in November. The conference, organized jointly by the Ministry of Health, the ADAI, and the ISAM, reflected Israel's active and growing involvement in various UN, WHO, and international forums and organizations dealing with substance abuse. (*Editors' note*: Conflict in the region between Israelis and Palestinians forced the cancellation of the conference.)

CONCLUSION

The significant growth in services for substance abuse in Israel shows the increasing concern for the problem of addiction shared by the ADAI, the Ministry of Labor and Social Affairs, and the Ministry of Health. In recent years, new services were opened and existing ones expanded. As a result, most substance abusers who seek treatment can be admitted promptly or within one month of their request.

Much has been accomplished in Israel through government and nongovernmental agencies to address the problem of substance abuse. The diversified and comprehensive nature of these efforts is, however, not without a number of shortcomings. For example, attention must be given to: (1) expanding methadone and other agonists maintenance programs; (2) promoting public awareness and acceptance of methadone as a treatment for addiction; (3) increasing government funding for substance abuse treatment services; (4) encouraging greater responsibility by local government for addressing substance abuse problems through resource allocation; (5) developing improved strategies for continuity of care, including relapse prevention; (6) improving integration of services across ministries; and (7) expanding the field to include tobacco and behavioral addictions.

NOTES

1. During the late 1960s and early 1970s, there were concerns that existing treatment programs were inadequate and that there were no rehabilitation services nor follow-up programs. Mayer (1977) described a pilot project involving a specialized unit for opioid addicts within a psychiatric hospital. He noted that while this specialized setting solved some of the more acute management problems, the project did not achieve its goals because of the lack of expertise among the staff and the absence of any aftercare or rehabilitation services in the community. Mayer recommended establishing specialized ambulatory and inpatient treatment centers for drug addicts and developing rehabilitation services. This plan of action was echoed by other mental health professionals active in the field of substance abuse at that time (Reiter, 1997). Eventually, it was adopted by governmental committees and became the basis for a comprehensive treatment service system that was developed a few years later.

2. The findings pertain to use "sometime during the preceding year," and suggest that 6.8 percent of adults (18–40) experimented with drugs, 3.2 percent used cannabis, 4.0 percent used psychotropic medication (not prescribed by physician), and 0.5 percent used opioid or hallucinogens (the categories not mutually exclusive). For youth (12–14), the results indicated that 6.4 percent experimented with drugs, 1.7 percent used cannabis, 5.4 percent used psychotropic medication (not prescribed by physician), and 1.5 percent used opioids or hallucinogens (the categories not mutually exclusive).

REFERENCES

Erdriech, M. (1977). Treatment trials in drug addicts in Acre. *Public Health, 19*(4), 406–408 (in Hebrew).

Falik, A. (1977). The problem of alcoholism. Special Issue: Drug Addiction and Its Treatment in Israel. *Public Health, 19*(4), 465–466 (in Hebrew).

Kersilovsky, D., & Yaglom, M. (1977). The problem of alcoholism in Israel. Special Issue: Drug Addiction and Its Treatment in Israel. *Public Health, 19*(4), 474–476 (in Hebrew).

Legarda, J., & Gossaop M. (1994). A 24-hour inpatient detoxification treatment for heroin addiction: Preliminary investigation. *Drug and Alcohol Dependence, 35*(2), 91–93.

Loimer, N., Presslich, D., Lenz, K., Pfersmann, D., Schmidt, R., Fodor, G., & Aschauer, G. (1989). Induced detoxification treatment of opiate dependent patients—A new therapy concept. *Weir Klin. Wocheuschr, 101*(13), 451–454.

Lowenthal, E. (in press). Ultra rapid detoxification as compared to thirty-days inpatient detoxification program—A retrospective follow-up study. *Journal of Substance Abuse.*

Mayer, R. (1977). From psychiatric hospitalization to a comprehensive treatment of the addicted. Special Issue: Drug Addiction and Its Treatment in Israel. *Public Health, 19*(4), 412–415 (in Hebrew).

Miller, L. (1971). The epidemiology of drug abuse in Israel. *Israel Annals of Psychiatry,* 9(1).

———. (1977). Introduction. Special Issue: Drug Addiction and Its Treatment in Israel, *Public Health, 19*(4), 381–382 (in Hebrew).

Rahav, G., Teichman, M., Gil, R., Rosenblum, Y., & Bar-Hamburger, R. (1990). *The use of psychoactive substances in Israel. An epidemiological survey, I.* Jerusalem: Anti-Drug Authority of Israel.

———. (1992–1998). *The use of psychoactive substances in Israel. An epidemiological survey, II* (1992); *Survey III* (1995); *Survey IV* (1998). Jerusalem: Anti-Drug Authority of Israel.

Reiter, M. (1977). Treatment of drug addiction. Special Issue: Drug Addiction and Its Treatment in Israel, *Public Health, 19*(4), 385–396 (in Hebrew).

Weiss, S. (1995). From a medical psychiatric, individual problem to public health-social problem: The development over time of the Israeli governmental alcohol treatment system. *Addiction Research, 3*(1), 49–56.

12

Outpatient Substance Abuse Treatment Using Scientifically Supported Treatment Manuals: A Strategy for Addressing Addiction among Palestinian and Israeli People

Jeanne Obert, Khuloud Khayyat Dajani, Sofia Borkin, Richard Rawson, and Abdul Aziz Thabet

INTRODUCTION

With few exceptions, there is agreement that meaningful attempts must be made to build bridges between the cultures, governments, and communities of Israel and Palestine. It is very possible to build cooperative activities that go far beyond symbol and ceremony. Both societies face problems that require solutions, and it is reasonable to assume that cooperative projects can synergistically strengthen both societies. One area of need common to both Israel and Palestine is the issue of drug abuse.

Policymakers, health care leaders, and criminal justice professionals believe that in both Israeli and Palestinian societies, drug abuse damages individuals and communities. Similarly, people in both Israel and Palestine want to reduce substance abuse and help those who have become addicted. There is little debate that the establishment of effective treatment services in Middle East communities would provide a major addition to the health care systems in the region. The desire to reduce drug use, associated infectious diseases (e.g., HIV, TB, and hepatitis), and drug-related crime is strongly held by all parties despite the fact that effective drug services are in short supply in the Middle East, as they are elsewhere. Recent research efforts in the United States, however, have created a body of knowledge that supports a number of specific drug abuse treatment protocols. This new knowledge and methodology, if properly exported to the Middle East and adapted to the needs of its substance-abusing populations, could provide a solid foundation for treatment systems in these communities.

The drug treatment protocol approach is only now being used in the U.S. substance abuse service delivery system. The strategy puts in place a state-of-the-art approach that can be modified and updated as new knowledge becomes available. Health care leaders and teachers in the region will have current knowledge to establish a system in their communities that can be adapted and improved over time. This chapter describes some of the treatment manuals developed with a scientifically sound foundation that are currently being used in U.S. treatment efforts. The strategic use of these manuals in Middle East training efforts may offer a perspective on how they can effectively improve the service delivery systems in that region. Furthermore, the use of the manuals and the modification process needed to adjust the materials for Palestinian and Israeli drug users provide a description of how these manuals can contribute to efforts that promote interaction and peace in the Middle East.

Drug Abuse Does Not Recognize Borders or Religion

Tremendous global resources are being focused on determining the causes, nature, and extent of addiction, to both alcohol and other drugs, and to developing effective prevention and treatment interventions. In the United States alone, the combined budgets of the National Institute on Alcohol Abuse and Alcoholism (NIAAA) and the National Institute on Drug Abuse (NIDA) are more than $822 million dollars annually (Epstein & Gfroereer, 1998). Federal dollars spent on substance abuse, both directly and indirectly, comprised nearly 10 percent of total spending on entitlements and 5 percent of the overall federal budget for fiscal year 1995 (Merrill & Fox, 1998).

Compelling research findings are beginning to reveal information on the genetic, biological, psychological, and sociological underpinnings of the disease of addiction. Many of the findings have called into question some of the traditional views of addiction to alcohol and other drugs. For instance, as a 1997 Institute of Medicine report states, "The stereotype that drug abusers could change their behavior if they were sufficiently motivated is inconsistent with understanding the complex, multiple factors involved in addiction" (Institute of Medicine, 1997). Addiction is no longer considered an indication of weakness, insanity, or moral deficiency by most treatment professionals. Staying abreast of the research findings, though, is a daunting task for treatment providers who are primarily concerned with the pragmatics of treatment delivery. It often takes years for drug abuse treatment practices to reflect research findings.

It is well understood that treatment works and can be used effectively by a society to diminish drug use in a cost-effective way (Caulkins, Rydell, Schwabe, & Chisea, 1997; Gerstein, Harwood, Fountain, Suter, & Malloy, 1994; Substance Abuse and Mental Health Services Administration [SAMHSA], 1997). Despite this understanding, many people in countries all over the world are not receiving the treatment they need, in part because knowledge regarding effective treatments is lacking. In the United States, for example, 80 percent of the approximately 9.4 million addicted and dependent individuals go without needed treatment services (Epstein & Gfroereer, 1998). The challenge, therefore, is to bring the benefits of drug abuse treatment research to treatment centers throughout the world.

DEVELOPMENT OF TREATMENT MANUALS

In the Institute of Medicine report, "Bridging the Gap between Practice and Research" (Institute of Medicine, 1998), the Committee on Community-Based Drug Treatment identified four factors that inhibit diffusion of drug abuse treatment knowledge: (1) the structure of treatment delivery systems; (2) the diversity of the clients, providers, and other stakeholders; (3) the stigmatization of people who are dependent on alcohol and other drugs; and (4) an inadequate base of knowledge about technology transfer specific to the field. The use of manuals in the delivery of treatment can be helpful in addressing at least three of these four issues. Carroll (1997) explains the usefulness of well-written, empirically based manuals in the following manner "Manuals define the theoretical underpinnings, goals, and differences among treatments. In addition, manuals describe the strategies the therapist uses to reach the treatment goals and articulate guidelines that direct the therapist through the treatment process." Some of the many purposes that manuals serve are to:

- provide a means for objectively comparing different types of psychosocialtreatment,
- aid in the training and evaluation of therapists,
- further the transfer of knowledge from research to practice,
- allow programs to replicate treatment in multiple settings,
- accomplish the task of prioritizing goals and objectives according to those deemed most important in research trials, and
- provide a way to evaluate individual components of a treatment model and to look at how they effect outcome (Kazdin, 1995; Luborsky & DeRubeis, 1984; Moras, 1993).

One of the first comprehensive substance abuse treatment manuals developed in the United States was compiled in 1989. The Neurobehavioral Treatment Manual (Rawson, Obert, McCann, Smith, & Scheffey, 1989) was created specifically for the purposes listed above. This original publication was the forerunner of a series of treatment manuals known as the Matrix Treatment Manuals (Rawson, Obert, Coleman, & McCann, 1999; Rawson, Obert, & McCann, 1995; Rawson, Obert, McCann, & Ling, 1991; Rawson, Obert, McCann, & Ling, 1992). The development of the Matrix Manuals was supported, in part, by NIDA and NIAAA. These U.S. research institutes are part of the National Institutes of Health. One of their mandates is the development of effective treatments for substance use disorders. During the early 1990s, NIAAA funded a research project, Project MATCH (Project MATCH Research Group, 1997), that was designed to see whether different types of alcoholics respond differently to specific therapeutic approaches. Three treatments were studied. These included a 12-step facilitation approach, a cognitive behavioral therapy model, and a motivational enhancement intervention. Each approach was philosophically distinctive, had demonstrated effectiveness, and was of the type that could be incorporated into a standard alcoholism treatment program. Each treatment orientation was outlined in a manualized format to be used as a treatment protocol during the research project. This was the first scientifically based, systematic comparison of substance abuse treatments using formalized treatment manuals. The treatment manuals from this project are now available to the public from NIAAA.

In April 1998, NIDA published the first of a series of treatment manuals that also describe specific treatment components that can be used by alcohol and other drug treatment programs to enhance their existing programs. Each of the manuals outlines psychosocial therapies designed specifically for cocaine abusers.

NIDA MANUALS

Cognitive-Behavioral Approach

The first NIDA Treatment Manual (Carroll, 1998) was developed specifically for use with cocaine abusers. It presented a cognitive-behavioral coping skills approach focusing on *how* patients might change their substance use habits. The approach is based primarily on Marlatt's Relapse Prevention (Marlatt & Gordon, 1985) cognitive-behavioral therapy. It also shares elements from Beck's Cognitive Therapy (Beck, Wright, Newman, & Liese, 1991) and the Community Reinforcement Approach (CRA; Azrin, 1976; Meyers & Smith, 1995). In this approach, clients are instructed on how to stop drug thoughts, learn new social skills, avoid high-risk situations, and improve employment status. The manual outlines 10 individual sessions during which the above topics are delivered in a nonconfrontational, client-centered style.

Community Reinforcement Plus Vouchers Approach

The specific goals of the Community Reinforcement Plus Vouchers Approach (Budney & Higgins, 1998) are to achieve abstinence long enough to learn new abstinence-sustaining life skills and to reduce alcohol consumption when it is associated with drug use (National Institute on Drug Abuse, 1999). The intervention described in the manual outlines 36 individual counseling sessions delivered over the course of 24 weeks. The sessions address issues within the context of marital therapy, vocational assistance, developing new social and recreational activities, learning new skills, and taking Antabuse, a substance used to inhibit alcohol intake. The Community Reinforcement Plus Vouchers Approach (Azrin, 1976) works with a system of contingency management that uses vouchers (points exchangeable for retail items) to reinforce clean urinalysis tests. The authors of this manual conducted five controlled trials documenting the efficacy of this approach (Higgins et al., 1991; Higgins et al., 1993; Higgins et al., 1994; Higgins et al., 1995).

Individual Counseling Approach

The individualized treatment approach grew out of the large NIDA-funded Collaborative Cocaine Treatment Study (Crits-Christoph et al., 1997). It combines use of the disease model of addiction with the spiritual dimension of recovery. Elements of this approach include monitoring drug use behaviors, encouraging abstinence and 12-step participation, and providing relapse prevention education.

THE MATRIX MODEL MANUALS

The Matrix Model treatment manuals were developed in a clinical setting using scientifically supported treatment principles, the input of patients, and the results of treatment. The original three manuals (Rawson et al., 1989; Rawson et al., 1991; Rawson et al., 1992) were designed specifically for use with patients dependent on cocaine, alcohol, and opiates, respectively. In these treatment manuals, the individual session materials are specific to a particular drug of choice, while the group session materials are designed to be delivered to mixed groups of both drug and alcohol users. Subsequent versions of the Matrix Manuals are more generic and are designed to be delivered in a setting employing more group and fewer individual sessions (Rawson et al., 1995; Rawson et al., 1999).

The interventions and underlying principles that make up the Matrix Model are based on empirical findings derived from the drug abuse research world. In developing the tenets of the model, treatment approaches were evaluated with regard to their practical utility rather than strict theoretical or ideological considerations. Many of the principles from the NIDA manuals and from other drug abuse research findings underlie the structure of the Matrix Model manuals. The key elements of effective outpatient treatment, as evidenced by research findings, constitute the basis of this treatment model.

Teaching Cognitive-Behavioral Concepts

Structure and expectations. During the first phase of treatment, the primary goal is to stop the drug use. Structure is an important element in supporting drug cessation. In the Matrix Model of Outpatient Treatment, structure is created through the help of the therapist, who, through interactions and lessons, coaches and encourages clients to organize their time. Scheduling, planning activities, and learning how to choose safe places and people are some of the ways patients are taught to accomplish this.

Positive collaborative relationship with the patient. The less confrontational, client-centered approach was first employed as an element of the Matrix Model in the early 1980s. At that time, the prevailing orientation of drug abuse therapists toward their patients was highly confrontational, very hierarchical, and often demeaning. The idea that a collaborative, non-judgmental attitude should be assumed so that the therapist can function as a coach or counselor when working with the patient was controversial. The client-centered, respectful attitude toward a patient was found in professional therapeutic relationships but not usually in the drug abuse therapist-client alliances. This style of interacting has since been extensively described and disseminated by Miller and colleagues (Miller & Rollnick, 1991), and termed "Motivational Interviewing." This style of therapeutic connection and allowing the patient to be responsible for his or her own recovery is central to the Matrix Model.

Involve and educate family members. Information regarding the recovery process and relapse helps both the patients and their families understand why particular interventions are being promoted (Carroll, 1998). By reducing the concerns about how and why the problem occurred and reducing recrimination and blame, clients and their families are better able to focus on remedying the situation in the present.

Positively reinforce desired behavior change. Contingency management research (Higgins et al., 1993) has confirmed the value of using positive reinforcement for desired behavior change. The application of positive reinforcement as a central element of the therapist-client relationship is key to the success of the Matrix Model. Social reinforcement as well as small tokens and acknowledgment certificates are a few of the ways this principle is applied in the Matrix Model.

Provide corrective feedback when necessary. Using the motivational interviewing style of interacting with clients does not mean that the therapist is never direct about the desired behavior change. Patients are given direct advice regarding new social networks, recreational activities, and skills to minimize drug use (Higgins et al., 1994). In fact, the client relies on the therapist to honestly provide professional feedback and opinions. Therapists often find it helpful to explain the supportive research findings to patients in the context of their recommendations. This style of teaching or coaching provides patients with the consistent, respectful message that the recovery process is theirs to enact.

Introduce and encourage self-help participation. Research demonstrates a strong association between Alcoholics Anonymous participation that occurs during or following professional treatment and improvements in achieving and maintaining abstinence. In general, self-help programs promote the ability of clients to develop appropriate social skills, create healthy social networks, establish healthy intimate relationships, and engage in substance-free healthy activities. They also provide opportunities to learn socially appropriate mores and norms, how to receive and give advice, and how to mentor others. Matrix patients are strongly encouraged both by the therapists and by peers to participate in self-help activities as part of the Matrix treatment experience.

Urinalysis to monitor drug use. Random urine testing conducted weekly is an important part of any outpatient treatment program. Drug testing is not intended to catch patients who may not be telling the truth about their drug use; rather, it is presented and employed as a supportive tool for initiating and maintaining sobriety

Figure 12.1
A Sample Program Schedule for a Four-Month Outpatient Treatment Program for Substance Abuse

INTENSIVE OUTPATIENT PROGRAM SCHEDULE

Week	Monday	Tuesday	Wednesday	Thursday	Friday	Saturday & Sunday
Weeks 1–4	6–7 P.M. Early Recovery Skills 7–8:30 P.M. Relapse Prevention		7–8:30 P.M. Family Education Group		6–7 P.M. Early Recovery Skills 7–8:30 P.M. Relapse Prevention	12-Step Meetings and Other Recovery Activities
Weeks 5–16	7–8:30 P.M. Relapse Prevention Group	12-Step Meeting	7–8:30 P.M. Family Education Group or Transition Group	12-Step Meeting	7–8:30 P.M. Relapse Prevention Group	
Weeks 17–52			7–8:30 P.M. Social Support			

Urine testing and breath-alcohol testing conducted weekly.
One individual session is included in each of the program phases.

and increasing structure. Positive tests should be viewed as indicators that the treatment plan needs adjusting, rather than serving as proof of treatment failure.

Treatment components. Building on the above principles, the Matrix Model manuals outline a program structure that includes individual sessions, early recovery groups, relapse prevention groups, family education sessions, and social support groups. The manuals explain in detail what the purpose of each component is, how each of these components should be delivered, and how the format of each session should be structured. Handout materials for each session guide the therapist through the process. Figure 12.1 shows a sample program schedule for a four-month outpatient treatment program. A short explanation of each of the components of the treatment follows.

Individual sessions. The individual sessions are important to develop constructive relations between the patient and the therapist. The positive, egalitarian relationship that is initially established in the first individual session is the vehicle through which the therapist, functioning as a teacher and coach, promotes the self-esteem, dignity, and self-worth of the patient.

Early recovery groups. These groups, used in the first several weeks of treatment, teach patients how to: (1) use cognitive tools to reduce craving; (2) schedule their time; (3) restrict the need to discontinue use of secondary substances; and (4) connect patients with community support services necessary for a successful recovery.

Relapse prevention groups. In the model pictured in Figure 12.1, the Relapse Prevention groups meet twice each week from the beginning of treatment through Week 16. They are the central component of the Matrix treatment package, and are sequenced at the beginning and at the end of each week. They include open groups that are formatted for a very specific purpose. These groups teach cognitive behavioral skills and coach patients in using the skills to stay "clean." Therapists specifically avoid allowing the groups to become confrontational or extremely emotional. Whenever possible, the use of a co-leader who has at least six months of recovery is employed. The co-leader serves as a peer support person who can share his or her own recovery experiences.

Family education sessions. The Family Education Groups are offered to patients and their families once a week for the first 12 weeks of treatment. The topics discussed include: (a) the biology of addiction; (b) conditioning and addiction; (c) medical effects of drugs and alcohol; and (d) addiction and the family. The information is delivered using slide presentations, videotapes, panels, and group discussions.

12-step meetings, social support groups (for program graduates), and urine testing. These essential elements round out the treatment components in each of the Matrix Model programs (see above). Each component of the program is important and critical for a successful treatment episode.

Use of Treatment Manuals in Palestinian and Israeli Communities

In November 1997, one of the authors (R. Rawson), a drug abuse research expert from the United States, was invited to lead substance abuse training efforts in Israel and the Palestinian territories. This project included community training sessions conducted in Khan Younis, Ramallah, and Beer Sheva with Palestinian and Israeli health professionals. The training was coordinated by the Economic Cooperation Foundation (ECF), the Palestine Council of Health (PCH), and the Regional Alcohol and Drug Abuse Resources Center (RADAR), Ben-Gurion University, with sponsorship by the United States Information Service (USIS).

In October 1998, Dr. Rawson with the senior author (J. Obert) returned to conduct a five-day intensive training at Al-Quds University at the Abu Dis Campus and a two-day training in Beer Sheva. Thirty-five senior health officials attended the Al-Quds workshops from the West Bank and Gaza, including Dr. Degani, Dr. Borkin, and others. The closing ceremony of the training session in Al-Quds was attended by Dr. Fati Arafat, representing the Palestinian Red Crescent Society, Haim Divon, Deputy Director General of the Israeli Ministry of Foreign Affairs, Dr. Sarri

Nusseibeh, the President of Al-Quds University, and Ron Pundik, Ph.D., Director of the ECF. In Beer Sheva, over 50 Israeli and Palestinian participants attended the two-day training, including the senior PCH health official and the Director of the Israel Ministry of Health, Department for the Treatment of Substance Abuse.

The clinical training at the locations named above focused on the possible establishment of outpatient substance abuse services in Palestinian and Israeli communities. The purpose of the training was to help operationalize how outpatient substance abuse treatment is structured and to illustrate the types of treatment content that are employed from the Matrix treatment manuals and materials. In the initial training sessions, the materials were in English and were used as a guide for the didactic and role-play sessions. In the second set of trainings, conducted with Palestinian professionals, the materials were translated into Arabic, which greatly facilitated the comprehension and acceptance of the approach. Copies of the translated Matrix materials were given to the Palestinian participants.

The use of the treatment manuals, and especially the use of the translated materials, appeared to tremendously increase the enthusiasm that the participants demonstrated for the training experience. Before the materials were employed, the abstract descriptions of treatment concepts and elements did not appear to be grasped effectively by participants. Prior knowledge about outpatient substance abuse treatment approaches among participants was very limited. Substance abuse treatment was something delivered in a residential setting. Describing how substance abuse treatment could be done on an outpatient basis and describing how this activity differed from general psychotherapy were quite difficult. However, the use of the client session handouts and the educational materials developed for family members concretely demonstrated what was done in treatment sessions and how these activities could promote drug cessation and abstinence.

The use of the treatment manuals for participants (including the translation of materials for non-English speaking individuals) was essential to starting the process of establishing outpatient services. After the intensive trainings in Abu Dis and Beer Sheva were completed in 1998, the materials were translated into Hebrew for use with Israeli clients and retranslated into "local" Arabic for Palestinian use. As of June 2000, the substance abuse treatment materials have been used in a number of the Israeli and Palestinian treatment service agencies.

Issues in Implementation

Translation of manualized treatment materials into the native tongue of an identified population is only the first step in making the treatment culturally congruent. The identified drug abusing populations and the treatment providers may begin their relationship with language barriers. For instance, the Hebrew translations do not address the needs of the Russian drug-abusing population (now about 25 percent of the country's addicts). The translation of the materials for use in the Palestinian territories and then in Israel needs to proceed in such a way that all the diverse language groups can identify with the materials and with the caregivers.

In addition to the need for language adjustments, the treatment materials will not be useful to the Israelis or the Palestinians without cultural adaptations. The Palestinians are planning to accomplish this by presenting the translated materials to a group of professionals from Gaza and the West Bank prior to their implementation. Their observations and suggestions will be incorporated to accommodate cultural deficiencies before the materials are distributed. Once the treatment model has been implemented, further evaluations of efficacy and relevance will be conducted, and the materials will continue to be adapted. Similar methods for improving the cultural relevance of the materials are being planned for the culturally diverse Israeli population.

One important issue to be addressed is the simplification of the materials intended for patient use. Many of the drug abusers seeking treatment in this region have a low level of literacy. Adapting the materials so that they are brief and easy to understand will be important. Graphics, pictures, and case examples will help the target audience understand and relate to the concepts being presented. Sample scripts that are culturally congruent can amplify the instructions for caregivers. Every effort must be made to ensure that the treatment providers clearly understand the concepts so that they can relay the information adequately to those they are attempting to assist. The degree to which the materials are understandable and the supervisors are helpful and supportive will largely determine the success of the information.

Several other problems might be expected to occur as this model of outpatient treatment is implemented in Palestinian and Israeli communities. For instance, the importance of the family unit in these cultures means that achieving family involvement in the treatment process is critically important to the success of the intervention. Families are often extremely disrupted by drug abuse, and getting the family's support, particularly initially, is a difficult task. The emphasis on viewing addiction as a medical condition rather than a moral issue can be very useful in this regard. If family members can be educated about the biology of addiction, progress can be made toward reducing the anger, shame, and guilt that impede recovery. Treatment professionals need to be instructed and supervised in employing creative techniques for achieving family involvement as early as possible in the treatment episode.

A related issue is improving access to treatment for women in these cultures. While many women may need help with drug abuse problems, the shame and denial about their condition will often keep them from seeking assistance. Again, the evidence-based, medical approach utilized in the Matrix Model of treatment can help reduce those barriers to treatment when the educational material is adequately disseminated.

Finally, treating addiction in an outpatient setting will be a new concept, particularly in Palestinian communities. Traditionally, substance abuse was treated in inpatient settings with little or no psychosocial "coaching" following discharge.

This outpatient intervention relies heavily on professional, supportive therapies that can be delivered by nonmedical, professional personnel. It is a new approach for many people in this region and will have to be proven successful before it will be trusted as an effective means of intervention.

REFERENCES

Azrin, N. H. (1976). Improvements in the community-reinforcement approach to alcoholism. *Behaviour Research and Therapy, 14*(5), 339–348.

Beck, A. T., Wright, F. D., Newman C. F., & Liese, B. S. (1991). *Cognitive therapy of cocaine abuse: A treatment manual.* Unpublished manuscript.

Budney, A. J., & Higgins, S. T. (1998). *A community reinforcement approach: Treating cocaine addiction.* Therapy Manuals for Drug Addiction, Manual 2. (U.S. Department of Health and Human Services Publication No. ADM 98-4309). Rockville, MD: National Institute on Drug Abuse.

Carroll, K. M. (1997). New methods of treatment efficacy research: Bridging clinical research and clinical practice. *Alcohol Health & Research World, 21*(4), 352–359.

———. (1998). *A cognitive-behavioral approach: Treating cocaine addiction.* Therapy Manuals for Drug Addiction, Manual 1. (U.S. Department of Health and Human Services Publication No. ADM 98-4308). Rockville, MD: National Institute on Drug Abuse.

Caulkins, J. P., Rydell, C. P., Schwabe, W. J., & Chisea, J. (1997). *Mandatory minimum sentences: Throwing away the key or the taxpayers' money?* Santa Monica, CA: RAND Drug Policy Research Center.

Crits-Christoph, P., Siqueland, L., Blaine, J., Frank, A., Luborsky, L., Onken, L. S., Muenz, L., Thase, M. E., Weiss, R. D., Gastfriend, D. R., Woody, G., Barber, J. P., Butler, S. F., Daley, D., Bishop, S., Najavits, L. M., Lis, J., Mercer, D., Griffin, M. L., Moras, K., & Beck, A. (1997). The NIDA collaborative cocaine treatment study: Rationale and methods. *Archives of General Psychiatry, 54,* 721–726.

Epstein, J., & Gfroereer J. (1998). *Changes affecting NHSDA estimates of treatment need for 1994–1996: OAS working paper.* Rockville, MD: Office of Applied Studies, Substance Abuse and Mental Health Services Administration.

Gerstein, D. R., Harwood, H., Fountain, D., Suter, N., & Malloy, K. (1994). *Evaluating recovery services: The California Drug and Alcohol Treatment Assessment (CALDATA).* Contract No. 92-00110. Sacramento: State of California Department of Alcohol and Drug Programs.

Higgins, S. T., Budney, A. J., Bickel, H. K., Badger, G., Foerg, F., & Ogden, D. (1995). Outpatient behavioral treatment for cocaine dependence: One-year outcome. *Experimental & Clinical Psychopharmacology, 3*(2), 205–212.

Higgins, S. T., Budney, A. J., Bickel, W. K., Foerg, F. E., Donham, R., & Badger, G. J. (1994). Incentives improve outcome in outpatient behavioral treatment of cocaine dependence. *Archives of General Psychiatry, 51*(7), 568–576.

Higgins, S. T., Budney, A. J., Bickel, W. K., Hughes, J. R., Foerg, F., & Badger, G. (1993). Achieving cocaine abstinence with a behavioral approach. *American Journal of Psychiatry, 150*(5), 763–769.

Higgins, S. T., Delaney, D. D., Budney, A. J., Bickel, W. K., Hughes, J. R., Foerg, F., & Fenwick, J. W. (1991). A behavioral approach to achieving initial cocaine abstinence. *American Journal of Psychiatry, 148*(9), 1218–1224.

Institute of Medicine. (1997). *Dispelling the myths about addiction: Strategies to increase understanding and strengthen research.* Washington, DC: National Academy Press.

———. (1998). *Bridging the gap between practice and research: Forging partnerships with community-based drug and alcohol treatment.* Washington, DC: National Academy Press.

Kazdin, A. E. (1995). Methods of psychotherapy research. In B. Bongar & L. E. Beutler (Eds.), *Comprehensive textbook of psychotherapy: Theory and practice* (pp. 405–433). New York: Oxford University Press.

Luborsky, L., & DeRubeis, R. J. (1984). The use of psychotherapy treatment manuals: A small revolution in psychotherapy research style. *Clinical Psychology Review, 4,* 5–15.

Marlatt, G. A., & Gordon, J. R., (Eds.). (1985). *Relapse prevention: Maintenance strategies in the treatment of addictive behaviors.* New York: Guilford Press.

Merrill, J., & Fox, K. (1998). The impact of substance abuse on federal spending. In W. J. Bukosky & R. I. Evans (Eds.), *Cost-benefit/cost-effectiveness research of drug abuse prevention: Implications for programming and policy.* (NIDA Research Monograph 176). Bethesda, MD: National Institutes of Health.

Meyers, J. J., & Smith, J. E. (1995). *Clinical guide to alcohol treatment: The community reinforcement approach.* New York: Guilford Press.

Miller, W. R., & Rollnick, S. (1991). *Motivational interviewing: Preparing people to change addictive behavior.* New York: Guilford Press.

Moras, K. (1993). The use of treatment manuals to train psychotherapists: Observations and recommendations. *Psychotherapy, 30,* 581–586.

National Institute on Drug Abuse. (1999, October). *Principles of drug addiction treatment: A research-based guide.* (National Institutes of Health Publication No. 99-4180). Rockville, MD: National Institute on Drug Abuse.

Project MATCH Research Group. (1997). Matching alcohol treatments to client heterogeneity: Project MATCH post treatment drinking outcomes. *Journal of Studies on Alcohol, 58,* 7–29.

Rawson, R. A., Obert, J. L., Coleman, G., & McCann, M. J. (1999). *The Matrix intensive outpatient program: An 8-week introduction to the treatment of stimulant abuse and dependency disorders.* Los Angeles: The Matrix Center, Inc.

Rawson, R. A., Obert, J. L., & McCann, M. J. (1995). *The Matrix intensive outpatient program therapist manual.* Los Angeles: The Matrix Center, Inc.

Rawson, R. A., Obert, J. L., McCann, M. J., & Ling, W. (1991). *The Matrix model of outpatient treatment for alcohol use and dependency.* Beverly Hills, CA: The Matrix Center, Inc.

———. (1992). *The Matrix model for the treatment of opioid addiction with naltrexone.* Los Angeles: The Matrix Center, Inc.

Rawson, R. A., Obert, J. L., McCann, M. J., Smith, D. P., & Scheffey, E. H. (1989). *The neurobehavioral treatment manual.* Beverly Hills, CA: The Matrix Center, Inc.

Substance Abuse and Mental Health Services Administration (SAMHSA). (1997). *National treatment improvement evaluation study.* Rockville, MD: Substance Abuse and Mental Health Services Administration.

13

Alcohol and Drug Abuse from an Islamic Perspective: Implications for Intervention*

Alean Al-Krenawi, John R. Graham, and Mahmud A. Sehwail

> O you believe! Strong drink, gambling and idols and divining arrows are an infamy of Satan's handi-work. Leave it aside in order that you may succeed. Satan seeks only to cast among you enmity and hatred by means of strong drink and gambling, and turn you from remembering Allah and from prayer. Will you then desist?
>
> —Koran, Surah v. verses 90–91

> The Prophet Muhammad said: "Allah has cursed al-khamr and cursed the one who brews it and the one for whom it is brewed, the one who drinks it and the one who serves it, the one who carries it and the one for whom it is carried, the one who buys and the one who eats (profits from) its price."
>
> —Ibn-Majah, 1975

Similar to the way culture and religion shape responses to illness and treatment, culture and religion influence drinking and drug use and attitudes toward individuals who develop problems with these substances (Orlandi, 1992). Attitudes toward alcohol and drug use vary widely among cultures, from seeing alcohol as essential and sacred to viewing it as dispensable and destructive (Mandelbaum, 1965). Some cultures reinforce abstinence as a norm; others approve of drinking only as part of religious ceremonies. Drinking, especially if it occurs in a group setting, may

*An earlier draft of this chapter, now revised, appeared in Al-Krenawi, A., & Graham, J. R. (1997). Nebi-Musa: A therapeutic community for drug addiction in a Moslem context. *Transcultural Psychiatry, 34*(3), 377–391. Particular thanks are extended to Sage Press and to the journal's editor, Dr. Laurence Kirmayer, for facilitating permission for this work to appear here.

symbolize solidarity or, if done alone, may be seen as individual gratification or self-indulgence (Stivers, 1976). Perceptions about alcohol and drug use may vary from religion to religion; however, every culture and religion has developed its own model of coping with alcohol and drug abuse when it begins to threaten community stability. In the Moslem world, religious leaders and traditional healers use religious and cultural strategies to treat alcohol and drug abuse, as we will elaborate in the present chapter.

In Malaysia, traditional treatment of substance dependence—mostly for opiate use but also for alcohol—is performed by Malay traditional therapists, Chinese-Taoist practitioners, and Hindu-Ayurvedic healers (Johnson, 1983; Lee, 1985). The clients of those healers who have established a reputation in drug rehabilitation are not limited to co-religionists. Adaptations of ritual procedures are made in a remarkably tolerant manner to accommodate patients of other religious persuasions. In the Malay-Islamic and Chinese-Taoist traditions, specialist healers have emerged in the detoxification and rehabilitation of substance-dependent people. Traditional treatment approaches to substance dependence appear well accepted by motivated addicts and by the community in Malaysia. These programs of treatment are met by the generally supportive attitudes of government health authorities, who tend to be well informed about the activities of traditional treatment centers (Werner, 1979).

The Koran and the Hadith (what has been said or done by the Prophet Muhammad) state clearly that alcohol is prohibited by Islam. In the absence of explicit textual references, religiously based proscriptions against drug use, in contrast, rely on Islamic scholars' extrapolation of sacred references to abstinence from alcohol. To be sure, the dangers of drug use are well represented in Islamic thought. As one Islamic scholar, Ibn-Tymiah, points out, "drugs are more dangerous than alcohol" (Al-Bar, 1998). In fact, such awareness has increased over time. Over the past 10 years, many books have been published and conferences held in Islamic countries warning against drug use (Bader, 1987). These warnings have been supported with references to the Hadith and the Koran (e.g., Koran Al-Infal, v. 22; Al-Baqra, v. 195). The present chapter examines drug use and abuse from an Islamic perspective, using one sacred site, Maqam Al-Nebi-Musa, as a case study on how ordinary Moslems may use their religion as a vehicle to recovery. Particular emphasis is placed on the therapeutic components of Islamic rituals.

This chapter therefore joins a small body of research on drug abuse in the Islamic world. It analyzes Nebi-Musa as a therapeutic phenomenon, conceptualizing the site as a five-stage treatment process and providing insight into its therapeutic significance in the context of the individual, family, group, and community. Although literature that examines addictions in a Moslem context is sparse (Al-Radi & Al-Mahdy, 1989; Bilal, 1989; Bilal, Kristof, Shaltout, & El Islam, 1987; Bilal, Makhawi, Al Fayez, & Shaltout, 1990), the Moslem-specific research that has been done has contributed to that small but growing number of publications on multicultural dimensions of drug rehabilitation (De-Leon, Melnick, Schoket, & Jainchill, 1993; Gillis, Tareen, Chaudhry, & Haider, 1994; Heggenhougen, 1984; Szalay, Canino, & Vilov, 1993).

Data for this chapter are derived from five days of ethnographic participant observation (Brooks, 1994; Glik, 1988; Pfleiderer, 1988) undertaken by one of the authors during 1994. Over the course of the participant observation, open-ended interviews ranging from two to four hours were conducted with each of five Sufi mystics. Other subjects provided data informally.

ISLAM

Islam is the world's fastest growing and second largest religion. In 1997, Moslems represented 19.4 percent of the world's population, numbering 1,126,325,000, and were found in 184 of the world's 262 countries (Encyclopedia Britannica, 1997). Moslems constitute a majority in more than 48 countries and are significant minorities in many others. Islam, as will be discussed, is theologically diverse. Approximately 83 percent of all Moslems are Sunnites, 16 percent are Shiites, and 1 percent belong to other traditions in Islam. Although the Arab world is often seen as the heartland of Islam, most Moslems, in fact, are found in Asia and Africa (Esposito, 1995). There are 300 million Moslems in Africa and 778 million in Asia (Encyclopedia Britannica, 1997). Moreover, in Western countries, as in non-Western countries, Islam is an increasing presence. By 1990, as an example, the Moslem community in the United States outnumbered its Jewish counterpart (Encyclopedia Britannica, 1996). Similarly, in Canada, there were more Moslems than Presbyterians (Bibby, 1987). In 1997 there were 5.53 million Moslems in North America, 32 million in Europe, and 1.35 million in Latin America (Encyclopedia Britannica, 1997). Moslem social institutions in the West have increased in like proportion. For example, by 1992 the number of North American Islamic mosques, schools, community centers, publishing houses, and media programming units totaled over 2,300 (Haddad & Smith, 1994).

The term "Islam," pronounced "al-Islam" in Arabic, refers to the religion based on the doctrine that Moslems believe was revealed in the year 610 A.D. to the Prophet Muhammad in the city of Mecca. People who adhere to the religion of Islam are called Moslems. Both terms derive from the Arabic root "Salam," meaning "peace" or "submission." The basis of Islam is the Koran, a Holy Book consisting of 114 chapters: "it is the eternal, uncreated, literal word of God, sent down from heaven, revealed . . . to the prophet Muhammad as a guidance for humankind" (Esposito, 1995, p. 243). A second valid religious authority is the Hadith, the tradition of the Prophet Muhammad's words and deeds as well as those of many of the early Moslems. Although originally transmitted orally, these texts have been written in direct, conversational prose (Esposito, 1995).

Social Consequences of Islam

In anthropological terms, Moslem society tends to be high context, meaning it emphasizes the collective over the individual, has a slower pace of societal change, and has a higher sense of social stability. Its opposite is a low context society, which is frequently found in the West and which reveres the individual over the collective, and for which transitions are fast paced (Hall, 1976). Not surprisingly, the Moslem religion reflects and reinforces the high-context disposition of its societies.

Social stability, for example, is understood by Moslems as the achievement of social peace. This imperative is reinforced by an emphasis on the collective over the individual—a mutually responsive brotherhood and sisterhood extending an ummatic bond to a global level. "Help each other in the acts of goodness and piety and do not extend help to each other in sinful acts or transgression behaviors" (Koran, 5, v. 2). The Prophet Muhammad also advised Moslems to "Help your brother [the Moslem] whether he is the oppressor or the oppressed."

When the Prophet was asked how to help him if he is the oppressor, he replied: "Hold his hand from oppression" (Al-Jawziyya, 1993). The prophetic Hadith points out that "Every one of you is a shepherd and each one of you is responsible for his flock" (Nagati, 1993).

This sense of collective responsibility is further reinforced by how the Moslem views his or her place within society. Islam, it should be emphasized, is not concerned with the welfare of the individual alone; it seeks to achieve a wider societal well-being. While ensuring the individual's freedom, it places equal stress on mutual responsibility. This principle, in turn, is two-dimensional. The individual achieves balance between thought and action (internal), while caring for the collective welfare of society (external) (Azmi, 1991; El-Azayem & Hedayat-Diba, 1994). But this internal individual-societal consonance is best realized by a third party: through total submission to the will and pleasure of God. As stated in the Koran: "My worship and my sacrifice and my living and my dying are all for Allah, Lord of worlds" (Koran, 6, v. 163).

The Islamic perspective of a person emphasizes selflessness, healthy altruism, perfection of self, and giving happiness to others (Al-Bostani, 1988; Al-Issawi, 1988). It has a high ideal of the ultimate good, but also a means of being within reach of all adherents, for Islam promises repentance to anyone who is committed to fulfilling its conditions: "He is the one that accepts repentance from His servants and forgives sin and he knows all that ye do" (Koran, 42, v.25). While the sin may not be condoned, the sinner is nonetheless provided an opportunity to turn from sin and to obtain spiritual purification (Mohamed, 1995; Rizvi, 1989). The following pages will provide insight into some of these Islamic mechanisms.

The Context of Nebi-Musa

The Nebi-Musa complex is on four acres of land. The compound itself is constructed of Jerusalem stone, is 4,500 square meters in area, and is surrounded by walls 10 meters in height and several meters thick. Five gates provide entry and exit (Asali, 1990). After a prolonged period of physical neglect, Nebi-Musa now enjoys a sense of renaissance. Thousands of pilgrims, many of them Palestinian, come to this place annually to pay homage to Moses and to seek his intercessions to God. Many arrive on their own or are accompanied by family members, although there are also more traditional group retreats ranging in size from extended families to entire communities. Participants follow several, if not all, of the established routines of Nebi-Musa: prayers five times a day, periods of individual meditation and contemplation, reading the Koran collectively and individually, seeking religious and temporal advice from spiritual mentors, and, most important of all, prayer at Moses' grave. According to long-established Moslem conventions, gender separation is strictly followed (Mass & Al-Krenawi, 1994). In addition, female visitors are accompanied by their families and never stay for more than several hours. Men's visits range from several hours, to several days, to several months. Of those staying for longer periods of time, an increasing number over the last four years were being treated for, and were recovering from, addiction to such psychoactive drugs as angel dust (i.e., PCP—a dissociative anestheic), cannabis, cocaine, crack, heroin, LSD, morphine, and opium.

In 1991, two Arab Moslem males, one in his early 40s, the other in his mid-30s, committed themselves to a spiritual journey to end long-standing abuse of psychoactive drugs. This included visits to numerous mosques in the vicinity of Jerusalem. When the two came to Nebi-Musa in 1992, they found it abandoned and in a state of unclean disrepair. They decided that they were called to stay there and to restore the site to its former physical and spiritual prominence. They became Sufis, described by Al-Ghazali as spiritual ascetics who have renounced property and have sought oneness with God through a lifelong commitment to meditation, mysticism, and spiritual discipline (Al-Ghazali, 1950). Within six months they were joined by three other Moslem Arab males who were recovering addicts, all in their 30s. Shortly afterward, the five established a program of drug therapy. Over the past five years, an increasing network of recovering addicts has become affiliated with these Sufis. Due to this process, Nebi-Musa joined several previously established drug programs found in mosques within Moslem countries such as Egypt and Saudi Arabia (Abu El-Azayem, 1987; Baasher & Abu El Azayem, 1980; Jilek, 1994).

Generally speaking, Nebi-Musa may be conceived as a four-tier institutional model. At the broadest perspective is the wider network of individuals who do not live on-site during the period of therapy and who may not have experienced the drug treatment program but who are familiar with and supportive of Nebi-Musa's religious mandate. At a second level is the entire population of Nebi-Musa retreatants, both drug and non-drug related. Among this population is a third subset who visit with the Sufis for a variety of religious and mental health reasons. They can, but are not obliged to, participate in the drug treatment program, and many within this subset are not recovering addicts. Among this subset is a fourth level of Sufi clients, the subjects of this chapter, who are recovering drug addicts and who live at Nebi-Musa for purposes of addiction recovery. Nebi-Musa's therapeutic community, in this sense, consists of a continuous flow of a core population of recovering addicts, but since the group is open ended, it also includes a flux of other retreatants who are not involved with addiction therapy. A social support network beyond the immediate compound itself also is significant to the recovery process.

At the time data were collected (over a five-day period), there were some 100 people at Nebi-Musa visiting for varying lengths of time. Among those living in the compound were 40 male recovering addicts. The duration of their stays ranged from two weeks to two months. The recovering addicts ranged in age from 25 to 40, the average being 35. All 40 were Moslems (although a small number of former participants had been Arab Christians). Most of the 40 were from Gaza, the West Bank, and other Arab areas of Israel. The average length of formal education was seven years. Nearly half had been employed as general laborers, although some had been merchants. Five had criminal backgrounds and three had served time in jail; in all instances the offenses were related to drug addiction. Thirty-five had tried other forms of drug rehabilitation that had been unsuccessful; these included in-hospital programs, in-clinic programs, and Narcotics Anonymous. Most were married and had children; none were divorced, although some were separated from their spouses. All discovered Nebi-Musa's treatment program through word-of-mouth and all voluntarily participated. Most were accompanied to the site by their families and extended families, although some came alone. Initial contacts were usually with family members, and subsequent visits, after individuals had reentered the secular world, were often unaccompanied.

The Treatment Program

As distinct from other retreatants, recovering addicts graduate through a five-stage treatment process. That process has evolved over the past five years, but it has followed a structure basically unaltered since its beginning. The first stage is initial contact, where one of the five Sufis interviews the applicant and assesses his readiness for the program. This takes place either with the family present and participating or on a one-to-one basis. Support from the family also is asked about, particularly regarding the provision of food for the duration of the applicant's stay and ongoing support once he has left Nebi-Musa and reentered the outside world. In addition to the interview, this first stage typically includes a tour of the site and a meal.

From the vantage point of Western therapy, the program thus incorporates established principles of interviewing the client, first to determine preparedness and readiness to participate in a drug treatment program (Toumbourou & Hamilton, 1993) and second to mesh client expectations and perceptions with the nature of the drug program itself (Oppenheimer, Sheehan, & Taylor, 1988). The Sufis seem to have considerable skills in reading a retreatant's "ecological map." Because of his high social status, as well as his ability to strike an alliance with the retreatants' family members, a Sufi is frequently able to utilize individual family members as sources of client motivation and support, particularly during difficult times over the course of treatment, when client morale and motivation may be low (Al-Krenawi, Maoz, & Reicher, 1994). One suspects that this level of familial participation may be far greater than that expected in a Western treatment model, reflecting the strongly interdependent notion of family common to Arab culture (Sayre, Cornille,

Rohrer, & Hicks, 1992). Incorporation of the family at the initial stage of assessment, and as a source of social support throughout the program and at discharge, also appears to conform to recent Western research into the relationship of family support to drug addiction program efficacy (Dembo, Williams, Wothke, & Schmeidler, 1994; Enders & Mercier, 1993).

Once the client has committed to the program, the helping relationship enters a second stage. One of the Sufis, in consultation with the others, assesses the client and determines whether he is able to begin the program within the compound, or whether he must first seek medical treatment from a hospital, clinic, or private physician before he is able to stay at Nebi-Musa. When the client is deemed able to commit to ongoing residency, the Sufi-client relationship is transformed. The Sufi assumes more authoritarian characteristics, and the client submissively agrees to having his head shaved and to staying for several weeks in a state of isolation, with 24-hour surveillance by a rotating combination of Sufi mystics and others who are in the latter stages of the program. Clients are subjected to an abrupt and sustained period of withdrawal, similar to the Western model of detoxification but unaccompanied by medication. In accordance with Islamic religious traditions, periods of craving are responded to with cold water showers, readings from the Koran, and massages of black cumin seed ointment (Al-Jawziyya, 1993). Much of the diet during this early stage of recovery consists of honey and milk (Koran, Suruh, Al-Nahal, v. 19). A typical day includes the religious discipline of praying communally in the mosque five times. Accompanied walks as far as 20 kilometers outside the compound and eating in the main dining area with the other retreatants closely parallel the Western emphasis on exercise and group socialization as means of recovery.

Various forms of client resistance, among them anger, denial, and wanting to leave the program characterize much of this stage. Resistance, which is fundamental to the therapeutic process (Allgood, Bishoff, Smith, & Salts, 1992), appears to decrease along with the physical reduction of craving, as the therapeutic environment provides a psychologically safe framework (Bernstein & Landaiche, 1992) and as individual relationships with the client increase in mutual cooperation, trust, and acceptance (King, 1992). Visits by the patient's family may well provide additional support through this troublesome part of therapy, as might the perception of, and actual reception of, group support.

There are obvious dangers at this stage, given current programmatic arrangements. The Sufis and other group members have little educational basis to assess whether medical treatment is indicated. It is not known how closely a client assessment is related to the duration, extent, and type of drug previously used. There are no trained medical professionals on site during periods of withdrawal. Proximity to hospital treatment is not close, and vehicles are not always readily available for emergencies. This is not to underestimate the considerable precautions that are undertaken, including the intensive nature of ongoing client observation and the network of Arab physicians that is readily available. It also should be noted that Nebi-Musa clients tend to have a non-Western view of professionals and are inclined, like other Arabs, to utilize medical personnel infrequently (Reiss, 1991; Stephen, 1992). In addition, according to an Arab proverb, insight into a particular medical problem—and thus the status of being a physician to treat a particular malady—is based on one's prior personal experience of having had that problem, and not on education. Sufi healers, in this sense, are "doctors."

During the program's third stage, the client adopts a more equal status. He is transferred from the isolation room to a room shared by as many as three others, lives communally with the other program participants, and immerses himself in Nebi-Musa's religious worship. A great deal of time is spent reading the Koran, discussing the Koran with the Sufis, and learning from the Sufis how to meditate and to incorporate Islamic thought into everyday life and into the process of recovery, in particular. Complete abstinence from drugs and alcohol is explained by the Koran, as is the redemptive force of God, as revealed in the process of undertaking righteous acts and rejecting sin (El-Azayem & Hedayat-Diba, 1994; Farsy, 1964). Various rituals at Nebi-Musa are intended to reinforce this spiritual process of recovery. Individual and group prayer and meditation take place at the grave of Moses at irregular intervals. The bathing process of Al-wdoa, which precedes every prayer, is particularly emphasized. Mosque prayer five times daily also becomes a well-established routine, as does the weekly practice of the Sufi ritual, the Dhikr, an invocation to God literally meaning "to remember, recall, mention, or utter" (Al-Ghazali, 1950), involving an extended, trance-like meditation accompanied by chanting, drum music, and dancing on a fixed spot. These practices of prayer, meditation, and other forms of religious devotion reduce anxiety and increase the client's sense of well-being (Azhar, Varma, & Dharap, 1994).

The introduction of sustained group interactions allows participants to universalize experiences, to share coping strategies, and to provide mutual support and encouragement, among other aspects typical of a therapeutic community's informal encounters (Bell, 1994; Rosenthal, 1989; Serok & Levi, 1993). Strong group cohesion tends to be reinforced by living arrangements, the leadership of the Sufis, the religious rituals, and by Islamic theology, including the exhortations to: "Hold fast together by the rope of Allah and not by being divisive among yourselves.... Believers are like a building, strengthening and supporting each other.... God helps he who helps his brother" (Koran, cited in Al-Radi & Al-Mahdy, 1989, p. 274).

Nebi-Musa's group dynamics approximate something of a family. The Sufis are proxy fathers, dispensing religious wisdom, providing role models for recovery, and encouraging a healthy group climate. This institutional framework of a therapy community with the therapist as parental surrogate and mentor is also common to the Western experience (Bratter, Bratter, Radda, & Steiner, 1993). By corresponding to Islamic norms and values, however, it permits successful group work with a Moslem population (Al-Krenawi, 1996; Banawi & Stockton, 1993).

On the individual level, Nebi-Musa's healing processes seem to conform to the gestalt and cognitive therapy ethos of replacing dysfunctional patterns of thinking, feeling, and interacting with their functional counterparts (Buchbinder, 1986). And like Western existential therapists providing psychotherapy to alcoholics, the Sufis encourage participants to focus on the essential issues of death, freedom, isolation, and meaninglessness as means of recovery (Flores, 1988; Johnson, Griffin-Shelley, & Sandler, 1987). Nebi-Musa thus may well cultivate a positive spirituality, healthy self-esteem, trust, and contentment with life, which as recent research indicates are important aspects of addiction treatment (Brown & Peterson, 1991; Corrington, 1989; Johnson, Sandler, & Griffin-Shelley, 1988; Nicholson et al., 1994). Its various religious rites are socially sanctioned vehicles for self-expression, catharsis, ventilation, self-satisfaction, and psychological release (Al-Krenawi & Graham, 1997). As well, the Koranic story of Moses contributes many distinctive facets for religiously based healing. The parallels between the suffering and endurance of a client with that experienced by Moses are readily evident. Moses' miraculous journey from Egypt to the Holy Land is an excellent metaphor for the journey of addiction recovery. And his resolute faith provides clients with inspiration to continue this arduous journey.

Thus, in retreating to Nebi-Musa, one enters the culturally specific symbolic and phenomenological universe of Islam. The Sufis perceive faith in God to be the fundamental basis of the helping relationship. This common cultural and religious background is an essential aspect of most modes of traditional healing (Asuni, 1990; Torrey, 1972; Umoren, 1990) and of establishing a therapeutic alliance (Davidson, 1992); also, it strongly parallels the importance of spirituality to the Narcotics Anonymous movement (and in particular its progenitor, the Alcoholics Anonymous movement) in the West.

Many of Nebi-Musa's drug addiction clients, it must be emphasized, appear to be radically transformed from a religious state varying between agnosticism to nominal adherence at the beginning of the program to strict religious adherence over the course of treatment. And so one encounters religion diachronically, in the sense of the immediate temporal and special context of treatment, but also synchronically, that is, in the transcendence of time and space and in the encounter of an omnipotent and omnipresent Deity. This assumption of religiosity, then, provides an opportunity for transcending one's historical circumstances, by making allowance for that "Ultimate Hope" that is the core of Islamic salvation (Al-Krenawi & Graham, 1997). On this basis, a theoretical frame of helping, often more meaningful to the client than any secular or Western counterpart, may well provide a powerful normative and intellectual framework encompassing virtually all aspects of addiction recovery (El-Azayem & Hedayat-Diba, 1994; Guessoum, 1986).

Throughout the five stages, beginning with the second, the client is motivated by the religious concept of an afterlife. Death anxiety is particularly prominent among Arab people (Abdel-Khalek & Omar, 1988; Templer, 1991). In individual sessions, but particularly in group sessions with clients, Nebi-Musa's Sufis discuss in considerable detail the Moslem tradition of the post-burial scenario, in which two angels appear to the dead. If the person led a virtuous life, the angels will treat the individual well, and will reveal a window depicting heaven—a foreshadowing of the place to which that individual will likely go at Judgment Day. If the dead person had led an immoral life, the angels will reveal a window of hell, and will torment and punish that person until Judgment Day.

In referring to such Moslem traditions, the Sufis appear to skillfully utilize the death anxiety as a therapeutic tool, and in so doing, cultivate client motivation to abstain from drug use—drug use being one of the possible reasons for eternal damnation. Moreover, clients are encouraged to view their lives as a totality of good and evil actions. Having previously abused drugs, an evil act, they are thus particularly motivated to compensate with good acts, such as abstinence from drug use.

The fourth stage, which is closely aligned to the third, sees the introduction of a regular routine of such communal tasks as caring for livestock, general maintenance and painting, cooking, and cleaning. Such activities certainly contribute to the institution's efficient functioning and provide the individual an important form of task-centered therapy or life skills training. Many, arriving at Nebi-Musa as low functioning people and with few work and psychosocial skills, leave the program with improved confidence, self-worth, discipline, work routines, and psychosocial skills. These attributes are positively reinforced by other members of the program. Thus, on balance, Nebi-Musa conforms to many of the characteristics common to Western therapeutic communities: a structured hierarchy, an implicit reward system, social learning, role modeling, maintenance of positive values, the healing power of a community of care, and established routines (Heit, 1993). And once a client leaves Nebi-Musa and reintegrates into the outside community, he has an important repertoire of skills and inner strengths for the fifth and final stage of aftercare.

Durations of stay at Nebi-Musa vary. Some leave the program early; relapse and multiple attempts at initiating the program are common, as in Western community therapy (Bleiberg, Devlin, Croan, & Briscoe, 1994; Condelli, 1994; De-Leon, 1990–1991). Of the 40 clients under consideration, five had previously gone through the program and had returned for brief periods of time, ranging from one day to two weeks, as part of an ongoing process of aftercare. The remaining 35 were thus in the program for the first time. The Sufis estimate that clients tend to stay an average of a little over two months, although retreats can be as short as one month and as long as six. Once released they are expected to maintain contact with Nebi-Musa and to undertake return visits. Many are said to retain close ties with their Sufis, consulting with them as spiritual mentors. According to the Sufis, visits vary in frequency from once every six months to biweekly, and in duration from a few hours to several days.

In accordance with Arab norms, virtually all of the residents go back to their home communities where they had been living prior to contact with Nebi-Musa. But their return is intended to be accompanied by significant changes to their social roles. They are expected to refrain from drug use, and to this end, to hold full-time permanent jobs where possible, to seek familial support, to stay in contact with Nebi-Musa, and to follow Islamic precepts devoutly. Some communities are known to contain spontaneous forms of self-help groups of former Nebi-Musa clients. And all clients, once in their home communities, are expected to be "ambassadors" of Nebi-Musa. In this sense, their personal formation resembles Narcotics Anonymous or Alcoholics Anonymous patterns. Some lecture to Arab high school students about their personal experiences with drug rehabilitation. Some provide community education to their former drug dealers or to current drug users. Most important of all, clients are expected to perceive their aftercare success in direct relation to their personal religious discipline.

A drug-free lifestyle is further reinforced by the client's improved social status within his community. Nebi-Musa's treatment program enjoys widespread community sanction, and the client's changed behavior and outlook provide much improved prospects for community acceptance. Nebi-Musa's deliberate incorporation of the family as an integral part of the aftercare support network is frequently supplemented by the religiously based support networks within the community, to which many clients are known to turn.

Pillars of Islam

Of particular theological significance are the five pillars of faith. These bear on the reciprocal relationships among an individual's physical, spiritual, psychological, and emotional well being (Azmi, 1991; El-Azayem & Hedayat-Diba, 1994). From a strictly individual perspective, there is an eschatological imperative for following Islam. Moslems hold that to deviate from the faith is tantamount to being less than a fully authentic human being. As stated in the Koran, oblivion occurs when humanity loses touch with this fundamental truth: "And be not like those who forgot God and He caused them to be oblivious of their own selves or souls" (Koran, 49, v. 19). And so a Moslem is required to adhere to the following pillars:

1. The Shahada, or profession of faith, is the belief that there is no other god but Allah and that Muhammad is His last prophet. Thus, Islam insists on the submission of the faithful to the oneness of God: "Say: He is God, the one and only" (Koran, 112, v. 1–4) is one of many Koranic verses emphasizing the monotheistic character of Islam.
2. The Salat is the imperative to pray five times daily: at dawn, noon, mid-afternoon, sunset, and evening. The prayers can be performed anywhere, and although individual prayer is allowed, group prayer is preferred.
3. The Zakat is the requirement to pay alms to the needy on behalf of one's family and business. "It was customarily calculated as an annual payment of two and one half percent of all capital assets, savings, and current income above a specified threshold" (Azmi, 1991, p. 223). The exact rate, however, can be flexible, in part according to the need established by the imam, or local Moslem cleric.
4. The Siam is the imperative to fast from food, drink, and sex during daylight hours during the month of Ramadan, which immediately precedes the celebration of the date on which Allah revealed the Koran to the Prophet Muhammad. Ramadan thus ends with

a three-day celebration, Id Al-Fitr, the breaking of the fast. Self-discipline and reflection, rather than abstinence and self-mortification, are emphasized.

5. The Hajj is a pilgrimage to Mecca, a holy city of Islam located where Allah revealed the Koran to the Prophet Muhammad. The pilgrimage should be undertaken at least once in a Moslem's lifetime, if he or she is financially, mentally, and physically so capable. The beginning of the pilgrimage season is the end of Ramadan, and the end of the season is the celebration of the Great Feast Id Al-Adha (see below).

Praying

Prayer five times daily, a main principle within the five pillars of Islam, assists the devotee to submit to Allah's will. While the individual can undertake daily prayer alone, it is preferable, if possible, to pray with others. An obvious place for this to occur is within the mosque, led either by the imam (Moslem cleric) or any other Moslem. In bringing an individual closer to God, the Hadith indicates that group prayer is 27 times more effective than praying alone (Al-Radi & Al-Mahdy, 1989). Group prayer likewise reinforces a sense of belonging to a single, worldwide community of believers. Larger assemblies of prayer, in mosques, are especially prevalent at noon on Fridays, the Moslem Holy Day. The prayer is preceded by a khutba, or sermon delivered by the imam.

Moslems also celebrate major and minor religious feasts in a group setting. These begin with group prayer in a mosque, and end in the sharing of a meal among family members. One of the two major feasts, as noted above, is the Id Al-Fitr, the feast at the end of Ramadan. In the mosque, it includes the corporate recitation of prayers and ends in people exchanging greetings; even enemies are encouraged to settle their differences and to exchange the peace.

The second major feast, the Al-Adha, commemorates the Koranic story where Abraham was told by Allah to slaughter his son Ishmael; as his knife was drawn toward the son's neck, by the will of Allah, the angel Gabriel intervened, putting a sheep in place of the son and thereby allowing the sheep to be sacrificed in Ishmael's stead. Each year, after mosque prayer, Moslems slaughter an animal and then consume it in a family meal, in honor of this event; if it is available, the animal is a sheep.

The Therapeutic Significance of Prayer and the Five Pillars

Mental health practitioners should comprehend the benefits, at several levels, of the above forms of prayers and the five pillars of Islam. All have a strong group element, reflecting and reinforcing Moslem society's high-context nature; as a popular Moslem saying has it, "God's hand [is] with the group." At the group level, emotional support and exchange of ideas or difficulties takes place, most often in the mosque, with other worshippers or with the imam. As emphasized by the Hadith, "The Prophet Muhammad remarked: Those who interact with people and express their hardships are better than those who do not interact with people and do not express their pains" (Ibn-Majah, 1975).

Group prayers help to create a sense of familiarity, friendliness, selflessness, and equality among the faithful. This is entirely consistent with the Hadith edict of equality of believers regardless of color, social strata, or wealth; the Prophet Muhammad said: "All the people are equal as the comb's teeth" (Nagati, 1993). Group prayers also reinforce a potential for natural support networks and provide a rationale for breaking down barriers that would normally interfere with the mutual exchange of social support. The group nature of prayer can thus influence the thought and behavior of their members in the context of group intervention (Yalom, 1975).

Group prayers mirror a wide range of instrumental and social support outside the mosque, such as family or marital advice, assistance with building a home or extension to a home, or assistance during times of sickness or other traumatic events. An excellent example is the in-mosque greetings of peace during major feast celebrations. Even enemies are compelled to be cordial. The feast seasons themselves often provide the context for settling instances of marital or family discord—at many times with the assistance of concerned family members, neighbors, or friends. Major feasts also include the imperative to visit relatives and close friends; visits are extended over a four-day period for the sacrifice holiday, and three days for the Id Al-Fitr. The feast periods preceding fasting periods are also associated with various good works, such as visiting sick friends or relatives, which themselves also provide the basis for natural social support.

On the level of the person in relation to the group, the practice catapults the praying individual into a worldwide body of believers, both dead and alive, thus reinforcing a sense of the integrity and strength of the religion. Group cohesion is reinforced by Moslem scholars, the religious rituals, and Islamic theology. The individual in Islam is also considered an independent member of the group who makes decisions to satisfy his or her needs and interests without hurting the group (Al-Radi & Al-Mahdy, 1989). The interests of the individual and the group, then, do not necessarily contradict one another; rather, they are supposed to be mutually reinforcing. The individual's voice is not silenced, and group members are always expected to express personal views (Al-Krenawi, 1995).

The recitation of the Koran during prayer, either silently or aloud, represents a continuous chain of teaching, listening, and memorizing Koranic sayings. On the individual level, the prayer is a reminder that a Moslem's daily life and faith are continuously intertwined. Praying can be viewed as an inexpensive psychological guard against anxiety and depression (Azhar et al., 1994; Nagati, 1982). The practice of prayer, meditation, and other forms of religious devotion can thereby lead to balance in the Moslem personality (Nagati, 1982), increasing the person's sense of well-being and relief, as well as reducing anxiety (Azhar et al., 1994). To put it in religious terms, the institutions of prayer and the Moslem five pillars "enable the believer to turn away from evil and to enhance his/her consciousness of God—an essential process in the actualization of human nature (fitrah)" (Mohamed, 1995, p. 14). On a final level, then, prayer itself, to the believer, allows the individual to encounter the omniscient wisdom and omnipotent healing powers of Allah (Abramowitz, 1993; Ranganathan, 1994; Saucer, 1991).

Sacred places also are important to Moslem spirituality. For instance, Moslems typically visit dead saints' tombs, which are holy places associated with stories of relieved personal anxiety, healed physical and mental ailments, and mediated requests to God (Al-Krenawi & Graham, 1996). There are particularly sacred maqam, or holy places—for example, the burial places of such prophets as Moses—where Moslems undergo recovery from addictions, among other forms of help for personal problems (Al-Krenawi & Graham, 1997). A highly important sacred place for Moslems is Mecca, the destination of the Hajj pilgrimage.

The Hajj to Mecca is not just a trip, but a journey to a particularly sacred and auspicious spot to obtain the spiritual gains of purification and redemption (Eliade, 1987; Turner, 1967). Before undertaking the Hajj, individuals have to reconcile with anyone with whom they have had a dispute; this in itself is yet another natural locus of conflict resolution. The pilgrimage often takes place together with a group, and once at Mecca, the supplicants ask God to forgive their sins and grant them His blessings. During the performance of the Hajj, Moslems help each other, gathering together for prayers.

During the Hajj performance, to expel evil forces, each pilgrim throws seven Jamrats [stones] at a site in Mecca called Iblis, named after the fallen angel who had been expelled from the Garden of Eden and who was the original source for all evil spirits (Koran, Surah Al-Hijr, v. 28–40). This process symbolizes a freeing of the self from guilt feelings and sins. Moreover, the process of tangible actions—of doing something—symbolizes and reinforces the overall sense of sin propitiation. From the Islamic perspective, after participating in the Hajj, a person is considered "born again," which means that all his or her sins are erased by God's will. This leads to satisfaction, relaxation, and release (Abramowitz, 1993; Al-Issawi, 1988); for many Moslems it can be the symbolic beginning of major life changes. For the rest of their lives, the pilgrim assumes the title Hajj, one who has undertaken the Hajj pilgrimage. Their social status consequently increases, and their personal conduct is expected to reflect kindness, devotion, and other virtuous attributes.

CONCLUSION

It must be emphasized that the findings presented in this chapter are necessarily tentative and preliminary. A number of researchers have written about the therapeutic significance of religion to psychotherapy (Azhar et al., 1994) and to psychiatric care with traditional populations (Bravo & Grob, 1989). A recent follow-up study found a Saudi drug treatment program integrating modern and religious components to be more successful than treatment programs having no religious components (Jilek, 1994, pp. 232–233). The former had success rates of 75 percent (Islam, 1993; Odejide, Ohaeri, Adelekan, & Ikuesan, 1989). Nebi-Musa's Sufis believe that their program has a success rate of 80 percent; quantitative research might substantiate this claim. Outcome research also could be used to compare Nebi-Musa's therapeutic success rate with therapeutic communities in Western societies (DeLeon, 1989a,b). Finally, several researchers provide evidence of the therapeutic benefits of integrating programs of modern and traditional healing (Mayers, 1989; Rappaport & Rappaport, 1981; Schwartz, 1985; Wessels, 1985). These principles could perhaps be applied aptly to Nebi-Musa's and other Moslem programs in the Middle East and around the world.

From a therapeutic viewpoint, as Jilek wisely observes, substance abuse clinicians working with non-Western populations "should inform themselves about culture-specific concepts of health and disease, attitudes towards substance use and abuse, and the views of prevention and treatment prevailing in this population" (Jilek, 1994, p. 249). And as West (1987) points out, "the notion that is held in the West about responsibility and the 'self-made' person takes on a different meaning in Islamic society." It is typical for Arab mental health patients to be resistant because many do not take responsibility for their problems. Moreover, they commonly "place the responsibility" on the mental health practitioner "to heal them" (West, 1987, pp. 105–106).

These factors enter into the Sufi-retreatant therapeutic alliance, with the Sufi taking on the role of a hakeem, that is, a "wise man and healer, not a physician in the Western sense but a professional working through the hands of Allah" (Machleidt & Peltzer, 1991, p. 105). Responsibility for defining a problem, and for problem solving, is therefore similar in nature to the NA/AA submission to a Higher Will. Some clients, it is true, become dependent on Nebi-Musa or on individual Sufi, although this may not, in all cases, be disadvantageous. As Machleidt and Peltzer (1991) imply in relation to Malawi patients, dependence on a healer can be therapeutically beneficial. And in a Moslem context, as El-Islam (El-Islam, 1967, 1982) points out, such dependence may reflect an enabling process of transference, whereupon the healer becomes a parent figure. In the case of Nebi-Musa, the retreatant assumes the role of religious devotee, prostrating himself before Allah, submitting to His will, and becoming a disciple of the Sufi healer. To understand the centrality of the Sufi healer and of religious devotion to Nebi-Musa's treatment program, then, is to appreciate its full therapeutic significance.

To this end, several guidelines may be used by professional practitioners to better appreciate, and integrate, an Islamic perspective in responding to alcohol and drug use and abuse in Moslem communities. These include, but are not limited to:

- Understanding Moslem family arrangements as more hierarchical and less flexible than those found in the West, with a communication style that tends to be implicit and indirect, rather than explicit and direct.
- Knowledge of Islam, including Shiite, Sunni, and Islamic movement traditions, as well as their common practices and social activities.
- Appreciation of the Moslem worldview on sociocultural and psychosocial phenomena, which may be encountered during intervention. Examples include social prohibitions against suicide and social constructions of sexuality that affirm heterosexual lifestyles.

- Comprehend the explicit link between a Moslem religious identity and that of the individual, and the symbiotic referencing to community identity of both.
- Appreciate the potential use of such natural support networks as spiritual or religious leaders and high-status members of society. Traditional healers in Moslem society, such as the Koranic healers, often operate with strong reference to the Koran and intercede in a wide variety of psychosocial and somatic complaints (Al-Krenawi & Graham, 1999a,b; Al-Krenawi & Graham, 2000).

REFERENCES

Abdel-Khalek, A. M., & Omar, M. M. (1988). Death anxiety, state and trait anxiety in Kuwaitian samples. *Psychological Reports, 63,* 715–718.

Abramowitz, L. (1993). Prayer as therapy among the frail Jewish elderly. *Journal of Gerontological Social Work, 19*(3/4), 69–75.

Abu El-Azayem, G. M. (1987). A psycho-social religious approach to contain substance abuse in Egypt. In *Congress Proceedings, World Islamic Association for Mental Health* (pp. 409–415). Lahore, Pakistan.

Al-Bar, A. (1998). *Drugs from Islamic perspective*. Syria: Daar Al-qlam (in Arabic).

Al-Bostani, M. (1988). *Studies in Islamic psychology*. Beirut: Dar Al-Blaah Press (in Arabic).

Al-Ghazali, A. H. (1950). *Ihyaa Uloom Al-Din [The revival of religious science]*. Cairo: Issa Al-Babi Al-Halabi Press.

Al-Issawi, A. R. (1988). *Islam and psychotherapy*. Beirut: Daar Al-Blaah Press (in Arabic).

Al-Jawziyya, I. Q. (1993). *Natural healing with the medicine of the Prophet*. (M. Al-Akili, Trans.). Philadelphia: Pearl.

Al-Krenawi, A. (1995). *A study of dual use of modern and traditional mental health systems by the Bedouin-Arabs of the Negev.* Unpublished doctoral dissertation, University of Toronto.

———. (1996). Group work with Bedouin-Arab widows of the Negev in a medical clinic. *Affilia: Journal of Women and Social Work, 11*(3), 303–318.

Al-Krenawi, A., & Graham, J. R. (1996). Social work and traditional healing rituals among the Bedouin of the Negev. *International Social Work, 3*(2), 177–188.

———. (1997). Spirit possession and exorcism in the treatment of a Bedouin-Arab psychiatric patient. *Clinical Social Work Journal, 25*(2), 211–222.

———. (1999a). Social work and Koranic mental health healers. *International Social Work, 42*(1), 53–65.

———. (1999b). Gender and biomedical/traditional mental health utilization among the Bedouin-Arabs of the Negev. *Culture, Medicine and Psychiatry, 23*, 219–243.

———. (2000). Culturally sensitive social work practice with Arab peoples in mental health settings. *Health and Social Work, 25*(1), 9–17.

Al-Krenawi, A., Maoz, B., & Reicher, B. (1994). Familial and cultural issues in the brief strategic treatment of Israeli Bedouins. *Family Systems Medicine, 12*(4), 415–425.

Allgood, S. M., Bishoff, R. J., Smith, T. A., & Salts, C. J. (1992). Therapist interventions: Do they really influence client resistance? *American Journal of Family Therapy, 20*(4), 333–340.

Al-Radi, O. M., & Al-Mahdy, M. A. (1989). Group therapy: An Islamic approach. *Transcultural Psychiatric Research Review, 26*(4), 273–276.

Asali, K. J. (1990). *Id Al-Nebi-Musa fe Flastien [The Nebi Musa Feast in Palestine]*. Amman: University of Jordan Press.

Asuni, T. (1990). Nigeria: Report on the care, treatment and rehabilitation of people with mental illness. *Psychosocial Rehabilitation Journal, 14*(1), 35–44.

Azhar, M. Z., Varma, S. L., & Dharap, A. S. (1994). Religious psychotherapy in anxiety disorder patients. *Acta Psychiatrica Scandinavica, 90*(1), 1–3.

Azmi, S. H. (1991). Traditional Islamic social welfare: Its meaning, history and contemporary relevance. *The Islamic Quarterly, 35*(3), 165–180.

Baasher, T. A., & Abu El Azayem, G. M. (1980). Egypt (2): The role of the Mosque in treatment. In G. Edwards & A. Arif (Eds.), *Drug problems in the sociocultural context: A basis for policies and programme planning*. Public Health Papers No. 73 (pp. 131–134). Geneva: World Health Organization.

Bader, A.M.C. (1987). *Social problems in the Arab world.* Cairo: Al-Maktab Al-Hadith (in Arabic).

Banawi, R., & Stockton, R. (1993). Islamic values relevant to group work, with practical applications for the group leader. *Journal for Specialists in Group Work, 18*(3), 151–160.

Bell, D. C. (1994). Connection in therapeutic communities. *The International Journal of the Addictions, 29*(4), 525–543.

Bernstein, P. M., & Landaiche, N. M. (1992). Resistance, counter resistance, and balance: A framework for managing the experience of impasse in psychotherapy. *Journal of Contemporary Psychotherapy, 22*(1), 5–19.

Bibby, R.W. (1987). *Fragmented gods: The poverty and potential of religion in Canada.* Toronto: Irwin.

Bilal, A. M. (1989). The Kuwait drug addiction scene: A changing pattern? *The International Journal of the Addictions, 24*(12), 1137–1144.

Bilal, A. M., Kristof, J., Shaltout, A., & El Islam, M. F. (1987). Treatment of alcoholism in Kuwait: A prospective follow-up study. *Drug and Alcohol Dependence, 19*(2), 131–144.

Bilal, A. M., Makhawi, B., Al Fayez, G., & Shaltout, A. F. (1990). Attitudes of a sector of the Arab Moslem population in Kuwait towards alcohol and drug misuse: An objective appraisal. *Drug and Alcohol Dependence, 26*(1), 55–62.

Bleiberg, J. L., Devlin, P., Croan, J., & Briscoe, R. (1994). Relationship between treatment length and outcome in a therapeutic community. *The International Journal of the Addictions, 29*(6), 729–740.

Bratter, B. I., Bratter, T. E., Radda, H. T., & Steiner, K. M. (1993). The residential therapeutic caring community. *Psychotherapy, 30*(2), 299–304.

Bravo, G., & Grob, C. (1989). Shamans, sacraments, and psychiatrists. *Journal of Psychoactive Drugs, 21*(1), 123–128.

Brooks, C. R. (1994). Using ethnography in the evaluation of drug prevention and intervention programs. *The International Journal of the Addictions, 29*(6), 791–801.

Brown, H. P., & Peterson, J. H. (1991). Assessing spirituality in addiction treatment and follow-up: Development of the Brown-Peterson recovery progress inventory (B-PRPI). *Alcoholism Treatment Quarterly, 8*(2), 21–50.

Buchbinder, J. (1986). Gestalt therapy and its application to alcoholism treatment. *Alcoholism Treatment Quarterly, 3*(3), 49–68.

Condelli, W. S. (1994). Domains of variables for understanding and improving retention in therapeutic communities. *International Journal of the Addictions, 29*(5), 593–607.

Corrington, J. E. (1989). Spirituality and recovery: Relationships between levels of spirituality, contentment and stress during recovery from alcoholism in AA. *Alcoholism Treatment Quarterly, 6*(3/4), 155–166.

Davidson, J. R. (1992). White clinician-Black client: Relationship problems and recommendations for change from a social influence theory perspective. *Journal of Multicultural Social Work, 1*(4), 63–76.

De-Leon, G. (1989a). Psychopathology and substance abuse: What is being learned from research in therapeutic communities. *Journal of Psychoactive Drugs, 21*(2), 177–188.

———. (1989b). Therapeutic communities for substance abuse: Overview of approach and effectiveness. *Psychology of Addictive Behaviors, 3*(3), 140–147.

———. (1990–1991). Aftercare in therapeutic communities. *The International Journal of the Addictions, 25*(9A–10A), 1225–1237.

De-Leon, G., Melnick, G., Schoket, D., & Jainchill, N. (1993). Is the therapeutic community culturally relevant? Findings on race/ethnic differences in retention in treatment. *Journal of Psychoactive Drugs, 25*(1), 77–86.

Dembo, R., Williams, L., Wothke, W., & Schmeidler, J. (1994). The relationships among family problems, friends' troubled behavior, and high risk youths' alcohol/other drug use and delinquent behavior: A longitudinal study. *The International Journal of the Addictions, 29*(11), 1419–1442.

El-Azayem, G. A., & Hedayat-Diba, Z. (1994). The psychological aspects of Islam: Basic principles of Islam and their psychological corollary. *International Journal for the Psychology of Religion, 4*(1), 41–50.

Eliade, M. (Ed.). (1987). *Encyclopedia of religion* (Vol. 13). New York: Macmillan.

El-Islam, M. F. (1967). The psychotherapeutic basis of some Arab rituals. *International Journal of Social Psychiatry, 13*, 265–268.

———. (1982). Arab cultural psychiatry. *Transcultural Psychiatric Research Review, 19*(1), 5–24.

Encyclopedia Britannica. (1996). *1996 Britannica book of the year.* London: Oxford University Press.

———. (1997). *1997 Britannica Book of the Year*. Chicago: Encyclopedia Britannica Inc.

Enders, L. E., & Mercier, J. M. (1993). Treating chemical dependency: The need for including the family. *The International Journal of the Addictions, 28*(6), 507–519.

Esposito, J. L. (Ed.). (1995). *Oxford encyclopedia of the modern Islamic world*. New York: Oxford University Press.

Farsy, M. S. (1964). *Islam and hygiene*. Leiden, Netherlands: E. J. Brill.

Flores, P. J. (1988). Alcoholics Anonymous: A phenomenological and existential perspective. *Alcoholism Treatment Quarterly, 5*(1/2), 73–93.

Gillis, J. S., Tareen, I.A.K., Chaudhry, H. R., & Haider, S. (1994). Risk factors for drug misuse in Pakistan. *The International Journal of the Addictions, 29*(2), 215–223.

Glik, D. C. (1988). Symbolic, ritual and social dynamics of spiritual healing. *Social Science and Medicine, 27*(11), 1197–1206.

Guessoum, A. (1986). Tolerance et psychiatrie (une vision Islamique). *Psychiatrie Francaise, 17*(4), 55–60.

Haddad, Y., & Smith, J. I. (1994). *Moslem communities in North America.* Albany: State University of New York Press.

Hall, E. (1976). *Beyond culture*. New York: Doubleday.

Heggenhougen, H. K. (1984). Traditional medicine and the treatment of drug addicts: Three examples from Southeast Asia. *Medical Anthropology Quarterly, 16*(1), 3–7.

Heit, D. S. (1993). Therapeutic communities for drug abuse: The contemporary scene in the U.S.A. *International Journal for Therapeutic and Supportive Organizations, 14*(3), 151–163.

Ibn-Majah, A. (1975). *Sunan Ibn-Majah*. (Vol. 2, p.1338, #4032). Cairo: Dar Ihya Atturath Al-Arabi (in Arabic).

Islam, R. (1993). Relapse following withdrawal of drug addiction. *British Journal of Psychiatry, 163,* 699.

Jilek, W. G. (1994). Traditional healing in the prevention and treatment of drug and alcohol abuse. *Transcultural Psychiatric Research Review, 31*(3), 219–256.

Johnson, R. A., Griffin-Shelley, E., & Sandler, K. R. (1987). Existential issues in psychotherapy with alcoholics. *Alcoholism Treatment Quarterly, 4*(1), 15–25.

Johnson, R. A., Sandler, K. R., & Griffin-Shelley, E. (1988). Spirituality and the regulation of self-esteem. *Alcoholism Treatment Quarterly, 4*(3), 1–13.

Johnson, S. H. (1983). Treatment of drug abusers in Malaysia: A comparison. *The International Journal of the Addictions, 18*(7), 951–958.

King, S. M. (1992). Therapeutic utilization of client resistance. *Individual Psychology: Journal of Adlerian Theory, Research, and Practice, 48*(2), 165–174.

Lee, R.L.M. (1985). Alternative systems in Malaysian drug rehabilitation: Organization and control in comparative perspective. *Social Science and Medicine, 21*(11), 1289–1296.

Machleidt, W., & Peltzer, K. (1991). The Chilopa ceremony: A sacrificial ritual for mentally (spiritually) ill patients in a traditional healing centre in Malawi. *Psychiatria Danubia, 3*(1–2), 205–227.

Mandelbaum, D. (1965). Alcohol and culture. *Current Anthropology, 6,* 281–293.

Mass, M., & Al-Krenawi, A. (1994). When a man encounters a woman Satan also is present: Clinical relationships in Bedouin society. *American Journal of Orthopsychiatry, 64*(3), 357–367.

Mayers, R. S. (1989). Use of folk medicine by elderly Mexican-American women. *Journal of Drug Issues, 19*(2), 283–295.

Mohamed, Y. (1995). Fitrah and its bearing on the principles of psychology. *The American Journal of Islamic Social Sciences, 12*(1), 1–18.

Nagati, M. A. (1982). *The Koran and psychology*. Beirut: Dar Al-Shorok Press (in Arabic).

———. (1993). *The tradition of the prophet and psychology*. Cairo: Dar Al-Shorok Press (in Arabic).

Nicholson, T., Higgins, W., Turner, P., James, S., Stickle, F., & Pruitt, T. (1994). The relation between meaning in life and the occurrence of drug abuse: A retrospective study. *Psychology of Addictive Behaviors, 8*(1), 24–28.

Odejide, O. A., Ohaeri, J. U., Adelekan, M. L., & Ikuesan, B. A. (1989). Alcohol treatment systems in Nigeria. *Alcohol and Alcoholism, 24*(4), 347–353.

Oppenheimer, E., Sheehan, M., & Taylor, C. (1988). Letting the client speak: Drug misusers and the process of help seeking. *British Journal of Addiction, 83,* 635–647.

Orlandi, M. A. (1992). The challenge of evaluating community-based prevention programs: A cross-cultural perspective. In M. A. Orlandi, R. Weston, & L. G. Epstein (Eds.), *Cultural competence for evaluators: A guide for alcohol and other drug abuse prevention practitioners working with ethnic/racial communities* (pp. 1–22). Washington, DC: Office for Substance Abuse Prevention, U.S. Department of Health and Human Services.

Pfleiderer, B. (1988). The semiotics of ritual healing in a north Indian Moslem shrine. *Social Science and Medicine, 27*(5), 417–424.

Ranganathan, S. (1994). The Manjakkudi experience: A camp approach towards treating alcoholics. *Addiction, 89*(9), 1071–1075.

Rappaport, H., & Rappaport, M. (1981) The integration of scientific and traditional healing: A proposed model. *American Psychologist, 36*(7), 774–781.

Reiss, N. (1991). *The health care of the Arabs in Israel.* Boulder, CO: Westview Press.

Rizvi, S. A. (1989). *Moslem tradition in psychotherapy and modern trends.* Pakistan: Institute of Islamic Culture.

Rosenthal, M. S. (1989). The therapeutic community: Exploring the boundaries. *British Journal of Addiction, 84*(2), 141–150.

Saucer, P. R. (1991). Evangelical renewal therapy: A proposal for integration of religious values into psychotherapy. *Psychological Reports, 69*(3, pt. 2), 1099–1106.

Sayre, L., Cornille, T. A., Rohrer, G., & Hicks, M. W. (1992). Family outreach residential addiction treatment: Changes in addicts' beliefs about social support. *Alcoholism Treatment Quarterly, 9*(1), 51–66.

Schwartz, D. (1985). Caribbean folk beliefs and western psychiatry. *Journal of Psychosocial Nursing and Mental Health Services, 23*(11), 26–30.

Serok, S., & Levi, N. (1993). Application of gestalt therapy with long-term prison inmates in Israel. *Gestalt Journal, 16*(1), 105–127.

Stephen, W. J. (1992). *Primary health care in the Arab world.* Somerset, England: Somerset House.

Stivers, R. (1976). Culture and alcoholism. In R. E. Tartarand & A. A. Sugarman (Eds.), *Alcoholism: Interdisciplinary approaches to an enduring problem* (pp. 573–602). Reading, MA: Addison-Wesley.

Szalay, L. B., Canino, G., & Vilov, S. V. (1993). Vulnerabilities and cultural change: Drug use among Puerto Rican adolescents in the United States. *The International Journal of the Addictions, 28*(4), 327–354.

Templer, D. I. (1991). Comment on large gender differences on death anxiety in Arab countries. *Psychological Reports, 69*(3), 1186.

Torrey F. E. (1972). What western psychotherapists can learn from witchdoctors. *American Journal of Orthopsychiatry, 42*(1), 69–76.

Toumbourou, J., & Hamilton, M. (1993). Perceived client and program moderators of successful therapeutic community treatment for drug addiction. *The International Journal of the Addictions, 28*(11), 1127–1146.

Turner, V. W. (1967). *The forest of symbols: Aspects of Ndembu ritual.* Ithaca, NY: Cornell University Press.

Umoren, U. E. (1990). Religion and traditional medicine: An anthropological case study of a Nigerian treatment of mental illness. *Medical Anthropology, 12*(4), 389–400.

Werner, R. (1979). Die behandlung von Malaysischen drogenabhaenigigen mit den methoden der traditionalten medizin. *Oeffentliches Gesundheitswesen, 41,* 332–343.

Wessels, W. H. (1985). The traditional healer and psychiatry. *Australian and New Zealand Journal of Psychiatry, 19*(3), 283–286.

West, J. (1987). Psychotherapy in the Eastern province of Saudi Arabia. *Psychotherapy, 24*(1), 105–107.

Yalom, I.L.D. (1975). *The theory and practice of group psychotherapy.* (2nd ed.). New York: Basic Books.

14

The Right Stuff: Key Personality Characteristics That Indicate Success in Overcoming Addiction in Israel

Rachel Lev-Wiesel

INTRODUCTION

Is it possible to predict the outcome of drug-free programs? What is the impact of personality characteristics (ego strengths) compared to social environmental factors in recovery from drug dependency? Should drug addicts acquire specific personality characteristics (the "right stuff") in order to recover? Should society invest only in those who have or acquire specific personal characteristics needed to recover from drug dependency?

Drug addiction is a worldwide problem. Governments make great economic and social investments to prevent people from using drugs as well as to treat those who become addicted. Regardless of the type of program implemented statistics indicate high rates of relapse (Rahav & Teichman, 1998). Factors contributing to addiction, including personal and environmental characteristics, have been studied; however, there is a lack of knowledge regarding factors that might promote recovery.

The drug problem was recognized by Israeli welfare authorities nearly 20 years ago as a result of the Israel-Lebanon War. In that period, the National Bureau for Decreasing Drug Use was established to develop treatment programs, such as therapeutic communities, hostels, and hospital departments (Riter, 1995) aimed at helping drug users to recover. According to current statistics, 10 percent of adolescents (60,000) between the ages of 12 and 18, and 8 percent of adults (160,000) between the ages of 18 and 40 use either hard or soft drugs (Rahav & Teichman, 1998). There are no exact statistics for those who underwent any of the recovery programs and remained drug free except for those published by Narcotics Anonymous (NA), which claimed that approximately 5,000 NA members, former drug addicts, managed to recover (become drug free) since 1986, when NA was first established in Israel. Most of the formal treatment programs in Israel demand that their clients join a local NA branch as part of the treatment process. Currently, 250 NA groups operate daily in all parts of Israel.

Millions of adults and young adults in the United States have undergone substance abuse treatment. However, relapse rates among these individuals are high and few have remained drug free.

Relapse—a breakdown or setback in a person's attempt to change a targeted behavior—has long been recognized as a frequent occurrence in most drug recovery programs, whether in institutional treatment settings, hostels, or self-help groups such as NA (Annis, Sklar, & Moser, 1998). Empirical studies indicate that regardless of the recovery program's elements and rationale, most substance users go through periods of intense drug use followed by periods of drug abstinence, which are followed by relapse (Longabaugh et al., 1995). The question that arises is: What drives this cycle and what may help to break it?

Various theories recognize the roles played by social, psychological, cultural, and situational factors (Chaney, O'Leary, & Marlatt, 1978; Marlatt & Gordon, 1985) in substance abuse, such as unresolved childhood trauma (Young, 1990), lack of social support networks (Humphreys & Noke, 1997), and low self-esteem (Weisz, 1996). Empirical studies have found that factors such as coping styles and coping responses contribute to continued abstinence or relapse among addicts (Annis et al., 1998; McCormick & Smith, 1995; Moser & Annis, 1996). Herman-Stahl and Petersen (1996) found that unsuccessful coping due to inadequate personal resources (social status and self-esteem) is implicated in the process.

This chapter examines the role of two personal resources—perceived potency and perceived social support—on the length of abstinence among NA members in Israel. This chapter also tries to determine whether the same resources or different ones are involved in different stages of the abstinence period.

Abstinent Behavior and Personal Resources

Remaining drug free after initial withdrawal is a notoriously difficult feat for most addicts. It requires coping with both external stressors, such as the pull of the previous substance-abusing peer group or a pathogenic family, and inner stressors such as the craving for drugs or the depression that drug use had covered (Baily, Hser, Hsieh, & Anglin, 1994). Many drug users rely on drugs to cope with unpleasant emotions, from boredom to frustration, anger, or depression, and abstinence means giving up this crutch, without an alternative source of emotional support.

In short, periods of abstinence are generally marked by considerable stress, which may lead the addict back to drugs for relief (Demas, Schoenbaum, Wills, Doll, & Klein, 1995). According to Hosen (1993), abstinence involves tradeoffs designed to obtain a preponderance of pleasant over unpleasant moments. It requires the addict to endure all the discomforts of being without drugs for the sake of psychological well being in the future.

According to stress theory, individuals' personal and social resources are instrumental to their ability to cope with stressful life events (Ben-Sira, 1991; Dohernwend & Dohernwend, 1974; Folkman & Lazarus, 1984; Sarason & Sarason, 1986). While adequate personal resources help people to maintain or regain their psychological homeostasis in times of stress, their lack may lead to difficulty coping and vulnerability to stress, breakdown, and disease (Folkman & Lazarus, 1984)—in short, to relapse.

Personal resources such as hardiness (Kobasa, 1979), sense of coherence (Antonovsky, 1979), socioeconomic status (Ben-Sira, 1985; Pearlin, 1982), and social support (Cox, 1978; Lin, Ensel, Limone, & Kue, 1979) have been found to play a crucial role in maintaining emotional homeostasis. More specifically, evidence indicates that the possession of personal resources such as self-esteem, self-efficacy, and social support can predict abstinent or relapse behavior (Gulliver, Hughes, Solomon, & Dey, 1995). Kingree (1995) found that relapsers have lower levels of self-esteem and family support than those who remain drug-free. Others found that perceived social support from friends significantly moderates the relationship between alcohol use and a family history of alcoholism (Feldman, 1968; Ohannessian & Hesselbrock, 1993). Meyers, Brown, and Mott (1993) and Ritcher, Brown, and Mott (1991) found that the quality of social support was related to substance use outcome following treatment, with abstainers having more support than relapsers.

Another personal resource that has been implicated in emotional homeostasis is potency (Ben-Sira, 1983, 1985; Lev-Wiesel, 1998; Lev-Wiesel & Shamai, 1998). Ben-Sira (1985) defines potency as a two-part quality consisting of: (1) enduring confidence in one's capacities, and (2) commitment to the social environment, which is perceived as basically meaningful, predictable, and marked by a reliable and just distribution of rewards. In operational terms, potency includes self-appreciation and mastery, on the one hand, and commitment to society and the conviction that society is meaningful and ordered, on the other. It is an experience-based confidence both in one's capacity to cope with stressors and the belief that things usually work out reasonably well. Recent studies that examine potency in specific populations such as child Holocaust survivors and adult survivors of childhood sexual abuse suggest that potency might also be based on genetic characteristics such as pain tolerance and the ability to withstand acute and ambiguous situations (Amir & Lev-Wiesel, in press; Lev-Wiesel, 1999).

Ben-Sira (1983, 1985) identified the quality of potency following his study of the success of rehabilitation among physically injured soldiers. He found that although many of the injured soldiers experienced high levels of self-control, sense of coherence, and other personal resources upon being injured, their levels of emotional homeostasis and adaptation differed over the rehabilitation process. This finding led Ben-Sira (1985) to suggest the existence of a mechanism, which he termed potency, that has the capacity to arrest the deleterious impact of stress over and above other personal resources. That is, potency is conceived of as a resource that is activated when other personal resources prove inadequate. Potency should be useful for understanding the ability to withstand the allure of relapse, because it involves the belief in one's capacity to recover even as one is in the midst of a crisis.

METHOD

Sample

The study sample consisted of 59 NA members (55 men, 4 women) recruited from an NA branch in a city in Israel. Narcotics Anonymous members were selected as the study population because of the popularity of the organization with addicts. Anonymous members were given a questionnaire before the start of one of their meetings, and the questionnaires were collected at the end of the same meeting. Four members refused to participate in the study.

The participants ranged in age from 26 to 45. All of them reported narcotics (heroin, cocaine) as their primary substance of abuse. Eighty-seven percent had been in prison more than three times in their adult lives. Thirty-three percent had only an elementary school education, 60 percent were high-school graduates, and 7 percent were university graduates. Forty percent were married, 24 percent were single, and 36 percent were divorced. All the participants had gone through periods of abstinence and relapse since they started abusing substances. The average age at which they started using drugs was 16.05 ($SD = 4.56$).

Instrument

The instrument consisted of a three-part questionnaire utilizing demographic and drug-related variables (e.g., age, family status, imprisonment experience, type of drugs used, age when drug use started, length of abstinence in past and present), potency, and perceived social support.

Potency was measured by the Potency Scale, developed by Ben-Sira (Longabaugh et al., 1995) and adapted for Israel. The scale consists of 19 statements covering four personal qualities: self-confidence (e.g., "I am able to do things as well as most other people"); mastery (e.g., "I have little control over things that happen to me, I feel that I am pushed around in life"); alienation, defined as the opposite of commitment (e.g., "Nowadays a person has to live pretty much for today and let tomorrow take care of itself; having the right connections is more important than talent for achieving something"); and anomie, defined as the opposite of a sense of meaning and justice (e.g., "Community leaders are indifferent to one's needs; my life goals are receding rather than being realized"). Respondents were asked to rate their agreement with each statement on a six-point scale, ranging from *not at all* (1) to *very much* (6). The Cronbach alpha was 0.82 for this scale, indicating high reliability.

Table 14.1
Correlations of Perceived Social Support, Potency, and Demographic Variables with Length of Past and Current Abstinence

	PSS	Potency	Past AP	Education	Current AP	Age of Start
PSS	1.00					
Potency	0.33*					
Past AP	0.13	0.45**				
Education	0.59***	0.23	0.29			
Current AP	0.45**	0.33**	-0.09	0.29*		
Age of Start	0.27*	-0.35*	-0.11	-0.50**	-0.17	1.00

PSS = perceived social support; AP = abstinence period.

*$p < .05$. **$p < .01$. ***$p < .001$.

Perceived social support was measured by the Perceived Social Support (PSS) scale developed by Procidano and Heller (1983). The scale contains two parts, perceived social support from family members and perceived social support from friends, each of which can be used separately. For the purpose of this study, only perceived social support from friends was used, for two reasons: most participants reported not having any relations with their family of origin for years, and 53 percent were either divorced or single. The scale consisted of 20 items addressing various expressions of perceived social support, including instrumental support (e.g.,"My friends give me all the support I need"), affective support (e.g., "My friends are sensitive and attentive to my personal needs and mood"), cognitive support (e.g., "I take my friends' advice"), and being the helper (e.g., "My friends turn to me for help in time of need," "My friends gladly listen to my advice"). The Cronbach alpha (0.85) for this scale indicates high reliability.

Results

The average length of the participants' current abstinence was 2.57 months (*SD* = 1.07). The average length of their longest previous period of abstinence was 9.85 months (*SD* = 3.43). Eighty-six percent of the participants were NA members during their prior periods of abstinence. Table 14.1 shows the correlations for the study variables. Potency was positively correlated with the lengths of both past abstinence (0.45, $p < 0.01$) and current abstinence (0.33, $p < 0.01$). Perceived social support was positively correlated only with the length of current abstinence (0.45, $p < 0.01$).

Among the demographic variables, only education was positively correlated with length of abstinence, and then only in the present (0.29, $p < 0.05$). Perceived social support, however, was correlated positively with education (0.59, $p < 0.001$), and negatively with the age that drug abuse commenced (0.27, $p < 0.05$). Potency

Table 14.2
Multiple Regression of Demographic Variables and Personal Resources on Length of Past and Current Abstinence

	Abstinence	
Variable	Past β	Current β
Education	0.09	-0.03
Age of start	0.05	0.25
Type of drug (hard/recreational)	0.22	-0.24
Imprisonment experienced	0.06	-0.26
Perceived social support	-0.02	0.53*
Potency	0.42*	0.17
F score	$F(1,26) = 5.58$	$F(6,21) = 2.17$
R^2	0.18*	0.38*

*$p < 0.05$.

(0.35, $p < 0.05$) and education (0.50, $p < 0.01$) were also correlated negatively with the age that drug use commenced (see Table 14.1).

Regression analyses were performed separately on current and past lengths of abstinence to determine the contributions of the variables. Demographic and drug-related variables were entered first (education, age of starting drug use, type of drugs used, and imprisonment experience), followed by the personal resources of potency and perceived social support, respectively.

Table 14.2 shows that although all the variables together predict 38 percent of the length of current abstinence ($R^2 = 0.38$, $F(6,21) = 2.17$, $p < 0.05$), only perceived social support made a significant contribution on its own ($\beta = 0.53$, $p < 0.05$). Regarding the length of past abstinence, all the variables together predicted 18 percent ($R^2 = 0.18$, $F(1,26) = 5.58$, $p < 0.05$), but only potency was found to contribute significantly on its own ($\beta = 0.42$, $p < 0.05$).

DISCUSSION

This study found that while both potency and perceived social support contributed to abstinence, perceived social support contributed the most to the relatively short period of current abstinence, while potency was found to contribute the most to the longer period of past abstinence.

A possible explanation for this finding stems from the tendency people have to attribute success to themselves and failure to others, while forgetting the difficulties involved in past successes (Kelly, 1955). Past abstinence is likely to be remembered as a success in which the person was able to overcome addiction, and its many difficulties forgotten. In contrast, current abstinence is replete with the day-to-day difficulties of refraining from drug use. The individual struggling with those difficulties is less likely to feel potent and more likely to feel that his or her accomplishment depends on social support.

A correlate of this explanation lies in the conscientious use of social support in the NA program. As participants in this program, all the subjects were receiving hefty doses of social support from the other participants. According to NA theory, this apparently enables them to identify with others who are coping with similar painful experiences and provides a buffer against the urge to return to drugs. Since not all the participants in the study were also members of NA during their past abstinence periods, some of them may not have received such social support then.

Another explanation for the importance attributed to potency in the longest period of abstinence has to do with the changing role of the abstainer in the NA group. New members in the group were given help by the others. The longer the person remained abstinent, the more he or she became involved in helping others to abstain. Acting as a helper and model for others and receiving their appreciation are likely to strengthen one's sense of worth, self-esteem, and potency. It may also be that the potency, related to lengthy abstinence, was contingent on the abstainers' perceived social support. Klein's theory of object relations (Segal, 1974) and Erikson's (1980) life cycle approach view basic trust in others as fundamental to self-identity, self-confidence, and self-esteem. The withdrawal and early abstinence phase of quitting substance abuse can be viewed symbolically as early childhood, in which the helpless and powerless individual depends entirely on others for support. In their studies of drug addicts, Knight, Cross, Giles-Sims, and Simpson (1995) found that parental absence in childhood predicted their psychosocial functioning in adulthood, whereas Baily and colleagues (1994) found that such absence was more prevalent among relapsers than recoverers.

Personal conversations with some of the participants in this study suggest that they perceived drugs as essential to their well-being. As one addict put it, "All day I worried, how am I going to get the next drug supply because I won't survive without it. . . . The thought of being without a drug supply frightens me." Without the drugs they have come to rely on, addicts in the first phases of abstinence rely on social support for their sense of security. As they receive that support, their self-esteem is enhanced, and this, in turn, increases their self-confidence and self-control, which Ben-Sira (1985) conceptualizes as potency. As the abstinence period becomes longer and the individual feels more potent, he or she may feel less need for social support.

The differential contributions of social support and potency support the understanding that this is not a uniform phenomenon; it has different permutations over time (Baily et al., 1994). According to stress theory, different demands require different resources (Folkman & Lazarus, 1984). The ordeal of withdrawal obviously requires resources such as physical care and moral support. The findings of this study suggest that the initial period of abstinence requires affective and cognitive social support to cope with the internal and external stressors noted above, whereas longer-term recovery requires a degree of life satisfaction, sense of meaning, and self-actualization. It may be that relapse occurs, after a relatively long abstinence, in response to the need that emerges to find meaning and satisfaction in life during the recovery stage. In this situation, potency rather than social support seems to be called for.

The findings seem to indicate that personality resources (both physical and psychological in nature), though latent, may be crucial to recovery. This possibility—prediction of recovery prospects according to the "right stuff"—potency—raises ethical problems: Should only those who have the "right stuff" be treated? Should society invest limited resources in drug addicts who have a certain degree of potency and ignore the others? Different questions may be raised concerning the effectiveness of treatment programs. According to this view, drug addicts who have the "right stuff" would recover no matter what type and cost of treatment were implemented as long as at the first stage of the program (physical recovery) they are prepared to accept social support.

To conclude, the findings seem to suggest that successful recovery may be based on the building or rebuilding of potency through social support. Indeed, high levels of self-confidence, self-esteem, and self-control may be the ultimate preventatives of addictive behaviors. As one NA member said: "To be saved, I need to find within myself strengths which I do not remember ever using. I keep asking myself if it is possible to transfer the strong will I had for getting the drugs into a will-power for staying clean."

REFERENCES

Amir, M., & Lev-Wiesel, R. (in press). Individual differences in post-traumatic stress disorder symptoms, psychological distress, personal resources and quality of life in Holocaust child survivors according to their Holocaust experiences. *Family Process*.

Annis, H. M., Sklar, S. M., & Moser, A. E. (1998). Gender in relation to relapse crisis situations, coping, and outcome among treated alcoholics. *Addictive Behaviors, 23*(1), 127–131.

Antonovsky, A. (1979). *Health, stress and coping*. San Francisco: Jossey Bass.

Baily, R. C., Hser, Y., Hsieh, S. C., & Anglin, M. D. (1994). Influences affecting maintenance and cessation of narcotics addiction. *Journal of Drug Issues, 24*(2), 249–272.

Ben-Sira, Z. (1983). Loss stress and readjustment. *Social Science and Medicine, 17,* 1619–1632.

———. (1985). Potency: A stress buffering link in the coping stress disease relationship. *Social Science and Medicine, 21*(4), 397–406.

———. (1991). *Regression, stress and readjustment aging*. New York: Praeger Publishers.

Chaney, E. F., O'Leary, M. R., & Marlatt, G. A. (1978). Skill training with alcoholics. *Journal of Counseling and Clinical Psychology, 46,* 1092–1104.

Cox, T. (1978). *Stress*. New York: Macmillan.

Demas, P., Schoenbaum, E. E., Wills, T. A., Doll, L. S., & Klein, R. S. (1995). Stress, coping and attitudes toward HIV treatment in injecting drug users: A qualitative study. *AIDS Education and Prevention, 7*(5), 429–442.

Dohernwend, B. S., & Dohernwend, B. P. (1974). *Stressful life events: Their nature and effects*. New York: Wiley.

Erikson, E. H. (1980). *Identity and life cycle*. New York: W. W. Norton.

Feldman, H. W. (1968). Ideological supports to becoming and remaining a heroin addict. *Journal of Health and Social Behavior, 9*(2), 131–139.

Folkman, S., & Lazarus, R. S. (1984). *Stress appraisal and coping*. New York: Springer.

Gulliver, S. B., Hughes, J. R., Solomon, L. J., & Dey, A. N. (1995). An investigation of self-efficacy, partner support and daily stresses as predictors of relapse to smoking in self-quitters. *Addiction, 90*(6), 767–772.

Herman-Stahl, M., & Petersen, A. C. (1996). The protective role of coping and social resources for depressive symptoms among young adolescents. *Journal of Youth and Adolescence, 25*(6), 733–753.

Hosen, R. (1993). A psychology of happiness and well-being and its relation to the psychology of addiction and dependence. *Psychology: A Journal of Human Behavior, 30*(2), 1–17.

Humphreys, K., & Noke, J. M. (1997). The influence of posttreatment mutual help group participation on the friendship networks of substance abuse patients. *American Journal of Community Psychology, 25*(1), 1–16.

Kelly, G. A. (1955). *The psychology of personal constructs*. New York: Norton.

Kingree, J. B. (1995). Understanding gender differences in psychosocial functioning and treatment retention. *American Journal of Drug and Alcohol Abuse, 21*(2), 267–281.

Knight, D. K., Cross, D. R., Giles-Sims, J., & Simpson, D. D. (1995). Psychosocial functioning among adult drug users: The role of parental absence, support, and conflict. *International Journal of Addictions, 30*(10), 1271–1288.

Kobasa, S. C. (1979). Stressful life events, personality and health: An inquiry into hardiness. *Journal of Personality and Social Psychology, 37*, 1–12.

Lev-Wiesel, R. (1998). Coping with stress: Possible forced relocation in the Golan Heights, Israel. *Journal of Applied Behavioral Science, 34*(2), 143–160.

———. (1999). Feelings of adult survivors of child abuse towards their offender parents. *Child and Adolescent Social Work Journal, 16*(4), 291–304.

Lev-Wiesel, R., & Shamai, M. (1998). Living under the threat of relocation: Spouses' perceptions of the threat and coping resources. *Contemporary Family Therapy, 3*, 271–295.

Lin, N., Ensel, W., Limone, R., & Kue, W. (1979). Social support, stressful life events and illness: A model and an empirical test. *Journal of Health and Social Behavior, 20*, 108–119.

Longabaugh, R., Wirtz, P. W., Beattie, M. C., Noel, N., et al. (1995). Matching treatment focus to patient social investment and support: 18-month follow-up results. *Journal of Consulting and Clinical Psychology, 63*(2), 296–307.

Marlatt, G. A., & Gordon, J. R. (1985). *Relapse prevention: Maintenance strategies in the treatment of addictive behaviors*. New York: Guilford.

McCormick, R., & Smith, M. (1995). Aggression and hostility in substance abusers: The relationship to abuse patterns, coping style, and relapse triggers. *Addictive Behaviors, 20*(5), 555–562.

Meyers, M. G., Brown, S. A., & Mott, M. A. (1993). Coping as a predictor of adolescent substance abuse treatment outcome. *Journal of Substance Abuse, 5*(1), 15–29.

Moser, A. E., & Annis, H. M. (1996). The role of coping in relapse crisis outcome: A prospective study of treated alcoholics. *Addiction, 91*, 1101–1113.

Ohannessian, C. M., & Hesselbrock, V. M. (1993). The influence of perceived social support on the relationship between family history of alcoholism and drinking behaviors. *Addiction, 88*(12), 1651–1658.

Pearlin, L. I. (1982). The social contexts of stress. In L. Goldberger & S. Breznitz (Eds.), *Handbook of stress, theoretical and clinical aspects* (pp. 303–315). London: Free Press.

Procidano, M. E., & Heller, M. (1983). Measures of perceived social support from friends and from family: Three validation studies. *American Journal of Community Psychology, 11*(1), 1–24.

Rahav, G., & Teichman, M. (1998). *Study report of the drug use in Israel, 1998, An epidemiological study*. Jerusalem: Israeli Drug Department.

Ritcher, S. S., Brown, S. A., & Mott, M. A. (1991). The impact of social support and self-esteem on adolescent substance abuse treatment outcome. *Journal of Substance Abuse, 3*(4), 371–385.

Riter, M. (1995). Treating drug users in Israel. In D. Green (Ed.), *Drugs: Facts, questions, problems* (pp. 405–375). Tel Aviv: Ministry of Defense and Ministry of Education (in Hebrew).

Sarason, I. G., & Sarason, B. R. (1986). *Social support theory research and applications*. The Hague: Martinus Nijhoff.

Segal, H. (1974). *Introduction to the work of Melanie Klein*. New York: Basic Books.

Weisz, C. (1996). Social identities and response to treatment for alcohol and cocaine abuse. *Addictive Behaviors, 21*(4), 445–458.

Young, E. B. (1990). The role of incest issues in relapse. *Journal of Psychoactive Drugs, 22*(2), 249–258.

15

The Evaluation of Treatment for Substance Use Disorders: Relevance to the Middle East

Maristela G. Monteiro

INTRODUCTION

According to the United Nations International Drug Control Programme (UNDCP), a growing drug problem has been emerging in the Middle East during the past five years, with Jordan becoming the main transit country for heroin to Israel and amphetamines to Saudi Arabia. The Bekaa Valley in Lebanon is considered to be a major opium-growing and heroin-producing area. Opium is also being cultivated in the Sinai peninsula despite law enforcement against it by the government of Egypt. Cannabis seizure and cultivation have increased in Egypt, and heroin from Afghanistan continues to flow into the region as well. This increase in the drug supply is expected to lead to an increase in drug use and related health consequences in the region.

Emerging drug use and associated adverse health and social consequences in the Middle East, as elsewhere, require the development of adequate responses, including treatment services. These services, however, need to reflect local conditions, build on existing resources and experiences, and involve the community and target groups in order to effectively address the health and social consequences of substance abuse. For example, HIV infection is now considered one of the major international public health problems of the last 30 years. Injection drug use has contributed to the rapid spread of HIV and other blood-borne diseases in several countries. HIV infection has been reported in over 130 countries around the world, with over 100 of those countries reporting that it has occurred through injection drug use. Appropriate services targeted to this population are essential to reverse the spread of HIV among those who inject drugs and to thwart its spread to the general population.

This chapter provides an overview of the planning and evaluation of drug treatment services. A first step in addressing this subject is to define what constitutes treatment—its philosophy, components, and goals. Evaluation of treatment services and systems should occur as part of a process and at multiple levels of service intervention—for example, from the early response phase to an identified need, to the determination of cost-effectiveness strategies of service provision, to the impact of the overall treatment system. Ideally, evaluation assessment (Why do we want to evaluate this program?) is an initial means for getting key stakeholders involved, followed by activities that assess needs and evaluate process, outcome, and economics. These stages of evaluation should each provide meaningful data for decision makers and program planners to develop, expand, or improve services.

WHAT IS TREATMENT FOR SUBSTANCE USE DISORDERS?

Definition

Treatment is the process that begins when psychoactive substance users come into contact with a health provider or other community service. Treatment is a comprehensive approach to the identification, assistance, health care, and social integration of persons presenting problems caused by the use of any psychoactive substance. Such contact may continue through a succession of specific interventions until the highest attainable level of health and well-being is reached (World Health Organization [WHO], 1998). The consequences of psychoactive substance use are regarded as health events that can be studied with scientific methods and dealt with by humane and sympathetic medical and psychosocial approaches. Details regarding the objectives and general principles of interventions follow:

Objectives

- To reduce substance use (ranging from total abstinence to functional use without problems in the case of some substances)
- To improve health and personal social functioning, including reductions in morbidity and mortality caused by or associated with the use of psychoactive substances
- To ensure that users are able to maximize their physical, mental, and social abilities, and have access to regular services and opportunities to achieve full social integration
- To reduce public health and public safety threats

Additional objectives include:

- To reduce criminal and other antisocial behavior

- To reduce costs to society.

General Principles of Interventions

- Interventions are useful to the extent that they respond to individual needs and situations.
- Adequate assessment of needs and available interventions—their applicability and acceptability—are essential for interventions to be effective.
- Professional treatment and nonprofessional interventions and support can effectively complement each other. Joint and comprehensive planning as well as monitoring of interventions increase their effectiveness.

SERVICE INTERVENTION

Public Health Approach

A public health approach to the treatment of substance use disorders should incorporate scientific knowledge about the nature and extent of specific drug problems. Effective primary and secondary prevention of harmful forms of substance use and the utilization of drug treatment rather than arrest and incarceration, for persons who have problems with illicit drug use should be emphasized. A public health approach should also emphasize the reduction of risks and serious adverse health consequences such as those related to unsafe injecting practices and needle sharing. The key elements of a public health approach are:

- Knowledge base: a scientific and administrative database providing a foundation of information on which decisions can be made.
- Political will: society's desire and commitment to develop and fund new programs and to support or modify existing programs. (This element depends on politicians, legislators, and citizens.)
- Social strategy: a plan to apply the knowledge base and political will, with the support of the public and social institutions, to improve or initiate programs such as services by health providers, structural interventions, and local activities for health promotion.

Systems Approach

Treatment systems for individuals with substance use disorders, particularly dependence, have developed in different ways in several countries around the world. Systems of treatment and care are not structures that are planned and created solely on the basis of scientific findings. Rather, systems of treatment and care grow, develop, and change gradually over several decades according to cultural, political, and other factors. They are often established as a result of attention being drawn to severe cases, sometimes as a result of national concerns about the increasing size of a problem, anxieties about its effect on the economy, or concern about its spread among young people. As a result, the structure, coverage, and content of treatment systems do not always meet the needs of potential clients and interest groups or the priorities set by public health officials, especially when trends in substance use and problems change in the target population. In many countries, these systems have never been evaluated, and this, in turn, has helped to promote the idea that treatment for substance use problems is ineffective.

Treatment approaches are complex and diverse, and may differ in modality, philosophy, stage specificity, setting, target, provider, time frame, efficacy, cost, availability, utilization, organizational characteristics, and financing. The treatments offered to people with drug and alcohol problems include a wide range of different interventions (World Health Organization, 1993a). Among the various interventions that have been used are medical detoxification, supportive counseling, brief interventions, videotaped self-confrontation, motivational interviewing, hypnosis, cognitive therapies, behavioral counter-conditioning treatments, relaxation therapy, prescriptions of various medications, drug-free rehabilitation houses, substitution therapies, self-help groups, acupuncture, and traditional healing. There are also a variety of settings in which people receive care. These include general hospitals, psychiatric hospitals, primary health care facilities, social service agencies, educational settings, rehabilitation services and half-way houses, and prisons and other correctional institutions.

To further understand the characteristics of national responses to alcohol and other drug problems, the World Health Organization conducted a key informant survey in 23 countries on treatment for substance use problems in 1993. That survey gives a rough idea about how services are organized at the country level, in both developed and developing countries. The 23 countries that participated were the Bahamas, Canada, Chile, Colombia, Congo, Egypt, Finland, Ghana, Hungary, India, Italy, Mexico, Nigeria, Norway, Pakistan, Poland, Russia, Spain, South Africa, Sri Lanka, Switzerland, Thailand, and Zimbabwe (World Health Organization, 1993b). Analyses of how substance use services are organized in these very different countries have revealed that treatment resources in most of them are scarce. The extent of drug and alcohol problems and the demand for treatment are much greater than the availability of existing treatment services. In addition, in many countries, the treatment services available are usually located in major cities and thus do not reach remote or rural areas where such problems also exist. Since treatment for substance use disorders has not been integrated into primary health care services in the vast majority of countries, a large population in need does not have access to treatment and care.

According to the WHO survey, psychiatrists were one of the professional groups most frequently involved in treatment. The location of treatment was often a psychiatric hospital, whether the service was provided for alcohol or other drugs, and whether the service was residential or nonresidential. Often, inpatient treatment was limited to detoxification for alcohol problems. Primary care services and personnel, including general practitioners, were not involved at all with treatment of drug and alcohol problems in many countries. Another observation common to most countries in the survey was the inadequate levels of staff training regarding the assessment, management, and treatment of drug and alcohol problems. The most common form of staff training consisted of their clinical experience alone; formal training or accreditation was an exception in the majority of countries surveyed.

Treatment Effectiveness

Confidence in the general effectiveness of treatment has been undermined by such suggestions as: results of treatment are poor and "do not work"; there are few differences in terms of effectiveness among various treatment approaches; and conventional treatment often appears no better than minimal interventions. Application of scientific methods and evidence-based medicine to the field of substance use disorders over the last 20 years is helping to change this pessimistic view about the effectiveness of treatment. For example, research on treatment effectiveness has now demonstrated that a continuum of interventions is required for the range of problems associated with substance dependence. Also, the treatment setting and the stages of treatment are important factors that need to be considered in planning services (Heather & Mattick, 1994; Institute of Medicine, 1990).

It is beyond the scope of this chapter to comprehensively review the effectiveness of all treatment approaches to the wide range of problems associated with substance use disorders. A brief overview is given here, but interested readers should rely on the international literature and recent reviews for specific information.

Overall, community-based (i.e., nonresidential non-inpatient) detoxification is the most efficient and cost-effective approach for detoxification for most patients with alcohol and benzodiazepine withdrawal. For opioid withdrawal, however, completion rates are higher in inpatient detoxification facilities. Inpatient detoxification is recommended for those patients likely to experience severe withdrawal and associated medical complications and who are at risk of death. Specialized facilities are preferable to beds on acute medical or psychiatric wards because specialized facilities are associated with higher admission rates, higher completion rates, and higher rates of ongoing abstinence than those found in general medical or psychiatric settings. When specialized facilities are nonexistent, however, the costs of developing such services need to be considered. If the costs prohibit the development of such services, then allocation of units within general wards might be the most cost-effective alternative.

A number of experimental trials of methadone are used for detoxification in community settings, with completion rates ranging from 10 to 30 percent. Inpatient opioid withdrawal using methadone has been evaluated extensively, with nonexperimental designs reporting completion rates of up to 80 percent. Such high completion rates are associated with increased use of medication to ameliorate withdrawal symptoms and to shorten the withdrawal period. Completion of inpatient withdrawal, however, does not typically prevent relatively rapid relapse among opioid-dependent individuals.

Since 1970, methadone maintenance treatment has become the dominant form of opioid substitution treatment throughout the world. Oral methadone is the most widely used substance for opioid agonist pharmacotherapy. Other less widely used but evaluated opioid agonist pharmacotherapies used are levo-alpha-acetyl-methanol (LAAM), a long-acting synthetic opioid taken orally, and buprenorphine, an opioid agonist and antagonist taken sublingually (Blaine, 1992). Oral methodone has been rigorously evaluated in several developed countries in well-controlled randomized trials, and numerous observational studies have demonstrated reduced illicit drug use and injecting practices, reduced criminal behavior, and improved physical, psychological, and social well-being. Also, methadone treatment has been proven effective in preventing behaviors linked to HIV infection. While there is a wide variation of dosing and effectiveness related to methadone treatment, research has shown that the prescription of higher doses of methadone (above 50–60 mg daily) is more effective in terms of treatment outcome, long-term maintenance is more effective than only detoxification, and ancillary and supportive services (including counseling, social, and medical services) as well as positive staff-client relationships are important factors in promoting the positive effects of methadone treatment.

In practice, even among developed countries, the goals, designs, delivery, and effectiveness of methadone maintenance programs vary considerably. Nevertheless, the measures of treatment effectiveness tend to remain constant. They include: less illicit opioid use and drug risk practices, reduced criminal activity, greater retention in treatment, and improved health status. Other factors that need to be considered are treatment effectiveness, acceptability, and the cost/benefits of interventions in different settings and conditions.

In terms of treatment effectiveness, such service provision must address the cultural, ethnic, and gender needs of clients. If it does not, poor treatment and outcomes will result. This is extremely important when new treatment approaches are developed based on experiences from other settings and conditions; also, care must be taken that treatment approaches are properly adapted to the local conditions, values, and beliefs of the community and the needs of various groups of clients.

Continuum of Treatment and Care

Evidence shows that quality treatment requires a comprehensive continuum of prevention and treatment services, from case screening and diagnosis to long-term rehabilitation and support interventions for clients and their families. A general list of the services include:

- Prevention/pretreatment
- Screening, assessment, diagnosis, intervention, and referral
- Outpatient counseling

- Psychiatric services
- Structured day treatment
- Short- and long-term residential treatment services
- Opioid substitution therapies, such as methadone treatment
- Outpatient- and community-based detoxification
- Hospital-based detoxification
- Case management services
- Rehabilitation and social services

It has been estimated that 75 to 85 percent of individuals with alcohol and other drug problems never receive formal treatment. It is important, therefore, that early problem identification and referral to treatment services be provided throughout the health and human services system. Early intervention and referral to outpatient services should be seen as a hallmark of quality alcohol and drug treatment since these steps lead to cost savings by reducing demands for health services that are needed to address the effects of long-term substance abuse.

Detoxification is often the initial and easiest phase of the treatment process. Detoxification involves management of physical and psychological symptoms of acute withdrawal and treatment of medical and mental health complications. Detoxification is often not complicated and can be dealt with in nonspecialized settings (sometimes even nonmedical settings), with appropriate social and psychological counseling, and pharmacological treatments for symptoms related to the withdrawal syndrome. The most critical step in treatment, however, may not be detoxification. Promoting motivation to maintain abstinence and prevent relapse tends to be a more important factor because of its relation to long-term outcomes.

Maintaining abstinence involves three components: continuing care, relapse prevention, and supportive living arrangements. Continuing care involves the provision of ongoing treatment to maintain gains achieved during early stages of treatment. Relapse prevention involves the use of specific methods to minimize the probability of relapse to drug use (pharmacological and behavioral methods). Supportive living arrangements involve interventions such as half-way houses and long-term residential care.

Various models of traditional healing and community support are used to help in the management of substance use problems, but most need to be evaluated. In many countries, voluntary mutual help organizations such as Alcoholics Anonymous and Narcotics Anonymous play a large role in supporting recovery from substance dependence. Their level of effectiveness is limited, but those organizations do reach a broad audience and have the advantage of being available without cost.

Therapeutic communities for the treatment of drug dependence have featured prominently in the drug abuse field since the early 1960s. These programs have a number of features in common including relatively long periods of residential treatment (6–18 months) and the holding of important functional and administrative roles by former substance users who have accepted the values of the community. The goal of the therapeutic community is to instill responsibility among the individual residents for their actions and to promote the therapeutic value of the group living environment. This is achieved and reinforced by group meetings, concrete rewards, and increasing social status for those exhibiting responsible behavior. The findings from evaluation studies show a high dropout rate, with fewer than 40 percent of patients remaining for more than three months. Those who participate for more than six months are more likely to remain substance free and to exhibit sharply reduced criminal behavior for many months or years after leaving the therapeutic community.

The single major drug-related cause of the increasing spread of HIV/AIDS is the shared use of needles and syringes, which transmits the virus more effectively than sexual behavior. Half of all AIDS cases in Spain, Italy, Portugal, Bahrain, and Yugoslavia are attributed to drug injection. Two-thirds of injection drug users (IDUs) in Thailand and close to one-third in Brazil regularly share needles. It is also known that HIV/AIDS can spread through drug-using populations with remarkable speed (Stimson, Des Jarlais & Ball, 1998). A growing body of evidence shows, however, that the HIV epidemic associated with injection drug use can be prevented, slowed, stopped, and even reversed. Key elements for success include: early implementation of prevention initiatives while HIV prevalence is low; community outreach for IDUs that provides HIV/AIDS information and helps to develop trust between IDUs and health care providers; and widespread provision of sterile injection equipment. IDUs do change their behavior toward safer injecting practices and may modify their sexual behavior as well. These services must also be evaluated when implemented in different settings.

EVALUATION RESEARCH

Definition

Evaluation is a necessary and continuous process that can lead to the improvement of treatment services provision. It is a means of acquiring feedback about the operation, outcome, and cost effectiveness of a program or a network of programs and services. It is an ongoing process that questions and gains information about the nature, extent, and impact of the services provided. It implies an attitude of continuously questioning and gaining information about treatment services.

Globally, there is a significant gap between what is known about effective treatment and what is being provided. Furthermore, much of what is being done is not evaluated. As a result, in many areas where treatment resources are scarce there may be major expenditures on less effective and more expensive treatments rather than more brief and cost-effective approaches.

Developing a healthy organizational response in support of evaluation requires educating and training program planners, managers, staff, researchers, and other key decision makers about the evaluation's importance and benefits in terms of improving services, including those related to increased treatment effectiveness and cost savings. The basis for any type of evaluation is, therefore, the involvement of all stakeholders to reach an agreement on what, why, and how evaluation should be done. Unless there is a clear understanding of what each partner can gain from working together to conduct the evaluation, the results of the evaluation are likely to become another paper or report on the shelves of libraries and archives.

Objectives

Programs or health care systems that are willing to use evaluation to improve services for substance use disorders can have a wide range of goals or objectives (Kushner & Moss, 1995). These goals or objectives may include improved access to treatment, quality of care, coordination with medical services, service efficiency, access to after care or rehabilitation and social services, outcome measurement, and cost effectiveness.

Service Levels for Evaluation

There are several levels to conducting evaluation of treatment for substance use disorders including single case, treatment activity, treatment service, treatment agency, and treatment system (World Health Organization, in press). Each is described as follows:

Single case evaluation is consistent with clinical practice in that it promotes a problem-solving approach to planning, implementing, and evaluating interventions tailored specifically to each client. Responsibility for getting feedback on the progress of each client rests with the clinician or therapist.

The evaluation of a *treatment activity* involves summarizing the involvement of a group of clients with a particular treatment modality (e.g., cognitive-behavioral therapy) and the progress they have made collectively toward reaching their objectives. A common approach is to identify objectives that all clients share while they are participating in the treatment activity, and to use these shared objectives to assess the progress of the overall group.

The evaluation of a *treatment service* also involves summarizing information about a group of clients. One treatment service (e.g., outpatient) can include more than one treatment activity or modality (e.g., cognitive-behavioral therapy, relapse prevention, social skills training). Because each client may be involved with many services, isolating the main factors contributing to changes in the individual and the group as a whole becomes difficult.

A *treatment agency* may offer more than one type of treatment service (e.g., detoxification, inpatient, outpatient, and continuing care). An evaluation at the agency level will summarize information about the involvement of a group of clients with the entire agency and their progress toward treatment objectives. Conclusions about the main factors contributing to positive change across the group are difficult to make at the agency level.

A community *treatment system* comprises various services, agencies, and treatment settings. It involves people with substance use disorders and includes both specialized and general services and agencies. An evaluation at the treatment system level examines the involvement of clients with various agencies and services and monitors their progress toward a number of objectives. At the system level, it is extremely difficult to attribute changes in client functioning to their involvement with any one element of the treatment network. Evaluation at this level, however, is helpful for examining changes in system functioning (e.g., decreased waiting periods, decreased dropout rates after referral, improved coordination and sharing of resources). The assumption is then made that the improvements to system functioning will translate into improved (or equivalent) client outcomes and more efficient use of system-wide resources.

Types of Evaluation

There are six main types of evaluation that can be planned and implemented within a treatment service, agency, or system:

- Needs assessment evaluation
- Process evaluation
- Outcome evaluation
- Client satisfaction evaluation
- Cost evaluation
- Economic evaluation

These evaluations may have a sequential relationship with one another. For example, needs assessment evaluations typically happen first and are often followed by process or outcome evaluations. Cost and economic evaluations often occur later, after process and outcome issues have been evaluated. There are no fixed rules about procedure, and some evaluations can be undertaken simultaneously.

Needs assessment is the first type of program evaluation. Ideally, needs assessment takes place before the program, or network of programs, is planned and implemented. This form of assessment addresses questions about how an existing program or community network of programs should be redesigned to address needs that are not being met. The following are examples of needs assessment questions:

- What type of treatment interventions should a program provide?
- What is the anticipated number of people who will use the services each year?
- What are the prevalence and incidence of substance use disorders in the community?
- What are the main gaps in the community treatment system?
- What is the projected demand for treatment in the community or the region as a whole?

Needs assessment is a formal and systematic attempt to determine and then close gaps between "what is" and "what should be." It involves documenting important discrepancies between current and desired outcomes and prioritizing these discrepancies for program planning and intervention. In this way, needs assessment involves both need identification and need prioritization.

Process evaluation seeks to determine the extent to which the program is operating as planned. The basic purpose of process evaluation is to describe what is happening in the program and the context in which it is operating. Questions such as the following are addressed in process evaluation:

- How many clients are treated each year?
- Are the types of clients being seen consistent with or suitable to the type of program or treatment system?
- Are people having trouble accessing the program? How long is the waiting list and how are people being managed while they wait?
- Are the staff who conduct client assessments appropriately trained and using effective methods?

At this stage, the evaluation questions do not ask about the changes in clients that may result from services being provided. Rather, the questions address "coverage" (i.e., Is the program or system reaching all those for whom it was intended?) and "process" (i.e., Has the program or system been implemented as intended and in an integrated manner?). Process evaluation seeks to determine the extent to which the program is operating as planned.

Client satisfaction assessment can add an important "consumer" perspective to evaluations of substance abuse treatment services and systems. This perspective is a critical feature of continuous quality service improvement. Without such a perspective, problems such as high dropout or low success rates might be related only to client factors when in reality these problems may reflect shortcomings in the services provided or in the treatment system as a whole.

The following are some of the questions that might be asked through a client satisfaction evaluation:

- Do the services address the clients' expressed needs?
- Are there aspects of the services that clients think could be improved?
- What is the perceived quality of care from the clients' perspective?

Client satisfaction questionnaires are available for general use and are appropriate for substance use treatment programs. Although some are brief and user-friendly and have demonstrated reliability and validity, the cross-cultural applicability is unknown in some instances. Other client satisfaction questionnaires can be developed to meet specific evaluation needs. Client satisfaction evaluation is an important component of quality services provision, so it is important to be cautious when interpreting the results. Client satisfaction is not a substitute for measuring other, more objective outcomes.

An evaluation of *treatment outcomes* should accomplish two things. First, it should measure how clients and their circumstances have changed. Second, it should show that the treatment experience has been a factor in causing this change. Some questions that might be asked in an outcome evaluation are:

- Have improvements been made in aspects of the person's life that were affected by alcohol and drugs?
- Has there been a reduction in the frequency and/or quantity of substance use?
- Are improvements related to particular characteristics of the clients and their social circumstances?
- What is the relationship between program or system participation and client improvement?

Outcome evaluation may be designed in one of a number of ways to measure change and show that change is attributable to participation in the program. The most widely praised strategy to measure change and infer causality is the randomized controlled trial. With this approach, patients are randomly assigned to receive one or more treatment options (e.g., inpatient detoxification vs. ambulatory detoxification; drug therapy vs. psychological therapy). Randomized controlled trials are considered the gold standard in the evaluation of treatment effectiveness. This is because the design allows for inference of causality. Another strategy that is relatively strong in its ability to allow causal inference is the quasi-experimental approach. Rather than randomly assigning clients to different alternatives, the individuals are selected in a systematic way. "Other outcome studies" examine changes for one group of clients over time. Clients are monitored in terms of changes before and after treatment and one can speculate about the role of treatment in producing these changes.

Regardless of which strategy is used for outcome evaluation, all outcome evaluations should include an "intent-to-treat follow-up" procedure. This means that an unbiased (random) sample of subjects is recruited at entry to a treatment program and all members are then sought for follow-up at one or more points during or after treatment.

When examining outcome, a number of strategies may be considered. They are, among others: alcohol and drug use frequency and patterns; consequences of substance use, including dependence; psychological functioning; physical health (including HIV status); social adjustment; family functioning; crime; and health care utilization. Whereas it is not necessary to measure all domains when evaluating a treatment approach, one should examine more than one domain given the broad scope of treatment objectives.

Whether the measurement strategy adopted in evaluation is quantitative or qualitative, it is important that the measures used are reliable and valid. In the context of program evaluation, outcome measures should be as brief and easy to administer as possible, while possessing acceptable validity and reliability credentials. Measures that have been developed in the public domain can be used without cost. Other instruments will require a payment to the publisher. In situations where more than one outcome measure is available, it should be reasonable to choose the measure of least cost. The importance of effective staff training must be stressed, as well as the need to ensure the quality of instrument administration.

Cost evaluation or cost estimates trace resources used under different circumstances. There are four broad questions that could be addressed. These are:

- What is the cost of treating substance use disorders?
- If alternative treatment approaches are producing equivalent outcomes, how do these approaches compare in cost?
- What are the different costs involved in the delivery of a service or service system?
- How do changes in costs relate to activity levels?

Answering these types of questions involves different approaches to cost analysis. Costs are defined as the economic resources used to provide a service. There are three categories of cost:

- Direct costs that measure the value of resources directly consumed. These costs can be health- or non-health-related.
- Indirect costs that reflect the value of lost or reduced productivity due to premature mortality or morbidity.
- Intangible costs, the most difficult to measure, that relate to the stress and isolation of those in ill health (in this case, drug dependence).

The major components of substance-use costs are:

- Health care costs
- Criminal justice costs
- Social-service costs
- Other external and hidden costs, such as those resulting from costs to people other than the individual (e.g., wife, children, parents, the community, who are affected by and relate to the isolation, stress, pain, and suffering of those affected by substance abuse)

Additional factors to consider related to cost evaluation of drug services can include prolonged life years, improved functioning and activity; relief from pain and anxiety or other distresses, greater capacity to work and earn, reduced health care costs, and enhanced quality of life.

Economic evaluations relate to the fact that limited resources exist in any community or region and choices must be made about resource use. Devoting resources to one activity may deprive another. Economic evaluations assist policy makers in deciding services to support. This type of evaluation involves identifying, measuring, valuing, and comparing costs and outcomes of alternative interventions.

Economic evaluations indicate the options that give the best value for the resources expended.

There are three broad questions addressed in economic evaluation:

- Is treatment worthwhile?
- Should investment (or further investment) be made in treatment A or treatment B?
- Should substance use interventions be chosen over other health or welfare interventions?

The question "Is treatment worthwhile?" compares the costs and consequences of a particular treatment or system of treatment against the do-nothing alternative. If the net benefits are greater than the costs, the policymaker would determine that the program is worthwhile from this monetary perspective.

For simplicity's sake, the question "Should investment (or further investment) be made in treatment A or treatment B?" is expressed as a choice between two options. More complex choices of different patterns of service provision also can be addressed. Answers to these types of questions involve comparisons across services with similar outcomes, for example, observed change in the frequency or quantity of use of a public service. This would result in a comparison of the costs across two program alternatives for achieving a given level of outcome.

Answering the question "Should substance use interventions be chosen over other health or welfare interventions?" generally involves comparing programs that have different outcomes and different population groups. This situation makes evaluation of alternatives difficult because there is unlikely to be any common unit of outcome to be compared. Economists therefore suggest the use of an outcome measure that reflects human well-being. These measures are sometimes referred to as measures of "utility." Most existing measures are based on changes in health and quality of life, across different types of health care interventions.

Cost-effectiveness analysis is another element worthy of consideration. This form of evaluation seeks to compare the costs of two or more different but comparable interventions that have the same benefit or outcome. The critical feature of cost-effectiveness evaluation is that the costs and consequences of treatment are assessed in relation to a primary outcome measure of a direct health gain that is valued by the individual client. These measures are used to construct a cost-effectiveness ratio that summarizes the net costs required for each unit of outcome. Given that the harms experienced by substance users lie in several domains of health and social function, a composite outcome measure may be required to understand the extent of change in several areas of concern to an individual. Consideration of the timing and duration of treatment benefits is also important. An important calculation is to convert all costs and benefits to a present value so that they can be compared (a process called *discounting*). While there is general agreement on discounting most resource consequences, there is less agreement on whether future health benefits should be discounted.

In *cost-utility analysis*, the individual's quality of life (usually expressed as *quality adjusted life years* estimated from a standardized instrument) is used as the primary benefit measure of treatment. In cost-benefit analysis, the outcomes themselves are measured in monetary units. These studies are less commonly used since there has been growing criticism of the appropriateness of outcome solely expressed in monetary terms. Full economic evaluations require two or more suitable alternatives to be evaluated. The most desirable design to determine robust effects is the randomized controlled trial (particularly for assessing a new treatment). Choice of design for an economic evaluation should be guided by the main questions being addressed.

Evaluation Assessment

Prior to starting one or more of the five main types of evaluation, a thorough preparatory assessment should be conducted. Evaluations, regardless of the type, may require the investment of substantial human and material resources, including the allocation of time to address the objectives that are established. Also, it may be important to consider the involvement of local expertise or consultants in the evaluation process for it to be successful.

The partners in an evaluation can include therapists, clinicians and other program workers, administrators and managers, researchers, government representatives, and community representatives. Discussions should be held with all relevant partners, and it is important to address any concerns that they may have about the planned study. Such discussions are a valuable means of identifying questions to be addressed. It should be recognized, however, that different groups may have different ideas about what to evaluate. Given the limited resources that are often available for evaluation, the primary intended users of the evaluation need to prioritize the issues to be examined.

Understanding Program Operation

It is important to have an understanding about how a program or system operates in relation to achieving its goals and objectives. A program logic model (PLM) can be a useful tool for this purpose (World Health Organization, in press). Essentially, a PLM is a schematic diagram of a treatment program (or set of programs) that charts the actual and theoretical relationships among processes, outputs, and intended outcomes. A detailed study protocol should also be developed that will describe the following:

- The aims of the study and the questions to be addressed
- Study design
- Research resources to be used (capital and human)
- Plans for subject recruitment, measurement, data management, data analysis, and report preparation
- Timetable and dissemination plan

Evaluation Research Ethics

Before participating in an evaluation, participants should receive an explanation of the purpose of the study and its procedures. It is essential that all participants understand the purpose of the evaluation and what will be required of them. Questions from potential participants should be addressed including issues of anonymity, confidentiality, and data protection. Also, participants involved in an evaluation should be asked to sign a consent form if they wish to participate. Confidentiality of gathered information from the participants should be achieved by a numbered reference system and maintained by the evaluation team. It is the responsibility of the team to ensure that all data gathered during the evaluation are kept secure. All studies that involve human subjects, including those of an evaluative nature, must receive approval by an appropriate ethics review body.

CONCLUSION

Changing trends and patterns of drug use, including the emergence of new drugs, are a challenge to drug policy and program decision makers. This is especially true in countries and regions such as the Middle East, where substance use is a relatively new phenomenon and where there may be insufficient expertise, will, or resources to address the problems. Given that limited resources are available to address the drug problem, policies and cost-effective treatments are indisputable priorities.

Evaluation research is not an academic exercise. It is an essential tool for shaping appropriate policy and refining service provision in terms of what needs to be done to address the drug problem.

REFERENCES

Blaine, J. D. (1992). *Buprenorphine: An alternative treatment for opioid dependence*. Research Monograph Series 121. Rockville, MD: National Institute on Drug Abuse.

Heather, N., & Mattick, R. (1994). The development of guidelines for drug and alcohol dependence treatment: Affecting policy and practice. *Drug and Alcohol Review, 13*, 119–126.

Institute of Medicine. (1990). *Broadening the basis of treatment for alcohol problems*. Washington, DC: National Academy Press.

Kushner, J. N., & Moss, S. (1995). *Purchasing managed care services for alcohol and other drug treatment: Essential elements and policy issues*. (U.S. Department of Health and Human Services Publication No. SMA 95-3040). Rockville, MD: U.S. Department of Health and Human Services.

Stimson, G., Des Jarlais, D., & Ball, A. (Eds.). (1998). *Drug injecting and HIV infection: Global dimensions and local responses*. London: UCL Press.

World Health Organization. (1993a). *Approaches to treatment of substance abuse*. WHO/PSA/93.10. Geneva: World Health Organization.

———. (1993b). *National drug and alcohol treatment responses in 23 countries*. WHO/PSA/93.15. Geneva: World Health Organization.

———. (1998). *30th expert committee report on drug dependence.* (Technical report series 836). Geneva: World Health Organization.

———. (in press). *WHO/United Nations drug control programme/European Monitoring Centre for Drugs and Drug Addiction workbook series on evaluation of psychoactive substance use disorders.* Geneva: World Health Organization.

PART V

Appendices: Treatment and Services Outlines

APPENDIX I

Department for the Treatment of Substance Abuse, Israel Ministry of Health: Responsibilities and Services

Jorge Gleser, David Elisha, Michael Reiter, and Anatoli Margolis

Treatment options for drug abusers began in Israel in 1975 with the establishment of two methadone centers and a drug-free rehabilitation center. A decade later, two inpatient units for detoxification of drug and alcohol abusers and an outpatient drug rehabilitation center were added. The treatment of substance abusers, however, remained a low priority in the Ministry of Health.

In 1990, the Department for the Treatment of Substance Abuse (DTSA) was established as part of the Division Mental Health in the Israel Ministry of Health. This action marked an important step in promoting the integration of the treatment of addictions into the medical and psychiatric fields. Prior to this, the treatment of alcohol and drug abuse in Israel was avoided by most medical and psychiatric institutions, and it constituted a rather marginal part of mental health services. Reflecting this situation were the facts that: (1) the treatment of alcohol and drug abuse was relegated exclusively to special treatment units, (2) the complexities associated with addiction warranted only a single national coordinator, and (3) the yearly budget allotted to this problem was quite limited.

Since 1990, the DTSA has seen a significant expansion of its professional staff. Moreover, the department's title was changed from Department for Detoxification from Alcohol and Drugs to Department for Treatment of Substance Abuse, thus reflecting a broader view of the problem and more comprehensive intervention strategies.

Currently, the DTSA is responsible for establishing service priorities and treatment policies, defining treatment and medical guidelines, and organizing efforts that monitor service provision for quality control. In addition, the DTSA is responsible for supervising the prescription of medications that are potentially addictive and for providing guidelines regarding addiction to medical staff and other professionals.

The significant growth in provision of services reflects the ministry's proactive approach to addressing addiction. New services have been made available and existing ones expanded.

Currently, as a result of the efforts made by the department, most substance abusers who seek treatment can be admitted either immediately or within one month of their request.

The service system offered by the Ministry of Health currently includes the following treatment centers and programs:

Ambulatory Services for Drug Addicts. Seven ambulatory centers are operating with a treatment capacity for over 1,000 patients. The ambulatory centers operate in a fashion similar to mental health clinics and are run by multidisciplinary teams. They provide diagnoses, individual and family counseling, and ambulatory detoxification. Rehabilitation treatment programs are offered in some centers, and plans are underway to expand the rehabilitation services.

Ambulatory Services for Alcohol Addicts. Together with the Ministry of Labor and Social Affairs, the DTSA operates 14 ambulatory centers that treat about 1,000 patients.

Inpatient Detoxification Units. Six inpatient units offer a total of 74 beds for detoxification of drug addicts; the length of stay ranges from 14 to 30 days. A special inpatient unit for alcohol detoxification has a 30-bed capacity. The treatment program includes physical detoxification, individual and group counseling for relapse prevention, social services, and milieu treatment.

Drug Maintenance Treatment Centers. Drug Maintenance Treatment Centers (DMTCs) in Israel are operated by the Ministry of Health. Current regulations do not permit privately run drug maintenance programs.

There are 11 regional DMTCs in Israel. Three mobile units operate in towns and villages in the north, center, and south of Israel and treat about 1,800 patients. The treatment program requires daily, on-site oral intake of methadone (Saturdays and religious holidays may be exempted), as well as participation in an on-site counseling program.

Youth Inpatient Units. The DTSA supports an eight-bed inpatient treatment unit for addicted juveniles in Jerusalem.

Dual Diagnosis Unit. Currently, a 16-bed unit in the Psychiatric Hospital in Beer Sheva and a five-bed unit in the Tirat Hakarmel Hospital in Haifa are available to address dual diagnosis patients (psychiatric disorders and addiction).

Newborns with Addiction Syndrome. Early in 1994, a pilot program to identify, supervise, and treat addicted pregnant women was established. General guidelines for all medical units regarding the treatment of addicted pregnant women and their newborns were developed. The DMTCs developed a special protocol for the treatment of pregnant women with methadone. In addition, a special treatment program was developed in a therapeutic community to treat addicted pregnant women and their newborn infants.

Children of Addicts. Currently the DTSA is developing a prevention program to at-risk children of addicts in all available ambulatory services.

Training Programs in Addiction. Postgraduate training programs for physicians and nurses have been offered since 1994. These programs are operated in conjunction with the Anti-Drug Authority and Tel Aviv University.

Data Collection. The DTSA developed a computerized system that includes a database for real-time clinical management as well as for quality control and research purposes. Also, the DTSA is currently planning a National Database Service together with the Ministry of Labor and Social Affairs and the Anti-Drug Authority.

Addiction in Primary Care. Guidelines and protocols for general practitioners have been developed with regard to tobacco smoking, alcohol use, and the abuse of medications. The guidelines address screening and detection, diagnosis of addiction and addiction potential, and primary intervention and referral.

Auditing and Licensing. One of the primary functions of the DTSA is to license and audit its treatment facilities. The department is mandated to do this under a law enacted in 1994. All auditing and licensing duties are performed jointly with the Anti-Drug Authority and the Ministry of Labour and Social Affairs. The DTSA has six medical inspectors assigned to the six Regional Health Centers. They are supervised by a Chief National Inspector.

Consulting Services. An important function of the DTSA to educate providers of health services and to provide consultation services to other national agencies. The Knesset (parliamentary) Substance Abuse Committee, the Anti-Drug Authority, and the Ministry of Justice are among the organizations that receive consultation services from the DTSA. The DTSA works together with government and public agencies to promote continuity of care. While the department sees its major function as supervising the medical aspects of drug and alcohol abuse treatment, it is clearly understood that, however important, this is just one aspect of a much broader problem.

Other Efforts. The DTSA is currently exploring the need to enlarge its scope of services to include tobacco addiction, behavior addiction, and performance-enhancing drug use in sports.

APPENDIX II

National Service for Drug Abuse Intervention, Division of Correctional Services, Israel Ministry of Labour and Social Affairs: Responsibilities and Services

Ariela Segev

INTRODUCTION

Drug addicts in Israel are referred for treatment and rehabilitation to the National Service for Drug Abuse Intervention (the Service). The goal of the Service is to carry out a policy of rehabilitation based on integration of the addict into the community. Personnel responsible for implementing tasks of the Service are social workers who have university degrees. Former addicts serve as counselors. The Service operates within the Division of Correctional Services in the Ministry of Labour and Social Affairs. The division coordinates the various services that are in charge of treating youth and adults who are in distress or socially deviant. By combining the various services under one division, a coherent, integrated policy is implemented, thereby contributing to the success of the therapeutic process.

The treatment approach utilized by the Service is based on social work practice methods including case, group, family, and community work. Trained personnel work with the client to promote the individual's strengths by developing individual, personal, and interpersonal skills. This includes the development of support networks involving family and friends. During the treatment process, personnel help the clients discover and develop the personal resources that might enable them to enhance their quality of life in such spheres as employment, leisure time, health, and housing.

At the local level, treatment of drug addicts is the responsibility of the municipal social services departments. More broadly, these local treatment programs constitute an important part of a network of nationwide services provided by the Ministry of Labour and Social Affairs.

The work of the Ministry's National Service for Drug Abuse Intervention includes far-reaching responsibilities for the treatment and rehabilitation programs of drug addicts. The Service is responsible for: (1) operating about 100 programs, through local service departments, and hiring 160 workers to address the needs of addicts; (2) providing a variety of therapeutic and rehabilitation services to addicts, their families, and children; (3) maintaining eight therapeutic communities that provide residential services to addicts for 6–12 months; (4) providing additional services for rehabilitation through cooperation and coordination among such agencies as the Vocational Training Division of the Ministry of Labour and Social Affairs, the Prisoner Rehabilitation Authority, and the Rehabilitation Projects Fund; (5) training professional staff through workshops, conferences, and courses; (6) formulating the Ministry of Labour and Social Affairs' treatment policy and publishing it in the Social Work Regulations; (7) coordinating the ministry's forum on drug abuse, as well as cooperating with other government units such as the Anti-Drug Authority and the Ministry of Health, Division for the Treatment of Drug Addiction; (8) initiating new legislation related to the treatment of addicts; and (9) supervising, with respect to relevant social institutions, the implementation of the Drug Users Institutes Law—1993.

TARGET POPULATION

The target population are adult and adolescent drug addicts who have applied to a local social service department for treatment and rehabilitation. Not included are chronic drug addicts who require methadone maintenance, addicts who need immediate medical attention, and addicts who suffer from mental illness, who are referred to other therapeutic facilities. Social workers currently counsel about 5,000 clients throughout the country as well as about 10,000 family members, including wives and children.

From data collected by the Service, it appears that about 50 percent of the clients who undergo detoxification remain drug free up to the final stages of rehabilitation. Data also indicate a steady rise in the number of addicts who come in for treatment, and that the Service is the largest therapeutic network for drug addicts in Israel.

MODES OF TREATMENT

From diagnostic evaluation to completion of treatment, clients are given service based on their needs as assessed by a social worker (see Table II.1). Treatment includes individual, group, or family therapy. From beginning to end, a social worker is with the client at every stage of the process, even when treatment is provided at a residential or ambulatory facility.

THERAPEUTIC STAGES

Diagnostic evaluation. After one or two meetings with the social worker, the purpose of which is to become acquainted and clarify expectations, the candidate is subjected to a comprehensive evaluation. This includes a probing discussion with the individual and his or her family. Additional evaluations are carried out as needed. The candidate is also referred for medical examinations and a urine test for the presence of drugs.

Referral to a diagnostic committee. A diagnostic committee meets to assess the information gathered and decides on the most appropriate treatment plan for the drug user and his or her family.

Physical detoxification. Following the recommendation of the diagnostic committee, the client undergoes physical detoxification. This can be undertaken in one of several contexts: (1) *in a hospital,* which lasts for about one month, after which the client returns to the social worker for continued treatment and rehabilitation in the community; (2) *in an ambulatory*

Table II.1
Treatment Model for Drug Abuse within the Social Service Departments

Referral to Drug Abuse Social Worker in SSDs	
Pre-Intake	• Information on the program • Elaboration of expectations
Intake (Assessment: 4–6 Weeks)	• Collecting personal information • Interviews • Home visits • Medical examinations • Psychological examinations

Diagnostic Committee
(Designs a treatment)
	• Participants
	  • Head of department
	  • Supervisor
	  • Social worker
	  • Client/family

Physical Detoxification 21–30 Days (Ministry of Health)	• Outpatient detoxification • Inpatient detoxification • Referral to methadone maintenance • Referral to therapeutic community
Recovery Period 3 Months	• Day center, individual, group, and family therapy

Rehabilitation Period
15–18 Months
	• Individual rehabilitation
	• Family rehabilitation
	• Normative rehabilitation
	• Vocational rehabilitation
	  • Vocational training courses
	  • On-the-job training
	  • Individual training
	  • Completion of studies
	  • Job placement by a worker or self-placement

Completion of Treatment	• Client leaves treatment for 3 months, or there are no further treatment goals for 3 months.
Follow-up	

setting, which is supervised by a physician who specializes in addiction. This setting is under the auspices of the Ministry of Health; or (3) *in a therapeutic community,* that is, a residential facility where drug addicts live for about a year. Therapeutic communities are equipped to supervise physical detoxification. Regardless of the setting, a person will not be accepted for physical detoxification without the approval and signature of a physician attesting to the candidate's ability to handle stressful circumstances.

Recovery period—a day center. The recovery period, which is devoted to preparing the client to return to the community, usually lasts about three to six months. The recovery process begins after successful physical detoxification. At this stage, the therapeutic relationship between client and social worker consists of casework treatment, participation in a support group, and family intervention. If space in a day center is available, the social worker arranges for the client's participation. Currently, there are 16 day centers, which are intensive comprehensive treatment facilities providing training in day-to-day skills, throughout the country.

Long-term treatment and rehabilitation. At the end of the recovery period, the process of rehabilitation begins. This lasts for about a year, during which time the client begins to cope with the psychological and social aspects of addiction. At this stage, emphasis is placed on the normative functioning of clients through individual, group, or family therapy. Moreover, efforts are made to provide addicts with skills that will enhance their ability to acquire employment when they return to the community.

The learning process. Before integrating the client into an educational setting, his or her basic knowledge of math and Hebrew, and learning, listening, and concentration abilities must be assessed. This proceeds with an understanding that many addicts have learning disabilities. Upon receiving the results of the tests, a decision is made as to which educational context to place the client into. If they are capable, clients may be referred to an intensive six-month study program. This program provides the addict with five full days of study per week taught by special education teachers. Taking into account the student's special characteristics, such as individual rate of learning, difficulty in concentration, deficiency in basic study skills, incapacity to organize material, anxiety at being tested, fear of failure, limited social experience, and quickness to lose composure, the emphasis is on individual learning.

Outside the classroom, the addict/student is supervised by a personal therapist who charts and assesses the client's progress and provides reinforcement, encouragement, and support over the course of difficult and frustrating months. Since there are many obstacles during the learning process, the therapists themselves often need the assistance and cooperation of the school, caseworker, family (children and spouse), and the other agencies involved. Periodically, throughout the learning process, the addict is given urine tests.

Vocational testing. Upon completing the learning process, the client undergoes a series of vocational tests, after which he or she and the counselors together will decide how best to pursue a vocational training track or employment. If needed, the clients undergo additional vocational testing, after which they will be referred to a rehabilitative vocational setting, vocational training (or a preparatory vocational training course), rehabilitation under the auspices of the National Insurance Institute, a job-search workshop, or, when possible and desirable, to search for a job independently.

Eight "technological preparation courses" are available for 100 drug-free clients at a time. These provide basic education for those who have completed 10 years or more of schooling, vocational testing, training, and job placement. The courses are sponsored by the Rehabilitation Project Fund and the Ministry's Division for Vocational Training and Rehabilitation

Services Administration. The experience of the past few years indicates that the percentage of clients entering the work force is very high (74 percent in three years).

NATIONAL INSURANCE INSTITUTE

An addict who has undergone detoxification and is clean of drugs may continue with a rehabilitative program and receive income maintenance from the National Insurance Institute (NII). Each month a drug abuse social worker updates the NII claims clerk on the condition of the addict in the rehabilitation program. According to an NII report, about 1,350 people receive income maintenance due to being in drug abuse rehabilitation, and 2,390 receive income maintenance who are "drug addicts."

SUPERVISION OF DRUG USERS' INSTITUTES LAW—1993

The National Service for Drug Abuse Intervention licenses and supervises institutions that treat drug users in accordance with the Supervision of Drug Users' Institutes Law—1993. According to this law, every institution that cares for three or more persons at the same time must apply for a license. These institutions need to apply for a license from a committee of the Anti-Drug Authority. Then, in accordance with the committee's decision, the license application is referred to the Ministry of Labour and Social Affairs or the Ministry of Health, so that the institution can be inspected and either awarded or denied a license. The Supervision Law enables the ministries to ensure professional care to drug users and to close any institution that does not meet the demands of the law.

GROUPS OF CHILDREN OF ADDICTS

As a result of living in a disrupted family environment where addiction prevails, children of drug addicts tend to suffer from many psychosocial problems. In response, the Service for Drug Abuse Intervention has, in conjunction with the Special Projects Fund of the National Insurance Institute, and the Israel Joint Distribution Committee's Department for Children at Risk, initiated a project to provide support groups for children of addicts. Thirty such groups have been established for children whose parents are receiving treatment for drug abuse. The groups, operated as part of the treatment programs for drug addicts, are run by local social services departments and led by two moderators, one an expert in child care and the other in drug abuse treatment.

The groups meet once a week for two hours. Once a month, a joint meeting is held with the parents. The main topics discussed in the groups include exposing the secret of the addiction, freely expressing feelings and problems, developing and acquiring tools to cope with the reality of a family in transition, and discovering and accepting missed childhood experiences. The group moderators play the role of adult models, and the group meetings provide an ongoing framework for self-discovery and mutual support. While the group meetings are highly structured and planned in advance, they are also flexible and open to matters raised spontaneously by participants in sessions. This is a nationwide project, operated through local social services departments, that responds to the needs of about 360 children.

Drug abuse victims, whose children participate in the groups, are undergoing a transforming process of treatment, rehabilitation, and change. From active addicts, they progress to being free of drugs and able to function on individual, family, and occupational levels. While the parents participate in ongoing therapy, they are constrained to cooperate with the treatment that, as part of the package deal, is rendered to their children. The parents freely describe the changes that occur at home as a result of their child's participation in the group: "My child taught me how to embrace; to this day I had not touched him." "My child told me that he was solely responsible for his body." "My child, who always kept quiet, has begun to talk."

TREATMENT PROGRAMS FOR ADDICTED YOUTH

The Ministry of Labour and Social Affairs is currently preparing a national program to treat addicted youth or habitual users at the local level. Surveys published by the Anti-Drug Authority point to a rise in the number of drug users among youth attending school. The rate rose from 6 percent in 1989–1990 to 9 percent in 1995 (representing some 52,000 youths), and to 10 percent in 1999. The percentage of adolescents who experiment with drugs is constantly rising. In spite of this finding, there are no community facilities in Israel run by a local authority that can provide services near to home. A small number of ambulatory centers and residential facilities treat addicted youth, including the Malchishua therapeutic community and two hostels.

The decision to employ a youth social worker in local social services departments comes from recognizing the importance of a coordinated approach to treating youth. There are other workers in the social services departments who may be involved in the therapeutic process such as those representing the Service for Girls in Distress, the Service for Youth and Young Adults, and the Youth Advancement Unit.

The goals of the treatment program are manifold: to identify and recruit drug-dependent youths and to enter them into a detoxification and treatment program and then a long-term therapeutic-rehabilitative process for about a year—all the while keeping them in their home and community. The program works with youths aged 12 to 18 who are addicts or habitual users, and who apply independently or are referred by a school counselor, parent, youth welfare officer, probation officer, social worker, or any other agency person for treatment. Particular emphasis is now being placed on opening a telephone "hot-line" through which clients can set therapeutic appointments as confidentially and discreetly as required.

ADDITIONAL DRUG ABUSE TREATMENT SERVICES OF THE DIVISION OF CORRECTIONAL SERVICES

As mentioned earlier, the Division of Correctional Services operates the following:

Adult Probation Service: The courts refer drug users, drug traffickers, property offenders, and persons accused of violence for evaluation and treatment.

Juvenile Probation Service: Minors who are involved with drug trafficking and sporadic drug consumption are referred to this service. Among the minors referred, many use drugs or are at serious risk of succumbing to drug use. According to recently published non-prosecution guidelines, a minor and his parents are summoned to a probation officer for evaluation immediately upon the opening of a police investigation.

Service for Youth and Young Adults: This service provides activities for young adults who are at high risk of sliding into drug use. These activities include preparation for army enlistment programs, sports (including a course at the Wingate Sports Institute), theater, video, and vocational training.

Service for Girls in Distress: This service deals with girls in distress, including sporadic drug users. Rather than targeting drug use per se, the treatment deals with the problems of adolescents.

Youth Protection Authority: The facilities of the Youth Protection Authority (YPA) provide care to youths in various states of distress and delinquency. In cooperation with the Ministry of Education, a long school day is provided that includes academic studies and extracurricular classes and activities. The YPA also supervises and counsels the therapeutic community for youth, a foster family program and hostel, and conducts prevention programs at various institutions.

Youth Rehabilitation Service: This service operates a nationwide network of special vocational schools for youths who have dropped out of school, and trains some of its workers to conduct drug prevention programs within the school.

Division for Manpower Training and Development: This division services 13,500 working and studying youths. Among its services are drug prevention programs. In support of this effort, the division holds in-service training and courses for teaching and counseling staff members, including lectures by experts, theatrical presentations, exhibits, and cultural events. The division is also involved with the vocational training of addicts belonging to the therapeutic community.

APPENDIX III

Anti-Drug Authority of Israel: Responsibilities and Services

Shlomo Gal

INTRODUCTION

The Anti-Drug Authority of Israel (ADAI), established in 1988 by a legislative act of the Knesset (national parliament), is the lead government agency responsible for addressing substance use and abuse in the country.

The ADAI has been mandated three distinct areas of responsibility: (1) the formation of national substance use and abuse policy; (2) coordination between the Ministries of Health and of Labour and Social Affairs, which are jointly responsible for the treatment and rehabilitation of drug addicts; and (3) the Ministry of Education, which has primary responsibility for prevention and the dissemination of information. Further, the ADAI maintains interministerial coordination between these front-line agencies and the Ministries of Interior, Justice, Internal Security, and the Treasury, all of which play secondary but vital roles in the ongoing campaign against drug abuse.

In addition, the ADAI initiates and maintains services and programs directed against drug abuse. These comprise prevention and public education, treatment and rehabilitation, law enforcement, human resources development, research, and volunteer organizations whose activities the ADAI coordinates, regulates, and supports. The ADAI strives to engender a public climate in which drug abuse is not condoned.

PREVENTION AND EDUCATION

The ADAI's most fundamental responsibility is to develop initiatives and implement programs to prevent youth at risk from becoming drug users and to help occasional users to stop using drugs. To this end, the ADAI has established an informational network that encompasses contact with the media, schools, parents, community groups, and a variety of informal means of communication. The strategy is to establish a healthy, normal lifestyle which would, of its very nature, eliminate the motivation for using drugs. Toward this end, a broad spectrum of community-based groups and programs receive ADAI support.

The personal stories of ex-addicts, recovered addicts, or prisoners—released from incarceration for the day in order to relate their life experiences—play an essential part of ADAI's prevention programs. To maximize the impact of these true stories on at-risk youth, the ADAI has developed special training seminars for the recovered addicts so that they can better determine which aspects of their life stories bear emphasis and sharpen their ability to communicate effectively.

Within the schools. In 1999, prevention programs were underway in more than 1,000 schools throughout the country. Among the most popular of these programs are the Peer Counseling Groups, in which adolescents are trained during intensive seminars to serve as educators and role models for their peers and younger children. This transpires within the context of a clearly defined substance abuse prevention program. The Peer Counseling Program was initiated eight years ago. In 1999, over 5,000 students received training as peer counselors.

In the general community. Outside the schools, prevention activity is primarily geared toward young people who, although perhaps part-time students, are already in the work force and to those who neither work nor attend school. In dealing with these youths at risk, the ADAI tries to encourage a fit between the skills of the youths and alternatives to drug abuse. One of the most successful of these projects is based on sports—"Yes to Sports! No to Drugs!" This project utilizes organized physical activities and sports as a means of creating an atmosphere that rejects drug use and advocates a healthier lifestyle by reinforcing the importance of coping under pressure and real-life skills. ADAI provides special training for physical education instructors who participate in this program.

Two other programs—Youth Teaches Youth and Youth Says No to Drugs—focus on the contribution of youths themselves in conveying an unambiguous message against drug abuse. The former was developed by the Israeli Psychological Consultation Service, and the latter was initiated by ADAI 10 years ago. Both programs provide a context for youth leaders to battle drug abuse in their communities.

Of special note is HALAS, the life without drugs program, which was introduced to high-risk, 14-to-18-year-olds in such community-based facilities as youth centers and vocational training facilities. The program operates in Hebrew, Arabic, and Russian so as to address the specific cultural and educational needs of the country's diverse youth-at-risk population.

Another successful approach is "Alternative," a mobile information campaign against drug abuse among youths. The program operates out of two buses that were uniquely designed to deliver credible information to young people. The bus functions as a mobile movie theater with special seating. One of the buses presents a film designed for young people who are not considered to be particularly at risk of succumbing to drugs. The other bus presents a different film for youths thought to be at far greater risk. Another critical target group is parents of at-risk youths, for which wide-ranging informational campaigns have been undertaken to heighten their vigilance and sensitivity to the problem.

Backpackers. Special information campaigns are conducted for backpackers who travel mainly to the Far East or South America, regions where drugs are inexpensive and freely available. Backpackers are informed about the dangers of the most popular local drugs and the drug policies of countries in these areas.

In the Israel Defense Forces (IDF). With the cooperation of the IDF Education and Youth Corps Command, the ADAI provides reliable drug prevention information to Israel's soldiers. In a series of talks, soldiers become acquainted with the army's approach toward drug abuse, enforcement methods, and punishment policy; learn about the specific harmful effects of different kinds of drugs; and are addressed by "a clean source" who recounts his personal story of drug abuse and rehabilitation. A special team has been trained to operate a mobile unit that provides information on remote army bases. Moreover, the ADAI has created "Coping," a unique prevention program designed to meet the needs of soldiers at particular risk, so-called "detached youth."

TREATMENT AND REHABILITATION

The ADAI, in view of its coordinating role among seven governmental ministries, provides funding, counseling, and technical assistance to a broad range of treatment and rehabilitation agencies, both governmental and voluntary, including: therapeutic communities, ambulatory and internal treatment facilities for youth, day centers, community treatment, detoxification, methadone treatment and rehabilitation facilities, and community-based detoxification units.

In general, taking into account both the degree of addiction and the living conditions of the drug abuser, a serious effort is made to adapt treatment to the individual needs of the drug victim. Further information regarding programs supported in part or whole by the ADAI may be found in the overviews provided by the National Service for the Treatment of Addiction of the Ministry of Labour and Social Affairs and the Department of Substance Abuse Treatment of the Ministry of Health.

LAW ENFORCEMENT

The ADAI furnishes financial support, technical assistance, and coordination among relevant law enforcement authorities, principally the police, prison services, military police, and the Finance Ministry's tax department.

COMMUNITY ORGANIZATION

The ADAI funds and offers professional planning assistance to local authorities, including community leaders, citizens, and the police, as well as others who work to promote values and attitudes that discourage the abuse of drugs.

VOLUNTARY BODIES

The ADAI supports a wide range of voluntary, anti-drug organizations, notably Al-Sam, MANAS (the organization of drug addict families), TELEM (a network of counseling clinics for youth run by the United Kibbutz Movement), Al-Tahara, and Al-Hilal (in the Arab sector).

RESEARCH AND INFORMATION

The ADAI conducts surveys and promotes research to determine the nature and extent of drug use in the country. From these efforts, a database has been developed that provides policy makers and program directors with critical, accurate, and up-to-date information, enabling them to respond rapidly and intelligently to shifts in patterns of substance use in Israel. Further, the ADAI conducts evaluation studies that help gauge the effectiveness of various prevention and treatment methods. Finally, through the Internet, the ADAI has developed an information system that renders its findings accessible to the general public.

HUMAN RESOURCES DEVELOPMENT

The ADAI provides vital support to universities throughout the country to promote interdisciplinary academic training and professional skills development in the field of addiction infrastructure of community and professional workers. The goal is to raise the staff's level of professional competence, self-esteem, and effectiveness in preventing drug abuse.

Index

Editors and Contributors

EDITORS

MOHAMMED AFIFI is Director of the Palestine Substance Abuse and Addiction Research Center (SARC-Palestine) and the Gaza Regional Alcohol and Drug Abuse Resources (RADAR) Center. He is founder of the Child Health and Community Research Association (CHCR), established in 1991, and he served as the Director of Health Promotion in the Palestine Ministry of Health from 1995 to 2000.

RICHARD ISRALOWITZ is Director of the Regional Alcohol and Drug Abuse Resources Center, Spitzer Department of Social Work, Ben-Gurion University. Professor Isralowitz has served as director, Graduate School of Applied Social Sciences' Research Center, Case Western Reserve University and director, Hubert Humphrey Institute for Social Research, Ben-Gurion University.

RICHARD RAWSON is an Adjunct Associate Professor and the Associate Director of the UCLA Integrated Substance Abuse Programs in the Department of Psychiatry at the University of California, Los Angeles. He is a founder of the Matrix Institute on Addictions and he has worked with the U.S. Department of State on numerous international drug abuse treatment and research efforts.

CONTRIBUTORS

ZIAD ABDEEN is Professor of Community Health and Dean of Scientific Research, Al-Quds University, East Jerusalem.

ISMAEL ABU SAAD is Senior Lecturer, Department of Education, Ben-Gurion University, Israel. He is former Director of the University's Center for Bedouin Studies and Development.

ALEAN AL-KRENAWI is Senior Lecturer, Spitzer Department of Social Work, Ben-Gurion University, Israel. He is presently Director of the university's Center for Bedouin Studies and Development.

MAHMOUD AL-ZUHEIRI, Deputy Director, Palestinian Anti-Narcotics General Administration (PANGA), has the rank of colonel in the Palestine National Authority Police Force.

THOMAS F. BABOR is Professor and Chairman of the Department of Community Medicine and Health Care at the University of Connecticut School of Medicine. He is a social psychologist who specializes in research on addictive disorders.

ANDREW BALL is Medical Officer in the World Health Organization Department of Child and Adolescent Health and Development. A drug and alcohol physician by training, Dr. Ball's main responsibilities relate to adolescent health, particularly in the areas of substance use, HIV/AIDS and sexually transmitted diseases, and, especially, vulnerable young people. He also has worked extensively in the development of rapid assessment and response methodologies for substance use.

PATRICK F. BOGAN is Executive Director of Friends Research Institute, Inc. (FRI) in Baltimore. He has been pivotal in the growth of FRI, which now administers studies in 22 states as well as in other countries.

SOFIA BORKIN is Research Associate, Israel Regional Alcohol and Drug Resources Center, Ben-Gurion University, Israel. Dr. Borkin has served as the director of the Negev Drug Detoxification Center and Negev Regional Inspector of Drug Services for the Israel Ministry of Health, Drug Treatment Services Unit.

KHULOUD KHAYYAT DAJANI is Assistant Professor and Associate Dean, School of Public Health, Al-Quds University, Jerusalem.

DAVID ELISHA is National Coordinator of Ambulatory Mental Health Services, Division of Mental Health, Israel Ministry of Health.

SALAH EL-SOUSI is Head of the Department of Pharmacy, Al-Azhar University in Gaza. His work addresses issues regarding substance abuse and pharmacology, including the abuse of legal drugs.

VIOLET FASHEH is Professor and former Dean (1991–1996) of the Faculty of Education, Bethlehem University. She has conducted research on youth and drug use issues as well as serving as an advisor to Palestinian drug treatment facilities and services.

SHLOMO GAL is Executive Director of the Anti-Drug Authority of Israel. He has served in a senior position (general, retired) in the Israel Police Force.

JORGE GLESER is Director, Department for the Treatment of Substance Abuse and Deputy Director, Mental Health Services, Israel Ministry of Health; President of the Israeli Society of Addiction Medicine (ILSAM); and Vice President of the International Society of Addiction Medicine (ISAM).

JOHN R. GRAHAM is Associate Professor, Faculty of Social Work, University of Calgary, Alberta, Canada.

ALBERT HASSON has worked in the substance abuse research and treatment field since 1977, with a special emphasis on directing clinical trials for cocaine and heroin addiction. He is the Administrative Director of the Matrix Institute on Addictions, a not-for-profit treatment organization in Los Angeles, California. He is a member of the planning group for the trilateral Middle East Drug Use Watch project.

RACHEL LEV-WIESEL is Senior Lecturer, Spitzer Department of Social Work, Ben-Gurion University, Israel.

ANATOLI MARGOLIS is Deputy Director, Department for the Treatment of Substance Abuse and Deputy Director, Mental Health Services, Israel Ministry of Health.

AHMAD MOHIT is the Regional Advisor for Mental Health and Substance Dependence in the Eastern Mediterranean Region of the World Health Organization. He is based currently in Cairo.

MARISTELA G. MONTEIRO is the coordinator of the progam on Management of Substance Dependence of the Mental Health and Substance Dependence Department at the World Health Organization (WHO) in Geneva. She is responsible for the area of alcohol and substance use epidemiology and treatment, capacity building for the evaluation of treatment and coordination of the WHO Injecting Drug Use Study.

JEANNE OBERT is a cofounder and Executive Director of the Matrix Institute on Addictions. The institute conducts treatment, research, and training in substance abuse disorders. Outpatient Matrix Model treatment services are delivered in five sites throughout the greater Los Angeles area as part of the UCLA Integrated Substance Abuse Programs as well as in other locations nationally and internationally.

GIORA RAHAV is Professor of Sociology, Tel Aviv University. He, along with Meir Teichman, are principle investigators of the epidemiological studies done for the Anti-Drug Authority of Israel.

MICHAEL REITER is Deputy Director, Department for the Treatment of Substance Abuse, Israel Ministry of Health.

GHAZI H. SAWA is Professor of Sociology, University of Jordan, Amman. Currently he is working as a senior research methodologist for the Institute of Public Administration in Riyadh, Saudi Arabia.

SHEKHAR SAXENA is Coordinator of the Team on Mental Health Determinants and Populations within the Department of Mental Health and Substance Dependence at the World Health Organization, Geneva. He has worked extensively in the area of substance abuse for the last 20 years, mostly with developing countries. His present responsibilities include coordinating prevention of substance abuse activities within the World Health Organization.

ARIELA SEGEV is Director of the National Service for Drug Abuse Intervention, Israel Ministry of Labour and Social Affairs.

MAHMUD A. SEHWAIL is Director of the Treatment and Rehabilitation Center for Victims of Torture, Ramallah, Palestine.

GARY SUSSMAN served as Program Coordinator for the Economic Cooperation Foundation, which is the nongovernmental organization credited for coordinating the Oslo Accord Agreement. Presently, he is pursuing a Ph.D. at the London School of Economics.

MEIR TEICHMAN is a Professor of Psychology and Head of Bob Schappel School of Social Work, Tel Aviv University.

ABDUL AZIZ THABET is a psychiatrist and a lecturer at the School of Public Health, Al-Quds University, East Jerusalem.

GUNDO WEILER is Head of the Medical and Policy Department, German National AIDS Organization, Berlin. His responsibilities include the development and implementation of national policies and programs for HIV/AIDS prevention and treatment.

SHOSHANA WEISS, an alcohol researcher, is the Director of Research in the Israel Society for the Prevention of Alcoholism, Ramat Gan, Israel, and the editor of *Alcohol in Israel—Interdisciplinary Scientific Journal.*

JOSEPH YANAI is Professor of Anatomy and Cell Biology, Hebrew University-Hadassah Medical School, Jerusalem.